Preparation and Revision for the DRCOG

For information on Churchill Livingstone titles, or to place an order, call:

UK: Freephone 0500 566 242
Europe: +44 131 535 1021
USA/Canada: +1 201 319 9800
Australia/New Zealand: +61 3 9699 5400

Preparation and Revision for the Diploma of the Royal College of Obstetricians and Gynaecologists

Janice Rymer MRCOG FRNZCOG
Senior Lecturer/Consultant in Obstetrics and Gynaecology,
Medical and Dental Schools (UMDS) Guy's and St Thomas' Hospital, London

Gregory Davis MD MRCOG FRACOG
Saff specialist/Lecturer, University of New South Wales,
Department of Obstetrics and Gynaecology, St George Hospital, Sydney

Adam Rodin BSc MRCOG
Consultant in Obstetrics and Gynaecology,
Wellhouse NHS Trust, London

Michael Chapman MRCOG
Professor of Obstetrics and Gynaecology, University of New South Wales,
St George Hospital, Sydney

SECOND EDITION

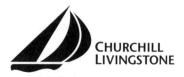

CHURCHILL
LIVINGSTONE

NEW YORK EDINBURGH LONDON MADRID MELBOURNE SAN FRANCISCO TOKYO 1998

CHURCHILL LIVINGSTONE
Medical Division of Pearson Professional Ltd

Distributed in the United States of America by Churchill Livingstone Inc., 650 Avenue of the Americas, New York, N.Y. 10011, and by associated companies, branches and representatives throughout the world.

© Longman Group UK Limited 1990
This edition © Pearson Professional Limited 1998

⬦ is a registered trademark of Pearson Professional Limited

First edition published 1990
Second edition published 1998

ISBN 0–443–05097-X

British Library Cataloguing in Publication Data
A catalogue record for this book is available from the British Library.

Library of Congress Cataloging in Publication Data
A catalog record for this book is available from the Library of Congress.

Medical knowledge is constantly changing. As new information becomes available, changes in treatment, procedures, equipment and the use of drugs become necessary. The authors and the publishers have, as far as it is possible, taken care to ensure that the information given in this text is up to date. However, readers are strongly advised to confirm that the information, especially with regard to drug usage, complies with current legislation and standards of practice.

The
publisher's
policy is to use
paper manufactured
from sustainable forests

Typeset by IMH (Cartrif), Scotland
Produced by Longman Singapore Publishers Pte Ltd
Printed in Singapore

Preface

The Diploma of the Royal College of Obstetricians and Gynaecologists is an examination to establish that a medical practitioner is adequately prepared to undertake obstetrics and gynaecology in a general practice setting. This book aims to provide basic knowledge of the syllabus and to assist the candidate to pass the examination. We begin by describing the structure of the examination in detail and devote a chapter to each section. The 'Clinical and Viva Examination' chapters have been replaced by 'Objective Structured Clinical Examinations' in accordance with the new DRCOG examinations. In these chapters advice on preparation is given and example questions are provided for practice. We emphasize in the text that the place to learn obstetrics and gynaecology is on the wards, in clinics and in the operating theatre. Discussion with colleagues and background reading is essential in obstetrics and gynaecology as there are many areas of controversy.

In covering the syllabus we have aimed for a 'common-sense' approach without dealing with minutiae. We have highlighted controversial areas and acknowledged that other views exist.

Each chapter commences with a section outlining the 'expectations of the examiners' to provide guidance for the candidate to concentrate on the core of the subject. The coverage is not definitive and should be augmented with other texts, as described in 'Suggested reading'.

We thank our eight contributors for providing their specialist expertise. Our greatest critics (the candidates) have demanded four new chapters, which have been included, on minimally invasive surgery, uterovaginal prolapse, obstetric and gynaecological emergencies and management of stillbirths. As this is the second edition assistance has been needed with updating certain chapters and we are particularly grateful to Philippa Kyle, Elizabeth Owen, Jennifer Higham, Alfred Cutner and Diana Hamilton-Fairley for their help with fetal medicine, infertility, menstrual disorders, urinary incontinence and recurrent miscarriage. We are also grateful to Jill Buxton and Roger Jackson from the Royal College of Obstetricians and Gynaecologists who have given us advice about the examination. In addition, we are indebted to Tracy Alderton, who has diligently typed the manuscript and coped with the never-ending alterations.

Every conception needs a father, and this book has had Dr Joe Rosenthal (general practitioner) who has painstakingly read and criticized every chapter. He has provided us with excellent consumer critique and we are eternally grateful.

It is our hope that this book will provide the medical practitioner with many of the necessary skills for passing examinations in obstetrics and gynaecology, and also a basic knowledge of the subject. We envisage that it will not only appeal to DRCOG candidates, medical students and MRCOG candidates but also have a place in the surgery of the general practitioner as a ready reference book for common problems.

London 1997   Janice Rymer

Contributors

Barry Auld MRCOG
Consultant in Obstetrics and Gynaeology, Buchanan Hospital, St Leonards-on-Sea

Simon Barton BSc MD MRCOG
Consultant Physician, Department of HIV/Genitourinary Medicine, St Stephen's Centre, Chelsea and Westminster Hospital, London

Michael Chapman MD FRCOG FRACOG
Professor of Obstetrics and Gynaecology, University of New South Wales, St George Hospital, Sydney

Gregory Davis MD MRCOG FRACOG
Staff Specialist/Lecturer, Department of Obstetrics and Gynaecology, St George Hospital, Sydney

Ann Duthie MD MRCP
Consultant in Paediatrics, Whipps Cross Hospital, London

Anthony Hollingworth PhD FRCS MRCOG
Consultant in Obstetrics and Gynaecology, Whipps Cross Hospital, London

Marie McDonald RGN, RM, ADM
Head of Midwifery and Gynaecology Nursing, Lewisham Hospital, NHS Trust, London

Ian Page MRCOG
Consultant in Obstetrics and Gynaecology, Royal Lancaster Infirmary, Lancaster

Adam Rodin BSc MRCOG
Consultant in Obstetrics and Gynaecology, Wellhouse NHS Trust, London

Jonathan Rosenthal BSc MSc MBBCH MRCGP DRCOG DFFP
Senior Lecturer in General Practice, Department of Primary Care and Population Sciences, Royal Free Hospital School of Medicine, London

Janice Rymer MD MRCOG FRNZCOG
Senior Lecturer/Consultant in Obstetrics and Gynaecology, United Medical and Dental Schools (UMDS) Guy's and St Thomas' Hospital, London

Christine Watson MD MFFP MRCH DRCOG DCH
Consultant/Senior Lecturer in Family Planning and Reproductive Health Care, Optimum Health Services and UMDS, University of London

Contents

SECTION I
THE EXAMINATION
1. General information   3
   J. Rymer
2. Preparing for the examination   8
   J. Rymer
3. The written paper   10
   J. Rymer
4. Objective structured clinical e0amination   27
   J. Rymer

SECTION II
THE SYLLABUS
A. Gynaecology
5. The menstrual cycle   37
   G. Davis
6. Menstrual disorders   44
   J. Rymer
7. Endometriosis, dyspareunia and pelvic pain   54
   G. Davis
8. Infertility   64
   M. Chapman
9. Congenital abnormalities of the female genital tract   69
   J. Rymer
10. Hirsutism and virilism   73
    M. Chapman
11. Bleeding in early pregnancy   77
    G. Davis
12. Benign conditions of the female genital tract   95
    A. Rodin
13. Gynaecological oncology   103
    A. Hollingworth
14. The menopause and hormone replacement therapy   117
    A. Rodin and J. Rymer

15. The premenstrual syndrome   124
A. Rodin
16. Urinary incontinence   127
J. Rymer
17. Uterovaginal prolapse   135
A. Rodin
18. Minimally invasive surgery   141
B. J. Auld

B. Obstetrics
19. Prepregnancy counselling and prenatal diagnosis   151
G. Davis
20. Antenatal care   160
G. Davis
21. Minor disorders of pregnancy   174
G. Davis
22. Infections in pregnancy   178
A. Rodin
23. Major complications of pregnancy   184

PART 1
Preterm labour   184
A. Rodin
PART 2
Hypertensive disorders   188
J. Rymer
PART 3
Rhesus isoimmunization   193
A. Rodin
PART 4
Intrauterine growth retardation   196
A. Rodin
PART 5
Antepartum haemorrhage   202
A. Rodin
PART 6
Maternal systemic disorders   207
A. Rodin

24. Labour—first stage   217
J. Rymer
25. Labour—second stage   223
J. Rymer
26. Labour—third stage   226
J. Rymer

27. Fetal monitoring in labour   230
    J. Rymer
28. Obstetric intervention   236
    J. Rymer
29. Breech presentation and transverse lie   244
    J. Rymer
30. Twin pregnancy   249
    J. Rymer
31. Obstetric analgesia and anaesthesia   254
    G. Davis
32. Puerperium and breast-feeding   264
    G. Davis
33. Obstetric and gynaecological emergencies   274
    J. Rymer
34. Home deliveries   283
    I. Page
35. Stillbirths   287
    M. McDonald
36. Maternity benefits   292
    I. Page
37. Statistics   296
    I. Page

C. Miscellaneous subjects
38. Neonatal medicine   309
    A. Duthie
39. Sexually transmitted infections in women   335
    S. E. Barton
40. Family planning   353
    C. Watson
41. Psychosexual counselling   375
    C. Watson

APPENDICES
  I.   Obstetric terms and definitions   382
 II.   Risk factors in obstetrics   384
III.   The fetal skull   386
IV.   Diameters of the normal female pelvis   387
 V.   Normal values in pregnancy   389
VI.   Partograms   390
Suggested reading   392
Index   393

The examination

1. General information

J. Rymer

DIPLOMA OF THE ROYAL COLLEGE OF OBSTETRICIANS AND GYNAECOLOGISTS (DRCOG)

The College awards a Diploma to registered medical practitioners who have appropriate postgraduate training and who satisfy the examiners. The Diploma is intended to recognize a general practitioner's interest in obstetrics and gynaecology and is not a specialist qualification.

The Royal College of Obstetricians and Gynaecologists produces a booklet entitled *Diploma Examination Regulations* which can be obtained from the Examination Secretary. The address is given at the end of this chapter.

You should obtain a copy of the Diploma Examination Regulations at the time of commencing your training.

Eligibility

The regulations state that:

1. The candidate must be *fully* registered as a medical practitioner in the register maintained by the General Medical Council or the Medical Council of Ireland.
2. The candidate must have held a recognized appointment for 6 consecutive months. (Recognized appointments are limited to the United Kingdom, Republic of Ireland, and HM Forces.)

If you want confirmation of your eligibility, return the form the College sends to you in the *Diploma Examination Regulations* with certificates confirming your recognized appointment, and your medical registration. The appointment certificate must state that the post is recognized by the College for the DRCOG examination.

Sample certificate

A sample certificate is shown in Figure 1.1

The College can refuse an application and does not have to give the reason for refusal.

SAMPLE CERTIFICATE

RECOGNISED APPOINTMENT FOR THE DIPLOMA EXAMINATION (DRCOG)

TO: The Examination Office
     RCOG

This is to confirm that Dr **
has completed/is expected to complete to my satisfaction a six
month **combined** appointment at the above hospital, recognised for
the purposes of the Diploma examination (DRCOG). The post
commenced on */*/** and terminated/will terminate on */*/**.

I further confirm that Dr **
is clinically competent to attempt the Diploma examination.

Signed .... FRCOG/MRCOG

Date..................... Hospital ....

RSJ/SD/8/96

Fig. 1.1 A sample appointment certificate.

If you withdraw your application after the closing date or fail to appear, then you will forfeit the examination fee.

DATES OF THE EXAMINATION

The examination is held in April and October. The closing date for applications should be obtained from the College. Late applications are not accepted. The multiple choice question (MCQ) papers and OSCE (Objective Structured Clinical Examination) are taken on the same day and you will be assigned to a centre chosen by the College. The entry fee (in sterling) must be sent with the application; the fee is subject to annual review. Details of the entry fee are available from the Examination Secretary.

Recognized appointments for the Diploma examination must have been completed by, or intended to have been completed by, the date of the examination. Evidence of having completed such training must be enclosed with the application.

EXAMINATION FORMAT

The examination is conducted in two parts:

1. *An MCQ paper of 2 hours duration.*
2. *An Objective Structured Clinical Examination (OSCE)* — this examination lasts approximately 2 hours and 15 minutes and consists of 22 stations, each station lasting 6 minutes.

You may not attempt the Diploma examination more than five times.

SUBJECT MATTER

The syllabus includes the following topics:

Obstetrics

1. Routine procedures in modern antenatal care
2. Epidemiology of maternal and perinatal morbidity and mortality
3. Complications of early pregnancy
4. Shared care and specialist referral
5. Prepregnancy counselling
6. Prenatal diagnosis
7. Methods of education for pregnancy, childbirth, and the newborn
8. The importance of social and emotional factors in childbearing
9. Antenatal and intrapartum infections
10. The roles of health care team members
11. The common conditions for which antenatal admission is required
12. The onset of labour
13. Normal labour
14. Pain relief in labour
15. Induction of labour
16. Physiology of uterine activity and oxytocic drugs
17. Fetal heart rate monitoring and acid-base studies
18. Abnormal labour
19. Abnormal presentations
20. Operative deliveries
21. Resuscitation of a shocked patient
22. Breech deliveries
23. Multiple pregnancies
24. Shoulder dystocia
25. The third stage of labour
26. Episiotomies

27. Breast-feeding
28. Puerperal infections
29. Puerperal disorders, both physical and psychological
30. Physiology of the normal puerperium
31. Maternal immunization with anti-D
32. Rubella vaccinations
33. Home deliveries
34. Indications for the flying squad.

Neonatal medicine

1. Examination of the newborn
2. Resuscitation of the newborn
3. Common diseases in the newborn infant
4. Normal development of the newborn
5. Congenital abnormalities in the newborn.

Gynaecology

1. Health education and preventive medicine
2. Gynaecological history
3. Gynaecological examination
4. Appropriate gynaecological investigations
5. Congenital abnormalities of the female genital tract
6. Psychosexual problems
7. Infertility
8. Abortions (miscarriages)
9. Menstrual disorders
10. Benign lesions of the genital tract
11. Gynaecological malignancies
12. Menopause
13. Urinary tract disorders
14. Vaginal discharge
15. Sexually transmitted diseases
16. Family planning
17. Medical records and clinical audit
18. Communication skills.

RESULTS

Each candidate receives a written result stating whether a pass or fail has been attained. The results are also posted on a board in the College approximately 2 weeks after the examination.

Successful candidates are required to pay a registration fee before being granted the Diploma of the Royal College of Obstetricians and

Gynaecologists. The amount of the current registration fee is available from the Examination Secretary.

WHEN YOU PASS

Once you have passed, and received your Diploma certificate, you are entitled to use the letters DRCOG after your name. The College has a register of diplomates, and you will receive details of College meetings, functions, and events. The College also has limited accommodation which is available to diplomates visiting London. Duplicate certificates cannot be provided in the event of loss or damage.

ADDRESSES

United Kingdom

The Examination Secretary
The Royal College of Obstetricians and Gynaecologists
27 Sussex Place
Regent's Park
London NW1 4RG
(Telephone: London 44 (0)171 262 5425)

Australia and New Zealand have similar examinations. The regulations can be obtained from the following addresses:

Australia

The Examination Secretary
The Royal Australian College of Obstetricians and Gynaecologists
254 Albert Street
East Melbourne
Victoria 3002
Australia

New Zealand

The Royal New Zealand College of Obstetricians and Gynaecologists
PO Box 1503
Wellington 6015
New Zealand

2. Preparing for the examination

J. Rymer

The Diploma examination is intended for general practitioners who have an interest in obstetrics and gynaecology. It is not a specialist qualification. The examiners will expect a 'common-sense' approach to problems, and management aimed at safe medical practice. To emphasize this we open each chapter in our syllabus section with 'Expectations of the examiners' to stress what important knowledge is to be acquired. It is very easy to waste time on minutiae when studying for such a broadly based examination as the DRCOG.

The following points are outlined to assist your preparation:

1. The best preparation for the DRCOG is an SHO post on a busy obstetric and gynaecological rotation with teaching from senior staff. Time spent on wards and in clinics is invaluable as the examination is so 'practically' orientated.
2. Ideally, reading should commence before the post starts, and the syllabus in this book provides a good basic knowledge. Thereafter consistent reading around subjects and conditions as they present on the wards will provide the substance of your learning. This is superior to reading a book from cover to cover.
3. It is advisable to plan a reading programme using the College guidelines for the DRCOG syllabus.
4. In all sections of the DRCOG the examiners will ask questions relevant to current practice. They are often particularly interested in current issues that are in the lay as well as the medical press. Therefore it is wise to keep up to date, and this is best achieved by reading the following journals:
    a. British Journal of Obstetrics and Gynaecology
    b. The British Medical Journal
    c. The Lancet
    d. The Diplomate
    e. Review articles in the British Journal of Hospital Medicine, Practical Therapeutics, and Hospital Update.
5. Journal clubs are a painless way of learning, and discussion around the topics is very valuable.

6. Each unit should have organized teaching sessions, and these are very worthwhile, especially if senior colleagues are present.
7. Revision courses for the DRCOG are good for consolidating knowledge, and for practising skills in OSCEs, especially if you have not been exposed to this format of examination previously. These are usually advertised at your hospital or in the British Medical Journal. It is important to realize that these courses do not cover the whole syllabus, but are valuable for identifying deficiencies in your knowledge, and allowing controversial areas to be discussed. When you only learn obstetrics and gynaecology in one unit it is easy to miss the fact that certain areas of management are controversial.
8. Senior colleagues have experience and a lot to teach. Listen to them!

In 1993 the RCOG published a document entitled 'Report of the DRCOG Working Party'. The working party defined three basic aims of training which are worthwhile keeping in mind during your preparation for the examination:

1. To ensure that doctors completing a defined programme of training have acquired knowledge, clinical skills, and attitudes to enable them to undertake the practice of obstetrics and gynaecology within the setting of primary health care.
2. To encourage the philosophy of updating knowledge and skills by means of further training or study.
3. To facilitate the integration of primary and secondary health care in relation to obstetrics and gynaecology.

3. The written paper

J. Rymer

GENERAL INFORMATION

The written paper consists of a multiple choice question (MCQ) paper lasting 120 minutes. The paper consists of 60 five part MCQs in book form.

MULTIPLE CHOICE QUESTIONS

A key word or introductory statement (the stem), is followed by five words or statements (parts) which relate to the stem. The candidate must decide whether each of the five parts is true or false. For each statement correctly answered true or false one mark is given and for an incorrect answer no mark is awarded.

The most important advice is to read the stem very carefully. Once you have done this read it again. You are allowed to write on the question booklet so you can mark your answers on it and put a question mark beside those of which you are unsure. You are advised to guess if you have no idea whether the statements are true or false, as there is no negative marking.

The first response to a question is more often correct than a later response, so it is unwise to alter the initial answers.

Remember to leave yourself time to complete the answer sheet.

Figure 3.1 is an example of a computer answer sheet.

Examples of multiple choice questions follow below.

Obstetrics

1. *In pregnancy:*
   A. the plasma volume increases more in singleton than in multiple pregnancies
   B. the blood pressure falls in the second trimester
   C. oxygen consumption rises
   D. the GFR decreases
   E. the fasting blood sugar levels rise.

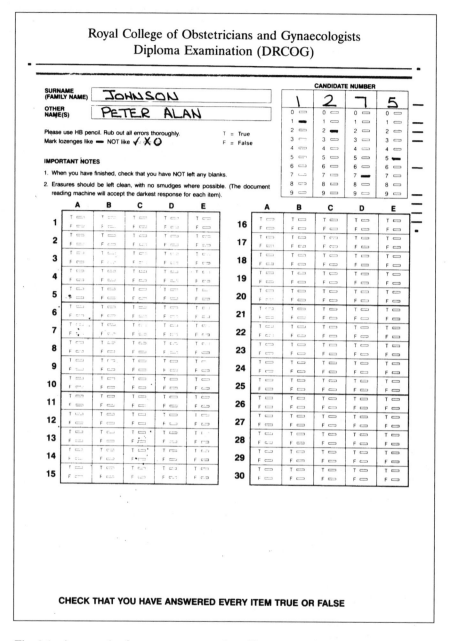

Fig. 3.1 An example of a computer answer sheet. You must mark either the T or F lozenge for each question, using an HB pencil.

2. *A raised maternal serum AFP may be associated with:*
    A. normal pregnancy
    B. trisomy 21
    C. threatened abortion
    D. twins
    E. anencephaly.

3. *Rhesus isoimmunization:*
    A. does not occur during the first pregnancy
    B. is no longer a problem in England since the introduction of anti-D prophylaxis
    C. may cause fetal ascites in a severely affected case
    D. may lead to Chadwick's sign being detected on ultrasound in early pregnancy
    E. 50 μg of anti-D following a first trimester abortion is sufficient.

4. *The following antenatal complications are more common in multiple than singleton pregnancies:*
    A. premature labour
    B. placenta praevia
    C. congenital abnormalities
    D. polyhydramnios
    E. pre-eclampsia.

5. *Relating to diabetes and pregnancy:*
    A. polyhydramnios complicates 60% of pregnancies in established diabetics
    B. pre-eclampsia is more common in diabetic pregnancies
    C. an IDDM patient with retinopathy should be advised to avoid pregnancy
    D. the glycosylated haemoglobin level gives an indication of diabetic control over the preceding weeks
    E. congenital abnormality is now the most important contributor to perinatal morbidity and mortality.

6. *A 20-year-old primigravida at 34 weeks presents to the antenatal clinic with a BP of 150/95 mmHg and proteinuria of 4 g/24 hours:*
    A. she should be told to rest in bed at home with daily visits from the community midwife
    B. a serum urate of 0.45 mmol/l is consistent with severe disease
    C. she may have thrombocytopenia
    D. delivery should always be by LSCS
    E. if she has oedema, the disease will be more severe.

7. *Preterm delivery:*
    A. preterm delivery accounts for 75% of all perinatal deaths

B. genital infection is not a risk factor
C. previous preterm labour is not a risk factor
D. by identifying at-risk patients (by risk screening) the incidence of preterm delivery can be reduced
E. tocolytic drugs delay delivery by a minimum of 1 week.

8. *The following are associated with a breech presentation:*
    A. placenta praevia
    B. multiple pregnancy
    C. an incidence of 3% at term
    D. Potter's syndrome
    E. Tay–Sach's disease.

9. *Non-stressed antepartum cardiotocography performed at 36 weeks:*
    A. can be interpreted using the same criteria as for a pregnancy at 26 weeks
    B. if the rate is 110/minute delivery should be undertaken as soon as possible
    C. deceleration in response to movement is a normal finding
    D. may show uterine activity
    E. if there is reduced variability for 20 minutes the fetus may be sleeping.

10. *The following are appropriate indications for chorionic villus sampling:*
    A. a woman aged 39 with a confirmed 12 weeks' gestation
    B. a woman aged 45 with a confirmed 8 weeks' gestation
    C. a woman who is known to be a translocation carrier
    D. a woman whose son has Niemann–Pick disease
    E. a woman aged 30 whose husband is aged 45.

11. *The following statements relating to vaccination in pregnancy are correct:*
    A. rabies vaccine is safe for use in pregnancy
    B. poliomyelitis vaccination is contraindicated in pregnancy
    C. inadvertent administration of rubella vaccination in pregnancy is an indication for termination
    D. tetanus vaccination carries no risk of intrauterine fetal infection
    E. human varicella zoster immunoglobulin should be given to the term newborn of a mother who has shown evidence of varicella zoster infection in the second trimester.

12. *The following features in a patient's history should alert the obstetrician to the possibility of systemic lupus erythematosus (SLE):*
    A. early onset severe pre-eclampsia
    B. second trimester intrauterine death
    C. early severe intrauterine growth retardation

    D. photosensitive skin rashes
    E. recurrent first trimester abortions.

13. *When a pregnant woman develops hepatitis B:*
    A. the course of acute hepatitis B is unaffected by pregnancy
    B. demonstration of hepatitis B e antigen in the mother's serum
       makes congenital infection unlikely
    C. caesarean delivery is indicated to reduce the risk of viral infection
       in the newborn
    D. most cases can be managed as outpatients
    E. transmission from mother to baby is commoner amongst Asian
       than Caucasian patients.

14. *The following statements about oral iron prophylaxis during pregnancy are
    correct:*
    A. diarrhoea and constipation can occur
    B. if prophylaxis is not given, iron deficiency will develop
    C. non-compliance of the mother occurs in less than 10% of cases
    D. maternal iron prophylaxis is recognized to reduce the incidence of
       infant iron deficiency anaemia
    E. oral maternal iron prophylaxis is associated with an increase in
       MCV.

15. *The following statements about severe pre-eclampsia are correct:*
    A. disseminated intravascular coagulation is a recognized underlying
       cause
    B. epidural anaesthesia is contraindicated if the platelet count is
       <100
    C. plasma volume is reduced
    D. diuretics are helpful in management
    E. the serum urate concentration is typically elevated.

16. *A patient at 38 weeks is found to have a uterine size of 32 weeks. The
    following ultrasound observations are suggestive of intrauterine growth
    retardation:*
    A. oligohydramnios
    B. an abdominal circumference on the 50th percentile for 32 weeks
    C. an anterior placenta
    D. a BPD on the 50th percentile for 38 weeks
    E. fetal tachycardia.

17. *Regarding labour:*
    A. induction of labour is not associated with an increased caesarean
       section rate
    B. prolonged labour in a multiparous woman is likely to be due to
       inefficient uterine action

C. Kjelland's forceps are associated with an increased incidence of neonatal cerebral irritability
D. the average length of the second stage in a nulliparous patient is 60 minutes
E. the minimum acceptable rate of cervical dilatation in the active phase of labour is 1 cm/hour.

18. *Puerperal psychosis:*
    A. occurs in about 1 in 1000 mothers
    B. is characteristically manic in type
    C. usually only results in a 2–3 weeks' hospital stay
    D. is not recurrent in future pregnancies
    E. is best treated by separation of the mother and the baby because of the risk of infanticide.

19. *Regarding forceps deliveries:*
    A. Wrigley's forceps have a cephalic curve, but no pelvic curve
    B. incorrect application of the forceps can result in cranial nerve palsies
    C. if the station of the head is −1 it is acceptable to use Kjelland's forceps
    D. a pudendal block can be used
    E. the patient does not need to be catheterized.

20. *Postpartum haemorrhage:*
    A. a previous postpartum haemorrhage is a risk factor for a subsequent postpartum haemorrhage
    B. can be prophylactically treated with an intravenous oxytocic with the delivery of the anterior shoulder followed by an intravenous infusion over 3 hours
    C. is defined as a blood loss of 500 ml within the first 12 hours
    D. can occur with morbid adherence of the placenta
    E. is the main cause of maternal deaths in the latest triennial report.

Statistics

21. *In the Confidential Enquiry into Maternal Deaths (England and Wales) for the period 1991–93:*
    A. hypertensive disease was the commonest cause of direct maternal death
    B. the death rate from ectopic pregnancy had fallen
    C. there was a maternal death rate of 14 per 100 000 total maternities
    D. about one-third of all maternal deaths were associated with caesarean section

E. death in association with abortion was included in the true
    maternal mortality rate.

22. *Concerning the 1991–93 Maternal Mortality Report:*
    A. the last report was published 5 years previously
    B. anaesthetic causes still claim the most lives
    C. direct mortality is lowest in women having their second baby
    D. genital sepsis remains a major cause of maternal death
    E. in deaths due to hypertensive diseases, the cause is usually
        cerebral haemorrhage.

23. *Concerning perinatal mortality in Britain:*
    A. the perinatal mortality rate includes stillbirths and first week
        neonatal deaths
    B. the three major causes are low birth weight, malformation and
        asphyxia
    C. the perinatal death rate decreases with increasing parity
    D. the lowest rate occurs in social class III
    E. if an infant is born before 24 weeks' gestation and shows signs of
        life, but then dies within the first 24 hours, it is not included as a
        perinatal death.

Neonatal medicine

24. *Babies of diabetic mothers have an increased risk of:*
    A. respiratory distress syndrome
    B. intrauterine growth retardation
    C. macrosomia
    D. anaemia
    E. hyperbilirubinaemia.

25. *In herpes neonatorum:*
    A. the majority of mothers have a history of herpes genitalis
    B. the herpes simplex virus (HSV) is frequently recovered from the
        amniotic fluid of infected infants
    C. Type I HSV is usually involved
    D. the presence of maternal antibodies is protective
    E. maternal viraemia is characteristically the cause.

26. *The following statements about neonatal resuscitation are correct:*
    A. an apnoeic baby at birth with a heart rate of less than 80
        beats/minute should be intubated
    B. in a baby who has been exposed to meconium inhalation it is
        important to visualize the cords
    C. drying and warming the baby together with simple stimulation
        normally corrects terminal apnoea

   D. the effects of pethidine given to the mother late in labour may be corrected during resuscitation of the newborn by the administration of naloxone (0.01 mg/kg) via an umbilical vein

   E. a diaphragmatic hernia is a recognized cause of a newborn failing to respond to resuscitation including intermittent positive pressure ventilation.

27. *Congenital cytomegalovirus is:*
   A. present in up to 20% of babies
   B. usual if the mother has a primary infection
   C. rare if the mother is immune prior to pregnancy
   D. usually symptomatic if the virus is recovered from the neonate at birth
   E. characteristically associated with significant neurological impairment following a primary maternal infection.

28. *Recognized complications of preterm birth include:*
   A. poor temperature control in the newborn
   B. transient tachypnoea of the newborn
   C. jaundice
   D. meconium aspiration syndrome
   E. apnoeic attacks.

29. *The normal infant delivered at term has:*
   A. a head circumference of 40 cm
   B. an impalpable liver
   C. a plasma glucose above 1.7 mmol/l
   D. brown adipose tissue
   E. no adult haemoglobin.

30. *Regarding fetal circulation:*
   A. the ductus venosus carries blood to the inferior vena cava from the umbilical artery
   B. the ductus arteriosus carries blood from the pulmonary artery to the aorta
   C the foramen ovale permits blood to pass from the right to the left ventricle
   D. the ductus arteriosus is contractile
   E. the umbilical vein becomes the ligamentum teres of the adult.

Gynaecology

31. *During a normal menstrual cycle:*
   A. the proliferative phase of the endometrium follows ovulation
   B. the plasma progesterone concentration rises following ovulation

   C. the average menstrual blood loss is 200 ml
   D. ovulation is dependent upon an intact hypothalamic pituitary
       portal circulation
   E. the blood loss is normally fluid because of the presence of
       fibrinolysins.

32. *The climacteric is usually associated with:*
   A. a reduction in the level of follicle stimulating hormone
   B. a reduction in circulating oestrogens
   C. an elevated serum 5-hydroxytryptamine level
   D. hyperprolactinaemia
   E. a reduction in the serum cholesterol concentration.

33. *The following statements about colposcopy are correct:*
   A. mild dyskaryosis on a smear should not be referred for
       colposcopy, but the smear should be repeated annually until a
       more significant change is detectable
   B. severe dyskaryosis on a smear always indicates CIN3
   C. an 'incomplete' colposcopic assessment can safely be followed by
       laser ablation providing a biopsy has confirmed CIN
   D. a mosaic pattern suggests intraepithelial dysplasia
   E. during prepuberty the transformation zone is more likely to be in
       the endocervical canal.

34. *The following statements concerning endometrial cancer are correct:*
   A. the risk of developing endometrial cancer is increased in diabetics
   B. postcoital bleeding is the classical symptom
   C. a dilatation and curettage is not required if the colposcopic
       assessment is normal
   D. the incidence is decreased in nulliparous women
   E. the incidence is increased in women who receive unopposed
       oestrogen therapy.

35. *Regarding ectopic pregnancies:*
   A. 95% occur in the fallopian tube
   B. PID is the most important aetiological factor
   C. ultrasound should always be performed prior to referral to
       hospital
   D. bleeding is usually the first symptom
   E. if the urine pregnancy test is negative the diagnosis is ruled out.

36. *The following investigations should be performed routinely on a woman who
   presents with symptoms of urinary urgency:*
   A. barium enema
   B. mid-stream urine (MSU)

    C. urodynamics

    D. abdominal X-ray

    E. pelvic examination.

37. *Concerning infertility:*

    A. AIH has been proven to increase the 'take home baby rate' in couples who have unexplained infertility

    B. clomiphene can be given to induce ovulation in anovulatory women

    C. if the postcoital test is normal then a semen sample is not needed

    D. GIFT is used in women who have tubal disease

    E. stress can cause anovulation.

38. *Concerning carcinoma of the cervix:*

    A. the peak age is 50–59 years

    B. it is the commonest malignant tumour of the genital tract

    C. early spread occurs via the venous system

    D. a microinvasive lesion has invaded the stroma to a depth of 3 mm and the lymphatics are involved

    E. it is more common in women who smoke.

39. *Polycystic ovarian syndrome:*

    A. clinical features include hirsutism, anorexia, and dysfunctional bleeding

    B. can be treated with clomiphene

    C. LH levels are usually raised

    D. women who have this disorder are at increased risk of endometrial cancer

    E. wedge resection of the ovaries is a common successful form of treatment.

40. *Therapeutic abortion:*

    A. mortality and morbidity increase with increasing gestational age

    B. uterine perforation requires immediate laparotomy

    C. secondary infertility is a recognized late complication of first trimester abortion

    D. the mortality rate of legal abortion is less than 1 per 1 000 000 maternities

    E. prostaglandins in an asthmatic can cause acute bronchospasm.

41. *Endometriosis:*

    A. can be treated with the CO_2 laser

    B. can be treated with danazol to create a 'pseudo-pregnancy'

    C. can cause Asherman's syndrome

    D. can cause dyspareunia

    E. if severe can cause infertility.

42. *Hirsutism:*
   A. polycystic ovarian syndrome and idiopathic hirsutism account for over 90% of cases
   B. is a side-effect of danazol
   C. is a side-effect of spironolactone
   D. shaving increases hair growth
   E. LH, FSH, and testosterone levels should be measured.

43. *Contraindications to oestrogen replacement therapy for postmenopausal women include:*
   A. cervical carcinoma
   B. past history of breast cancer
   C. past history of DVT
   D. diabetes
   E. past history of endometrial cancer.

44. *Infertility:*
   A. the incidence of unexplained infertility in infertile couples is about 10–15%
   B. there is a decline in fecundity with age
   C. if the husband is identified as having 'poor' sperm then investigations in the partner can be abandoned
   D. azoospermia is associated with small testes and a low FSH level
   E. GIFT can be used in women with unexplained infertility.

45. *Genital prolapse:*
   A. can be caused by vaginal delivery
   B. vaginal narrowing can occur after colporrhaphy
   C. vaginal hysterectomies have less postoperative morbidity than abdominal hysterectomies if prophylactic antibiotics are used
   D. cannot occur in a nulliparous woman
   E. can become worse after the climacteric.

46. *Hydatidiform mole:*
   A. can produce ovarian enlargement and breathlessness
   B. can present with pre-eclampsia before 20 weeks
   C. when complete is totally maternally derived
   D. if partial, has more chance of being followed by choriocarcinoma than a complete mole
   E. can be treated by hysterectomy in the older woman.

47. *The vagina:*
   A. the anterior wall is longer than the posterior wall
   B. the normal epithelium contains mucus secreting glands
   C. is related in its lower third to the bladder base

D. the pH is acidic during the reproductive phase of life
E. ovarian function can be assessed by the cytology of vaginal wall smears.

48. *A 25-year-old nulliparous woman is referred from her general practitioner with an abnormal smear:*
    A. a smear should always be repeated before referral
    B. menstruation is the best time to perform colposcopy as the transformation zone is easily seen
    C. ideally ectocervical cells should be seen on the smear
    D. colposcopic assessment may be incomplete
    E. at colposcopy bizarre vessel branching suggests CIN.

49. *Ovarian cancer:*
    A. 30% have metastases beyond the pelvis at the initial diagnosis
    B. can be properly staged using a Pfannenstiel incision
    C. the mortality rate has significantly changed over the past 20 years
    D. laparoscopy is acceptable as a 'second-look' operation
    E can present with vague symptoms of dyspepsia, tiredness, and abdominal distension.

50. *Dysfunctional uterine bleeding:*
    A. is a diagnosis of exclusion
    B. a dilatation and curettage is therapeutic
    C. the endometrial curettings are abnormal
    D. danazol can be used as treatment
    E. laser ablation of the endometrium is acceptable treatment.

Sexually transmitted infections

51. *Trichomonas vaginalis:*
    A. can be diagnosed by colposcopy
    B. causes clue cells on microscopy
    C. on a wet mount, preparation may reveal motile flagellated protozoa
    D. can be treated with metronidazole
    E. classically produces a thick white discharge.

52. *Regarding AIDS:*
    A. vertical transmission appears to occur in 30% of infants delivered to HIV infected women
    B. transmission of HIV to the fetus has been proven to occur in the first trimester
    C. is caused by a retrovirus
    D. nosocomial exposure is an important mode of spread
    E. the diagnosis of HIV in children is difficult due to passive acquisition of maternal HIV antibodies.

53. *Hepatitis B infection in a pregnant woman:*
    A. carries a 1.8% chance of mortality
    B. is associated with congenital abnormalities
    C. infection in a pregnant woman carries a 60% increase in preterm delivery
    D. in the third trimester the risk of vertical transmission is 20%
    E. newborns of HBsAg positive mothers should have hepatitis B immunoglobulin at birth.

54. *The lesions of syphilis include:*
    A. perivascular inflammation
    B. cranial nerve lesions
    C. aortic aneurysm
    D. vulval ulceration
    E. condylomata acuminata.

Family planning

55. *The combined oral contraceptive pill is protective against:*
    A. ovarian cancer
    B. endometrial cancer
    C. cervical cancer
    D. ectopic pregnancy
    E. pelvic inflammatory disease.

56. *Regarding IUDs:*
    A. menorrhagia is an absolute contraindication
    B. encrustation of a copper device is associated with failure
    C. actinomycosis may be seen with prolonged use of IUDs
    D. are contraindicated in women who have had a caesarean section
    E. IUDs inserted within 5 days of unprotected intercourse can act as postcoital contraception.

57. *Sterilization:*
    A. the failure rate is 1–5 per 1000 procedures (in females)
    B. vasectomy is safer than female sterilization
    C. in males is deemed successful if two postoperative seminal specimens are 'sperm free'
    D. postoperatively menstrual loss should decrease
    E. the failure rate is increased if performed at the time of abortion.

58. *Regarding the combined oral contraceptive pill:*
    A. it should not be prescribed to women over the age of 37 years
    B. if diarrhoea occurs, the pill may not be absorbed
    C. in higher doses it can be used as the morning after pill

D. it is associated with an increased incidence of pulmonary embolism

E. it should not be prescribed in diabetic women.

ANSWERS TO MULTIPLE CHOICE QUESTIONS

The correct answers are given below.

Obstetrics

1. B.C.
2. A.C.D.E.
3. C.E. Rhesus isoimmunization has dramatically decreased in incidence but has by no means disappeared. Chadwick's sign is a clinical sign of early pregnancy.
4. A.B.C.D.E. This question emphasizes the fact that nearly all antenatal complications are more common in multiple pregnancies.
5. B.D.E. Polyhydramnios complicates 25% of pregnancies in established diabetics. Diabetic retinopathy, diabetic vascular disease, and neuropathy are not adversely affected by pregnancy.
6. B.C.
7. A. There is no evidence that identification of risk factors reduces the incidence of preterm delivery. Tocolysis has not been shown to reduce perinatal morbidity or mortality.
8. A.B.C.D.
9. D.E. At 26 weeks the variability may be reduced. If there are no other adverse features, a fetal heart rate of 110/minute is normal. Decelerations in response to movements are an ominous sign. Fetuses do have sleep cycles of 20 minutes, so a CTG must be continued for longer than 20 minutes to see if it becomes reactive.
10. A.C.D. CVS is not normally performed at less than 11 weeks due to possible risk of limb defects.
11. A.D. If vaccination is required in pregnancy, live vaccines should be avoided. Passive immunization is available with anti-rabies human immunoglobulin. The Salk inactivated virus is used for poliomyelitis vaccination in pregnancy.
12. A.B.C.D.E.
13. D.E. Acute maternal infection with hepatitis B virus may result in congenital hepatitis and the risk depends on the trimester in which maternal infection occurs, being highest at term.
14. A.E.
15. B.C.E. Severe pre-eclampsia can result in DIC. As the plasma volume is reduced in these women, diuretics are contraindicated.
16. A.B.

17. C.E. In the active phase of the first stage of labour the cervix dilates at up to 3 cm and 6 cm/hour in primigravidae and multigravidae respectively (the minimum acceptable rate is 1 cm/hour). The average length of the second stage in primigravidae is 40 minutes, and in multigravidae, 20 minutes.
18. A.
19. B.D.
20. A.B.D. A postpartum haemorrhage is defined as a blood loss of $\geq$ 500 ml within the first 24 hours after delivery. Hypertensive diseases of pregnancy were the main cause of maternal deaths in the latest triennial report.

Statistics

21. A.B.E. For the period 1991–93, the death rate from ectopic pregnancies has almost halved, despite an increase in the incidence of ectopic pregnancy. The maternal death rate per 100 000 total maternities was 60. Nine out of 103 deaths were associated with caesarean section.
22. C.D. The report on confidential enquiries into maternal deaths in England and Wales is performed every 3 years. The major cause of death in cases of hypertension was previously cerebral haemorrhage but in 1991–93 ARDS was the commonest cause.
23. A.B. The perinatal mortality rate is the number of stillbirths and first week deaths occurring from 24 completed weeks of pregnancy to 7 days after birth per 1000 total births, but if an infant is born before 24 weeks' gestation and shows signs of life but then dies within 7 days, it is to be included as a perinatal death.

Neonatal medicine

24. A.B.C.E. Severe diabetics are at risk of IUGR.
25. A.
26. A.B.D.E.
27. A. CMV is the most common viral infection during pregnancy. By the time an infant is born with the stigmata of congenital CMV infection, damage has occurred in utero and therapy at birth is not effective. There are currently no therapies or immunization practices.
28. A.B.C.E. The passage of meconium is rare in preterm infants, and if it occurs, listeriosis should be considered.
29. C.D.
30. B.D.E.

Gynaecology

31. B.D.E. The average menstrual blood loss is about 40 mls.

32. B. FSH and LH levels rise, and oestradiol levels fall.
33. D.E.
34. A.E. Intermenstrual bleeding is the classical symptom of endometrial carcinoma, and postcoital bleeding is suggestive of cervical carcinoma. A postmenopausal woman who has bleeding should be referred for endometrial biopsy.
35. A.B.
36. B.C.E.
37. B.E.
38. A.E. Cervical cancer is second to ovarian as the commonest malignant tumour of the genital tract. The incidence of cervical cancer has fallen but the peak age is still 50–59 years, and the incidence has doubled in women under 40 years. The lymphatics are not involved in a microinvasive lesion.
39. B.C.D.
40. A.C.E. If uterine perforation occurs during the procedure, a laparoscopy should be performed and the completion of the evacuation performed while another operator is watching through the laparoscope. Laparotomy is carried out if the uterine tear is actively bleeding.
41. A.D.E. Danazol creates a 'pseudo-menopause'.
42. A.B.E. Spironolactone is used in the treatment of hirsutism.
43. B.E.
44. A.B.E. It is common in cases of 'infertility' to have 'subfertility' in both partners. Men with azoospermia have small testes and high FSH levels.
45. A.B.C.E.
46. A.B.E. Complete hydatidiform moles are totally paternally derived.
47. D.E.
48. D.E. A smear showing severely dyskaryotic cells demands colposcopic referral and a smear showing malignant cells demands urgent referral.
49. D.E. 75% of women with ovarian carcinoma have stage III or stage IV disease at time of presentation. A vertical incision is essential for correct staging. Laparotomy is usually performed, but laparoscopy is acceptable and this is done at 1 year postoperation.
50. A.D.E. A dilatation and curettage is a diagnostic procedure.

Sexually transmitted diseases

51. A.C.D. *Trichomonas* is easily diagnosed by colposcopy and typical Y-shaped vessels are seen. Clue cells are usually associated with *Gardnerella vaginalis*. The classical discharge of *Trichomonas* is usually profuse, offensive, and greenish-yellow.
52. B.C.E. Vertical transmission occurs in approximately 15%.

53. A.E. Hepatitis infection in pregnancy is associated with a 20% increase in preterm delivery. In the third trimester the risk of vertical transmission is 66% and less than 10% if the virus is acquired earlier.
54. A.B.C.D.

Family planning

55. A.B.D.E.
56. B.C.E. Beware of questions that say 'absolute'.
57. A.B.C.E.
58. B.C.D.

4. Objective structured clinical examination

J. Rymer

Objective structured clinical examinations (OSCEs) are well established as a method of student assessment and are gradually being introduced into postgraduate assessment. In 1994 the RCOG commenced OSCEs for the Diploma examination. Major weaknesses were identified with the previous form of assessment, namely clinicals and vivas. OSCEs have been developed because they are valid, reliable, have high fidelity and are a feasible method of assessment. The examination consists of a circuit of 22 stations of which 20 are marked. At each station the candidate has to perform a task and these stations may test knowledge, skills, communication, or problem-solving ability. Depending on the type of station there may be a role-player, a patient, a photograph, or a clinical scenario. The stations will be laid out in a clockwise direction 1 to 22 and on your entrance card will be the station number and circuit number at which you start. The invigilator will instruct you as to when to proceed to your station number. When you sit down it is important that you check that you are at the right station and there will be an answer book on the desk with your name and candidate number on it. Again you need to check that this is correct and, if not, alert one of the invigilators. In the answer books it is imperative that you only write within the boxes and you must use the pencil provided.

At each station you will have 6 minutes and then a bell will sound. When this occurs you move in a clockwise direction to the next station. There will be two rest stations within the OSCE. You can use this time for a rest and to check your answer sheet.

KNOWLEDGE OR FACTUAL STATION

These stations are purely assessing your knowledge regarding certain subjects. The material provided may be a photograph, results of investigations or a clinical scenario. The answer sheets are designed so that you only write within the boxes — only one answer within one box. The columns on the right hand side are for the examiners only so do not write within them as they are optically read and erroneous marks may mean incorrect marking. The following are examples:

27

Station 1

For Examiner's Use Only	
Correct	No Mark
Total	

1. What common gynaecological procedure has been carried out in the laparoscopic picture illustrated?

> < | > <

2. Give three important facts that your patient should be aware of about the procedure and which you should discuss with her.

> < | > <

> < | > <

> < | > <

3. What is the usual failure rate of this procedure?

> < | > <

4. Is the procedure shown in the photograph an appropriate procedure to carry out in the week following delivery?

> < | > <

5. State a reason.

> < | > <

6. Name the metal structures used for this procedure.

> < | > <

7. If the patient had had her LMP 6 weeks prior to the procedure, what investigation would you do?

> < | > <

8. What medium has been used to distend the abdomen?

> < | > <

Station 2

For Examiner's Use Only	
Correct	No Mark
Total	

Name the sutures and fontanelles that are marked on this specimen. Numbers 1–6.

1.
2.
3.
4.
5.
6.

>	<	>	<
>	<	>	<
>	<	>	<
>	<	>	<
>	<	>	<
>	<	>	<

Define denominator

7.

>	<	>	<

What is the denominator of the following presentations: vertex, breech, face?

8.
9.
10.

>	<	>	<
>	<	>	<
>	<	>	<

CLINICAL SKILLS STATION

As with the pre-existing clinicals you may be asked to examine a patient.

(You may be asked to examine a pregnant patient, although this is unlikely due to the feasibility of having pregnant patients within an OSCE circuit. It would be more likely to be a plastic model, or a role-player. Your instructions as to what to examine will be quite clear.)

The following are guidelines for examination:

General examination

Observe the patient's facies, demeanour, and nutritional state. Ask yourself, 'does the patient look well?' A pregnant patient should have 'the bloom of pregnancy' due to vasodilatation and increased blood volume. Start by looking at the patient's hands. The blood pressure can then be taken, in the seated semiprone or lateral position. Check the conjunctivae for evidence of anaemia. If the patient is hypertensive remember to examine the optic fundi but do not spend too much time on this aspect. Look for thyroid enlargement, and inspect and palpate the patient's breasts. The heart and lungs should be auscultated. Sacral oedema and pretibial oedema should be tested for. The legs should be inspected for varicosities, and the reflexes must be tested.

Abdominal examination

As with every medical examination, remember: inspection, palpation, percussion, and auscultation.

Inspection

Observe for striae gravidarum. Is the swelling symmetrical? Are fetal movements seen? Are there any scars present (particularly look for a laparoscopy scar)?

Palpation

Firstly, palpate the upper margin of the uterine fundus and measure the symphysiofundal height with a tape measure. Then feel for the presenting part and determine whether it is engaged or not. (The examiner may ask you to express this in fifths palpable above the brim.) Then palpate the uterus to determine which side the fetal back is on. If you are unable to determine the presentation, don't panic, as in some cases this may be difficult.

Percussion

Is seldom necessary.

Auscultation

You must listen for the fetal heart in the appropriate place. (You may be asked to demonstrate the fetal heart with the sonicaid.)

Vaginal examination

In the context of an OSCE, this would more likely be with a pelvic model and you may be asked to pass a speculum, take a cervical smear or swab and then do a bimanual examination. Marks could be given for technique and dexterity. In this situation it would be appropriate to talk to the model as if it was a live patient.

The following is an example of a clinical skills station relating to an obstetric patient.

Prior to a skills or communication station you may have a rest station where information will be given to you for the actual communication station. This will give you time to prepare. The marking system will not be given to you, but a sample marking system is given here.

Station 3—Rest Station

At the next station you will meet Mrs R. T. She is a 34-year-old primigravida and is currently at 37 weeks' gestation. You need to check her BP, examine her abdomen, and check for oedema.

Station 4

Marks awarded for:	Marks
Examiner to mark	
1. Introducing yourself	1
2. Taking BP correctly (positioning etc.) and getting the correct BP	1
3. Observing abdomen and detecting scar	1
4. Measuring symphysiofundal height	1
5. Assessing presentation	1
6. Determining engagement of head	1
7. Determining lie	1
8. Testing for oedema adequately	1
Role-player to mark	
1. Rapport	1
2. Not hurting patient during examination	1

COMMUNICATION STATION

Remember that at these stations communication is being assessed and knowledge is often secondary. The purpose of these stations is to assess your ability to communicate with the patients, so you must always treat the patients as individuals and be considerate. You want to convey to the examiner that you are a kind, compassionate and discerning clinician. As soon as you arrive at this station introduce yourself to the patient or role-player. Remember that some patients are excellent historians and some are not. The role-player may have been briefed not to communicate well and therefore the station is assessing your skill to extract information. If there is a role-player at the station she will have been briefed to give the same scenario to each candidate. Remember the role-player or patient may well be awarding some marks.

The following is an example of a communication station, and how the marking may be awarded. In this case the information is given to you at the rest station preceding the station where the patient/role-player is.

Station 5

This is a rest station. At the next station you will be seeing a patient. Please read the following scenario to prepare yourself for the next station:

> Mrs Trihard is a 27-year-old woman who has been trying to become pregnant for 2 years. This is the first time she has come to see you (you are her general practitioner). Please take a relevant history from her and explain to her that you wish to arrange for a day 21 progesterone and semen analysis.
>
> *Remember you will only have 6 minutes.*

Role-player information (information not given to candidate)

You have been trying for a pregnancy for 2 years. You are rather embarrassed about the subject but it is very important to you, and your husband is not very helpful. You have been taking your temperature for 18 months and you are finding it all very stressful. You are having intercourse twice a week but it is all becoming rather forced especially at the appropriate time. You have regular periods and have no history of pelvic infection. It does worry you that your husband may be having an affair with his secretary.

Your answer sheet will be blank apart from the marking columns, but the allocation of marks is shown here for your information.

Please hand this sheet to the examiner

Station 6

	For Examiner's Use Only	
	Correct	No Mark
	Total	
Candidate introducing his/herself	> <	> <
Making patient feel comfortable	> <	> <
Extracting appropriate information	> <	> <
Listening to patient	> <	> <
Explaining the serum progesterone test	> <	> <
Explaining the semen analysis	> <	> <
Checking if patient has any questions	> <	> <
Future plan of management	> <	> <
Role-player to mark confidence of candidate	> <	> <
Role-player to mark rapport	> <	> <

SUMMARY

An OSCE ensures that each candidate is exposed to the same examination questions and environment. Therefore the marking is very rigid and standardized.

Station 1—Answers   Marks

1. Laparoscopic sterilization with clips   1
2. Failure rate
   Relative irreversibility
   That it may require an open operation
   Anaesthesia
   Ectopic risk
   Postoperative regret   3
3. 1 : 200–1 : 500   1
4. No   1
5. Tubes too thick, therefore higher failure rate   1
6. Filschie clips   1
7. Pregnancy test   1
8. CO_2 1

Station 2—Answers   Marks

1. Frontal suture
2. Anterior fontanelle (bregma)
3. Coronal suture
4. Sagittal suture
5. Posterior fontanelle
6. Lambdoidal suture   6
7. The denominator is a defined point of the presenting part and
   is used to describe the fetal position   1
8. Cephalic—occiput
9. Breech—sacrum
10. Face—mentum   3

The syllabus

A. GYNAECOLOGY

5. The menstrual cycle

G. Davis

Expectations of the examiners

A basic knowledge of the menstrual cycle is essential to the understanding of most gynaecological disorders and hormonal methods of contraception. Examiners will not expect a detailed knowledge of the endocrinology of the menstrual cycle but could ask about the basic principles.

HYPOTHALAMUS–PITUITARY–GONAD (HPG) AXIS

In the fifth month of intrauterine life, primordial follicles in the ovary of the female fetus reach their maximum number (approximately 6–7 million per ovary). From then on, follicles continue to grow and become atretic until the menopause. This process occurs independently of gonadotrophin stimulation and under all physiological circumstances including ovulation, pregnancy and periods of anovulation. As most women ovulate 400–500 times in their life, it is the fate of the vast majority of these follicles to become atretic.

No full development of the follicle occurs until the onset of puberty. At puberty, changes in the sensitivity of the HPG system result in the pulsed secretion of gonadotrophin releasing hormone (GnRH) from the hypothalamus. This in turn causes a similar pulsed release of the gonadotrophins, follicle stimulating hormone (FSH) and luteinizing hormone (LH), from the anterior pituitary. Thereafter, FSH and LH are secreted in pulses every 70–220 minutes depending on the phase of the cycle. This pattern of release is modulated by the steroid feedback on the hypothalamus and pituitary.

Follicular phase

At the beginning of each cycle, FSH stimulates further growth in follicles which have reached a critical stage in their development. In normal cycles, the development of one follicle outstrips the others (dominant follicle). The production of inhibitory factors by the dominant follicle and the falling levels of FSH in the mid-follicular phase lead to atresia in the remaining follicles. As the dominant follicle grows, oestrogen production within the follicle increases dramatically leading to the rising levels of oestradiol seen in the peripheral blood during this phase. LH promotes conversion of cholesterol to androgens in the theca cells. These androgens are then converted to oestradiol by the action of aromatase.

Ovulation

It is the rising levels of oestradiol in the peripheral circulation which trigger the LH surge from the pituitary which leads to ovulation approximately 36 hours after the initial rise in LH. The mid-cycle surge of LH (and to a lesser extent FSH) stimulates the completion of meiosis in the oocyte and the production of progesterone and prostaglandins in the follicle. The prostaglandins and enzymes activated by the LH/FSH surge free the oocyte from its attachments to the surrounding granulosa cells and cause lysis of the follicular wall to release the oocyte. The follicular phase varies but is usually 14 days or longer.

Luteal phase

With the release of the ovum, the follicle shrinks and the granulosa cells produce a yellow pigment which gives the corpus luteum its name. The corpus luteum produces all three classes of sex steroids: androgens, oestrogens, and progestins, but it is the production of progesterone which distinguishes the luteal from the follicular phase. The massive secretion of progesterone is important in preparing the endometrium for implantation and also suppresses the growth of new follicles past the preantral stage. The lifespan of the corpus luteum is 9–11 days, after which it regresses and steroid levels fall unless pregnancy intervenes. Human chorionic gonadotrophin (hCG) from the implanting pregnancy maintains the production of steroids from the corpus luteum until the 14th or 16th week of gestation, by which time placental steroidogenesis is well established. As the menopause approaches the follicles become more and more resistant to stimulation. The pituitary responds to the low oestradiol concentration by increasing the amount of FSH released. Finally, despite high concentrations of FSH there are no further responsive follicles and amenorrhoea (the menopause) ensues.

ENDOMETRIAL CYCLE

Proliferative phase

This corresponds to the follicular phase in the ovary. The most obvious response to oestradiol in the endometrium is cell division (hence the name 'proliferative phase'). Mitosis occurs in both stromal and epithelial cells

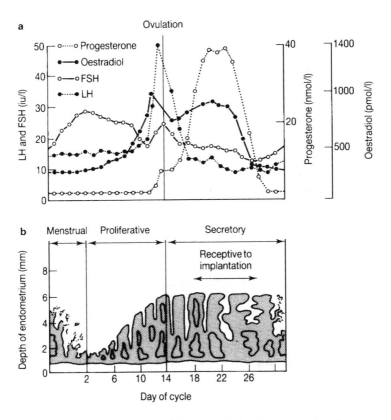

Fig. 5.1   (a) Hormonal and (b) endometrial changes during the menstrual cycle.

leading to growth of the glands and thickening of the endometrium from 0.5 mm in the menstrual phase to 3.5–5 mm in height at the end of the proliferative phase.

Secretory phase

Microscopically, the first sign of the effect of progesterone on the endometrium is the appearance of vacuoles at the base of the epithelial cells lining the glands which displace the nuclei towards the gland lumen. Mitotic activity ceases but the glands and spiral arterioles continue to grow, becoming progressively more coiled and tortuous. The glandular cells, presumably full of secretory products, bulge into the glands and the glands become dilated with secreted material.

The stroma becomes oedematous in the mid-secretory phase and stromal cells undergo decidualization. They change from being thin fibroblast-like cells to the large polyhedral cells seen in true decidua in pregnancy.

Menstrual phase

Falling levels of oestradiol and progesterone at the end of the secretory phase cause cyclical constriction and dilatation of the spiral arterioles in the endometrium. These spasms are successively more intense and prolonged, leading to generalized vasoconstriction, ischaemia and cell disintegration with release of lysosomal enzymes. Neutrophil leukocytes infiltrate the endometrium and breakdown continues until rising concentrations of oestradiol in the subsequent menstrual cycle initiate healing.

LOWER GENITAL TRACT CHANGES

Cervix

Cervical changes during the menstrual cycle are of major importance in fertility. Their use to predict ovulation has largely been superseded in the treatment of infertility by more reliable measures but they still form the basis of the symptothermal method of contraception.

The cervical mucus becomes more profuse, fluid and less viscous as oestradiol increases in the follicular phase. Immediately prior to ovulation (2–3 days) when oestradiol peaks, the mucus demonstrates the capacity to be drawn out into a long thread without losing its continuity (spinnbarkeit). This change is evident on scanning electron microscopy as an increase in the pore size of the honeycomb-like appearance of the mucus and facilitates sperm migration through the cervix. In the luteal phase and under the influence of exogenous progesterone the pore size is decreased and the mucus is less fluid and more viscous.

The changes in cervical mucus can also be observed by drying mucus on a microscopy slide. As ovulation approaches the mucus develops a characteristic 'ferning' pattern in which the dried mucus assumes the appearance of a fern frond. The other observable cervical change is that the os is more open around the time of ovulation which also improves sperm transport.

Vagina

Vaginal secretions are increased in response to oestradiol but the most striking change in the vagina is in the morphology of the vaginal epithelium. Oestradiol stimulates the growth and maturation of superficial cells in the stratified squamous epithelium of the vagina. Therefore, in smears taken from women just prior to ovulation superficial cells are dominant, while more intermediate cells are seen in smears early in the cycle or later in the cycle in the presence of progesterone.

'PHYSIOLOGICAL' TREATMENTS IN GYNAECOLOGY

Infertility

Steroids

Progesterone supplementation to support the luteal phase of the cycle is controversial. It is used on the basis that it helps prepare the endometrium adequately, thereby increasing the chances of successful implantation and reducing subsequent miscarriage.

In women with premature menopause wishing to conceive, sequential therapy with oestrogen followed by oestrogen and progesterone (mimicking a natural cycle) has been used successfully to prepare the endometrium for the implantation of fertilized donor eggs.

Clomiphene

Clomiphene is thought to have many different actions. As an antioestrogen it binds to oestrogen receptors in the pituitary but does not activate them. This blocks the binding of oestradiol preventing feedback inhibition of FSH secretion. More FSH is therefore secreted by the pituitary increasing the stimulation of ovarian follicles. A side-effect of this is to increase the incidence of multiple ovulation and subsequently multiple pregnancy. Clomiphene will not induce ovulation in conditions associated with low oestradiol concentrations, e.g. hypogonadotrophic hypogonadism, weight-related anovulation, etc. It should mainly be used for women with ovulatory disorders associated with polycystic ovarian syndrome (PCOS).

FSH/LH

An alternative method of inducing ovulation is to bypass the pituitary completely and to give either FSH alone or in combination with LH. The latter (human menopausal gonadotrophins, hMG) is commonly used but as it is derived from postmenopausal women's urine there is a move towards biosynthetic production of FSH. This 'recombinant FSH', as it is known, is pure but very expensive. The oestradiol concentrations are lower because there is less LH stimulation of the essential precursors, androgens. Monitoring using oestradiol is therefore more difficult. Whatever the type of gonadotrophin used monitoring with ultrasound scanning of the size and number of follicles is essential. In anovulatory infertility, when clomiphene has failed, low doses of hMG are used over several weeks. For superovulation, either in combination with intrauterine insemination (IUI), or prior to in vitro fertilization (IVF), larger doses are used over a shorter period of time. In this regimen, the pituitary may also be bypassed by giving hCG to mimic the LH surge and induce ovulation. LH and hCG are structurally similar but hCG is used as it is cheaper because large quantities are extracted from the urine of pregnant women. In IVF treatment cycles injections of hCG are continued through the luteal phase to maintain the corpus luteum until pregnancy or the next period supervenes.

GnRH

In women who have absent or abnormal hypothalamic GnRH secretion, pulsed GnRH can be artificially delivered by means of a small, battery-driven pump. This pulsed GnRH allows a normal pituitary ovarian response and is therefore usually associated with a single dominant follicle and singleton pregnancy. This has remained largely a research tool and most women with this condition wishing to conceive have gonadotrophins as described above.

GnRH analogues

More recently, synthetic GnRH analogues which have a longer half-life than natural GnRH have been used to abolish a woman's endogenous cycle. These act by initially causing an outpouring of LH and FSH but then down-regulation of the gonadotrophin secreting cells in the pituitary leading to very low levels of LH and FSH. An artificial cycle is then imposed using LH/FSH and hCG as before. Improved pregnancy rates in IVF have been reported using this method. These agents have also been used experimentally in other hormone-dependent conditions such as uterine fibroids, endometriosis, and breast, endometrial and prostatic carcinoma.

Contraception

Hormonal contraception

The two major contraceptive actions of the combined oral contraceptive pill are to prevent ovulation and to make the cervical mucus resistant to sperm transport. Ovulation is prevented because the constantly elevated levels of oestrogen and progesterone inhibit gonadotrophin secretion, preventing follicle development and the LH surge. The effect on the cervical mucus is a result of progesterone and is the main contraceptive action of the progestogen-only pill.

Irregular bleeding

Anovulatory bleeding

This is a common cause of irregular bleeding particularly at the extremes of a woman's reproductive life and associated with PCOS. Failure to ovulate leads to prolonged endometrial stimulation and irregular, incomplete shedding. It is treated by replacing the absent cycle regulator, i.e. the corpus luteum, with exogenous progesterone for 10–14 days to achieve endometrial maturation and subsequent shedding after progesterone is withdrawn.

Prolonged bleeding

In the short-term management of this condition, continuous oestrogen, or, more commonly, progesterone will usually stop the bleeding. Following hormone withdrawal, menstruation will ensue. When pathology has been excluded, cyclical therapy for 3–6 months is often necessary to regulate the cycle.

SUMMARY

The menstrual cycle is the product of complex hormonal and target organ interactions. The length of the cycle is regulated by ovarian events, but normal menstruation requires intact functioning of the whole axis: hypothalamus, pituitary, ovary and endometrium. The cyclical production of the steroids from the ovary (follicular/luteal phases) leads to the cyclical changes in the endometrium (proliferative/secretory phases) whose major goal is the preparation of a suitable environment for the implanting embryo.

6. Menstrual disorders

J. Rymer

Expectations of the examiners

The candidate will be expected to have a basic knowledge of the physiology of the menstrual cycle. Menstrual disorders are common, and the initial assessment and management of these disorders are within the scope of general practice. However the candidate is also expected to understand what specialist referral will involve and the subsequent management that would occur in hospital.

MENORRHAGIA

Definition

Excessive menstrual bleeding that occurs with regular or irregular cycles. Median menstrual blood loss is 30–40 ml in total per period; >80 ml = pathological.

Interesting facts

There has been a tenfold increase in the number of periods that women experience during their reproductive life (reducing family size, less lactation, early menarche, late menopause).

If menstrual loss is >60 ml/month, a negative iron balance will potentially develop on a normal Western diet.

In routine clinical practice, objective measurement of menstrual blood loss is not used, so clinicians rely on the woman's assessment which has been shown to be inaccurate in approximately half of cases.

Pathophysiology

Menstrual bleeding can be ovulatory or anovulatory. In general, regular, painful periods are associated with ovulation, and irregular, painless periods with anovulation. The latter is more common in the extremes of menstrual life. There is now evidence that in women with proven menorrhagia, there are elevated levels of prostaglandins in the

44

endometrium, and these women have an altered responsiveness to the vasodilator PGE_2. Progesterone inhibits prostaglandin production and oestradiol increases prostaglandin production. Ovulatory bleeding is associated with normal levels of these peripherally circulating hormones, so it is thought that altered prostaglandin synthesis is responsible for the increased menstrual loss. In particular the ratio of PGE_2 and prostacyclin to PGF_{2a} is significant, the former causing vasodilatation and inhibition of platelet aggregation and the latter promoting vasoconstriction and platelet aggregation.

In anovulatory cycles, oestrogen and progesterone levels are variable, causing irregular shedding of the endometrium.

Aetiology

1. Physiological, i.e. normal loss but interpreted as excessive. This commonly occurs in women who stop the oral contraceptive pill. Having been used to painless, light periods while taking the pill, they then revert to normal periods which are more painful, and heavier.
2. Dysfunctional uterine bleeding (hormonal). This is a diagnosis which is made after pelvic pathology has been excluded.
3. Congenital, e.g. increased endometrial surface area of which an example is a bicornuate uterus.
4. Traumatic, e.g. IUD.
5. Infective, e.g. chronic pelvic inflammatory disease.
6. Neoplastic, e.g. fibroids, endometrial polyps.
7. Metabolic, e.g. thyroid dysfunction.
8. Psychological factors.
9. Adenomyosis.
10. Blood dyscrasias.
11. Iatrogenic, e.g. drug ingestion as seen in women on long-term anticoagulation.

'Physiological' and 'dysfunctional uterine bleeding' account for 50% of all cases of menorrhagia.

Assessment

History is notoriously inaccurate but it is essential to distinguish menstrual bleeding from non-menstrual bleeding. The number of pads/tampons used does not equal amount lost, and a history of flooding or clots is unreliable. Objective measurement is impractical. Despite these limitations the diagnosis is based on the patient's own assessment of her menstrual loss.

Examination should include measurement of weight, a search for signs of endocrine disturbance, and a pelvic examination, including a cervical smear if indicated.

Investigations

1. Full blood count: if anaemia is present iron supplementation should be considered with medical treatment.
2. Thyroid function tests if any other stigmata of dysfunction exist.
3. Further tests are determined by history and examination: e.g. clotting disorders—clotting profiles, pelvic infection—endocervical swabs.
4. Vaginal ultrasonography—transvaginal scanning can measure the thickness of the endometrium and detect abnormalites of the cavity, e.g. endometrial polyps. As the vaginal probe is so much closer to the pelvic organs, the uterus and ovaries can be more easily scanned.
5. Endometrial biopsy. This should be performed if the menorrhagia is a recent phenomenon, if the woman is over 40 years of age, or if there is any intermenstrual bleeding. There are various techniques available. Outpatient endometrial sampling is becoming more popular and this involves a small diameter (2 mm) plastic cannula which is inserted through the cervical canal into the endometrial cavity. The inner plastic tube is withdrawn, creating a vacuum, and endometrial tissue is drawn into the plastic cannula. Dilatation and curettage has been largely replaced by hysteroscopy where the endometrial cavity can be visualized and biopsies appropriately directed. It must be remembered that whatever form of endometrial biopsy is performed, the procedure is diagnostic, not therapeutic, although some women may experience a few months of lighter periods after a formal dilatation and curettage.

Treatment

Any pathology that is found should be appropriately treated. One is then left with the treatment of dysfunctional uterine bleeding.

Anovulatory

In adolescents and premenopausal women the oral contraceptive pill can be prescribed, making the periods lighter, regular, and less painful. Cyclical progestogens (e.g. medroxyprogesterone acetate 10 mg daily for 10 days) can be used to induce regular withdrawal bleeds. Likewise, in perimenopausal women, once the endometrium has been sampled, cyclical progestogens can also be used to induce regular withdrawal bleeding. If no withdrawal bleeding occurs, then there has been no oestrogenic stimulation of the endometrium which indicates no ovarian function, and the 'menopause' has occurred. If the woman is experiencing climacteric symptoms with menorrhagia, then it is appropriate to put her on hormone replacement therapy, remembering that she needs progestogens for at least 12 days of each calendar month.

Acute arrest for heavy bleeding. Start with a high dose of a progestogen and decrease, e.g. norethisterone 30 mg b.d. for 3 days, 20 mg b.d. for 3 days, 10 mg b.d. for 3 days, 5 mg b.d. for 10 days. Cessation of treatment will be followed by a withdrawal bleed.

Ovulatory

1. *Non-steroidal anti-inflammatory drugs.* These inhibit biosynthesis of the prostaglandins, and reduce menstrual flow by about 30% in most women with menstrual blood loss greater than 80 ml/day. The advantage of this treatment is that it is only taken for a few days of each cycle, i.e. during menstruation.
2. *Antifibrinolytic drugs.* These probably act by reducing enhanced fibrinolytic activity found in the uterus in women with excessive menstrual blood loss. Reductions are in the order of 50%. Side-effects are common, e.g. nausea and dizziness.
3. *Oral contraceptive pill.* The absolute contraindications must be ruled out, and the relative contraindications considered. Ovulation is suppressed, and the oestrogen levels remain constant. This inhibits endometrial growth reducing menstrual loss.
4. *Danazol.* The mechanism is uncertain but it induces atrophy of the endometrium as a result of low levels of circulating sex steroids. Normal dose is 200 mg daily. Disadvantages are that it requires daily dosage and has side-effects, e.g. weight gain, virilizing effects.
5. *Hysterectomy.* This is the definitive treatment but involves the risks associated with major pelvic surgery, e.g. pelvic thrombosis. Controlled trials have shown that postoperative psychological morbidity is similar to that seen preoperatively.
6. *Endometrial ablation or resection.* The endometrium is visualized hysteroscopically and destroyed with the laser or resectoscope. Some women become amenorrhoeic and the majority have reduced menstrual loss. Some women require further surgery as the long-term results can be disappointing.
7. *Hormone releasing IUD.* The progestogen released from these devices affects the endometrium making it atrophic. After 1 year of use most women have only scanty spotting of blood.

Summary

Menorrhagia is a common symptom which is difficult to assess objectively. As a generalization, heavy irregular bleeding is anovulatory and occurs in the extremes of reproductive life, and heavy regular bleeding is usually ovulatory. In dysfunctional uterine bleeding, hysterectomy should only be considered after failure of conservative medical treatment.

DYSMENORRHOEA

PRIMARY

Definition

Painful periods for which no organic or psychological cause can be found.

Pathophysiology

There is an abnormally high production of endometrial prostaglandins which cause excessive uterine contractions. Generally associated with ovulatory cycles.

Assessment

History is important, as pain occurs with onset of menstruation and then declines. Examination must exclude obvious pathology.

Investigation

If diagnosis is made on history then no further investigation is needed. If treatment fails to improve symptoms then a laparoscopy is needed to exclude pathology.

Treatment

1. Non-steroidal anti-inflammatory agents are prostaglandin synthetase inhibitors and will decrease pain and reduce menstrual loss.
2. Oral contraceptive pill will inhibit ovulation. Primary dysmenorrhoea is usually associated with ovulation, thus the pill will relieve primary dysmenorrhoea.

SECONDARY

Definition

Painful periods where an organic or psychosexual cause can be found.

Aetiology

1. Pelvic inflammatory disease
2. Endometriosis
3. Ovarian tumour
4. Previous pelvic or abdominal surgery
5. Misplaced IUD
6. Past history of sexual abuse
7. Other psychological problems.

Assessment

History is important and may take time if psychosexual problems are present. Pelvic examination must be performed, and swabs taken if indicated. Restricted mobility or fixed retroversion of the uterus suggests the presence of adhesions secondary to endometriosis, pelvic inflammatory disease, or previous surgery.

Investigations

These will be guided by history, but laparoscopy is indicated in most cases.

Treatment

This depends on the cause. Often reassurance that the pelvis is normal is treatment in itself.

POLYCYSTIC OVARIAN SYNDROME

Definition

A common disorder that is almost always associated with either menstrual disturbance or hyperandrogenism.

Interesting facts

It was previously thought that anovulation was an essential feature of this syndrome but more than 80% of women who have hirsutism and regular cycles have PCOS on ultrasound.

Aetiology

Controversial, but recent evidence points to a gonadotrophin-dependent, intraovarian androgen excess. This is thought to be either due to a primary inherited abnormality of P450c17 α (enzyme in steroid pathway) or secondary to inherited or acquired hyperinsulinaemia.

Biochemical investigations

Testosterone and androstenedione are characteristically raised. A higher body mass index (BMI) is associated with increased serum testosterone and an increased prevalence of hirsutism. Hyperinsulinaemia is a prominent feature in obese patients with PCOS, and this enhances ovarian androgen production and inhibits hepatic synthesis of sex hormone binding globulin (SHBG), thereby increasing the exposure of hair follicles to free testosterone.

Hyperinsulinaemia also has an adverse effect on cardiovascular risk factors, e.g. decreased HDL, increased triglycerides and glucose, and raised blood pressure.

Appearance

The ovaries are typically enlarged, thickened, pearly white with sclerotic capsules and subcapsular follicular cysts. Bisection shows numerous cysts in the cortex, and on ultrasound scan a peripheral ring of follicles is seen.

Management

Hyperandrogenism

The mainstay of therapy is a combination of ethinyloestradiol with the antiandrogen cyproterone acetate, or a combined oral contraceptive pill containing non-androgenic progestogen. These will give cycle control, reduce hyperandrogenic symptoms and provide contraception. Other therapies include:

1. Spironolactone 50 mg b.d.
2. Flutamide 250 mg b.d. days 5–25 of the cycle. (A non-steroidal pure antiandrogen.)
3. Finasteride 5 mg daily—a prototype inhibitor of 5 α reductase, the cutaneous enzyme responsible for the conversion of testosterone to the more bioactive dihydrotestosterone.
4. LHRH analogue and addback therapy. Endogenous gonadotrophins are suppressed and then oestrogen and progesterone are 'added back'.

Anovulation

The management will depend on whether the woman wishes to conceive or not. If she does not then either the oral contraceptive pill or cyclical progestogen administration is suitable. If she wishes to conceive then initial treatment should be achievement of normal BMI, then clomiphene, and then gonadotrophin stimulation.

Ovarian electrodiathermy has produced promising results with regard to inducing ovulation and significant conception rates. However, more experience is needed.

Summary

PCOS is a complex and common syndrome and is a spectrum of disease from mild symptoms e.g. hirsutism with regular cycles, to severe symptoms, e.g. hirsutism, obesity and amenorrhoea. These women may also be insulin resistant and hyperinsulinaemic.

AMENORRHOEA

PRIMARY

Definition

No menstruation by 14 years with growth failure or absence of secondary sexual characteristics, i.e. breast development and pubic hair growth, or no menstruation by 16 years when growth and sexual development are normal.

SECONDARY

Definition

Absence of menses for 6 months (or six cycles) in a previously menstruating woman.

Aetiology

The causes can be divided into compartments:

1. Target organ and outflow tract dysfunction
2. Gonadal failure
3. Pituitary dysfunction
4. Hypothalamic dysfunction
5. Thyroid or adrenal dysfunction.

Assessment

The history should involve specific questioning about galactorrhoea, weight change, hirsutism, life crisis, possibility of pregnancy, recent gynaecological surgery, and cyclical pain.

Investigations

1. Serum prolactin level ($\times$ 2)
2. Thyroid function tests if indicated
3. Serum FSH, LH, testosterone, and SHBG levels.
4. Karyotype if phenotype abnormal
5. Ultrasound scan of pelvis.

Treatment

See Figure 6.1. If the prolactin level is high then refer to a specialist centre for a CT scan of the pituitary fossa and bromocriptine or carbergoline if a microadenoma is present.

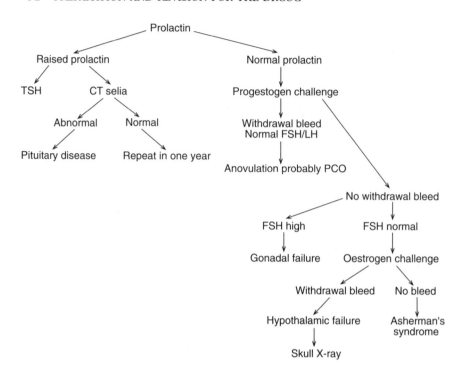

Fig. 6.1 Amenorrhoea – management plan.

Thyroid disease should be treated appropriately. If both thyroid and prolactin levels are normal, then specialist referral would be appropriate at this stage. Management will involve a progestogen challenge test, e.g. 5 mg medroxyprogesterone acetate b.d. for 5 days. If this is followed by a withdrawal bleed, then anovulation is the diagnosis, most likely secondary to polycystic ovarian syndrome. In the absence of a withdrawal bleed, a raised FSH level indicates gonadal failure (i.e. menopause). If FSH is normal then an oestrogen challenge test is performed, e.g. 2.5 mg conjugated oestrogens daily for 21 days, with the above medroxyprogesterone acetate regimen for the last 5 days. If there is no withdrawal bleed, then there is an outflow tract disorder, i.e. Asherman's syndrome, or cervical stenosis (assuming that the rest of the genital tract has been adequately examined and found to be normal). If there is a withdrawal bleed, then the problem is hypothalamic, but a CT is performed to check the pituitary fossa.

INTERMENSTRUAL BLEEDING

Definition

Vaginal bleeding occurring in between menstruation.

Aetiology

Although classically associated with endometrial carcinoma, intermenstrual bleeding may also occur with cervical carcinoma. Regular mid-cycle bleeding can occur in association with ovulation or the combined oral contraceptive pill.

Assessment

History is important, as a recent onset of intermenstrual bleeding is more suspicious of endometrial carcinoma (see Ch. 13).

Investigations

1. Cervical smear.
2. Endometrial biopsy is indicated in most cases, except those where changing the oral contraceptive pill rapidly corrects the disturbance.

Treatment

If on the oral contraceptive pill, take two pills on the days when the breakthrough bleeding is occurring, or change to a different pill preparation with a lower oestrogen content or a higher progestogen content.

POSTCOITAL BLEEDING

This is the classical symptom of cervical carcinoma so the cervix must be inspected and cervical smear taken. Further management depends on the cytology result (see Ch. 13).

7. Endometriosis, dyspareunia and pelvic pain

G. Davis

ENDOMETRIOSIS

Expectations of the examiners

Endometriosis is a common condition which causes pain and infertility. The examiners will expect the candidate to have a sound knowledge of its presentation and methods of treatment.

Definition

The presence of functioning endometrial tissue outside the uterine cavity. Histopathological examination must confirm the presence of glands and stroma.

Interesting facts

The reported incidence of endometriosis varies widely but is probably about 10% of menstruating white women and 30% of women presenting with infertility. It may be asymptomatic and an incidental finding at abdominal surgery for other reasons, or it may cause severe, chronic pelvic pain. The severity of the pain may often be disproportionate to the extent of the disease.

Endometriosis may be present outside the uterus or within the myometrium (adenomyosis) but not usually both. This suggests that the two have different underlying causes. Adenomyosis is a histological diagnosis made after hysterectomy, usually for menorrhagia, and will not be discussed further. Conventionally, endometriosis has been described as presenting in infertile white women aged between 30 and 45 years of higher socioeconomic status. As the use of laparoscopy has become more widespread, this description has become less accurate. Users of the combined oral contraceptive pill have a lower incidence of endometriosis.

Pathophysiology

Aetiology

Classically there are three theories concerning the pathogenesis of endometriosis:

1. *Retrograde menstruation.* Viable fragments of endometrium are known to reach the pelvic cavity during menstruation. In susceptible individuals these may implant, leading to intrapelvic distribution of endometrial deposits. However, retrograde menstruation is common and this theory does not explain the development of endometriosis at distant sites.
2. *Lymphatic or vascular spread.* Small, viable endometrial 'emboli' can be recovered from the lungs and provide an adequate explanation for the presence of endometriosis at peripheral sites.
3. *Metaplasia of coelomic epithelium.* It is proposed that the repeated inflammatory insult of menstrual fluid may lead to a redifferentiation of the primitive coelomic epithelium which constitutes the visceral peritoneum.

No single theory adequately explains the distribution of endometriosis and it is likely to be a combination of the above factors. It is not known what determines a woman's susceptibility to developing endometriosis but it is probably a result of immunological and physical components. In addition, direct 'inocculation' may occur during surgery leading to the development of endometriosis in hysterotomy, hysterectomy and caesarean section scars. Heredity is thought to play a major part.

Site

Endometriosis commonly occurs in the dependent part of the pelvis: uterosacral ligaments, pouch of Douglas, ovaries. It is less commonly seen on other peritoneal surfaces of the abdominal cavity, in the bowel and bladder and in the umbilicus or scars from abdominal surgery. It has also been described in distant sites, e.g. lung, thigh, vulva.

Pathology

Commonly endometriotic deposits consist of multiple small (< 1 cm), raised blue-black nodules which appear as if ink has been injected under the peritoneum. In more severe disease the nodules may be larger with variable amounts of surrounding fibrosis. If the ovary becomes involved then an endometrioma (or chocolate cyst) may form. In chronic endometriosis there is extensive pelvic damage due to fibrosis and adhesion formation.

Microscopically, glands and stroma are present together with a variable amount of bleeding and fibrosis. These deposits may be out of phase with the woman's menstrual cycle but decidualize during pregnancy like normal endometrium.

Assessment

Women may present with symptoms due to the local effects of endometriosis or through the complications that have occurred as a result of the disease. Forty per cent of women with endometriosis present with the combination of dysmenorrhoea, dyspareunia, and infertility.

History

Pain. Classically, endometriosis is associated with secondary dysmenorrhoea. The pelvic pain is directly related to the onset and duration of the menses and is usually progressive unless treated.

Dyspareunia. Intercourse may be painful on deep penetration throughout the menstrual cycle. (See 'Dyspareunia' below.)

Complications

Infertility. Endometriosis may cause infertility in the absence of other symptoms. Minimal disease is associated with infertility but does not 'cause' the infertility itself as pregnancy rates are the same with and without treatment. More severe disease associated with adhesion formation and pelvic distortion prevents successful fertilization and implantation.

Lower genital tract. Uncommonly deposits in the vagina or vulva may give rise to bleeding or dyspareunia.

Bowel. Endometriosis involving the bowel may cause cyclical rectal bleeding, stricture or rarely obstruction.

Bladder. The bladder is rarely affected but cyclical haematuria may occur if it is involved.

Abdominal wall. Deposits in the umbilicus or abdominal wounds cause cyclical swelling and pain at the affected site.

Examination

Abdominal examination may reveal the presence of a mass (endometrioma), but more commonly there is tenderness in the lower abdomen. Abdominal wall deposits are usually tender and the diagnosis is made on the history and histology after excision. Pelvic examination may reveal nodules in the vagina which can bleed. On bimanual examination the uterus may be tender and fixed in retroversion by adhesions, and nodules on the uterosacral ligaments may be palpable.

Investigations

The diagnosis is usually confirmed by laparoscopy. Involvement of other systems is investigated in the appropriate manner, e.g. cystoscopy and biopsy if bladder involvement is suspected. The extent of the disease is usually classified as mild (minimal), moderate or severe. The American Fertility Society has produced a scoring system to assess the severity based on the size and extent of the lesions and the amount of adhesion formation.

Treatment

Minimal disease should only be treated if pain is a problem. The treatment of asymptomatic women with infertility is controversial, as treatment does not improve their chances of future pregnancy. Symptomatic or severe disease can be treated medically or surgically.

Medical

Medical treatment is based on the prolonged inhibition of ovulation and was introduced because of the improvement in endometriosis that supposedly occurs during pregnancy. It is suppressive rather than curative.

Danazol. 200–800 mg/day for 6–9 months. The actions of danazol are complex and it primarily prevents the mid-cycle surge of gonadotrophins. It is an androgen derivative and produces a high androgen, low oestrogen environment which does not support the growth of endometriosis. Side-effects occur in 80% of women and are a result of: (1) low oestrogen—decreased breast size, hot flushes, vaginitis; or (2) high androgen—acne, oily skin, weight gain, hirsutism. Only 10% of women find the side-effects sufficiently troublesome to stop the drug but it should be stopped immediately if there is any deepening of the voice as this is irreversible. Shorter courses are useful to induce amenorrhoea before a switch is made to progestogens.

Combined oral contraceptive. This is given continuously for 6–9 months. Weight gain is a more prominent side-effect than when the pill is given cyclically, but otherwise the side-effects are similar.

Medroxyprogesterone acetate 30 mg/day is as effective as danazol, is cheaper and has fewer side-effects. Breakthrough bleeding is a common problem which is treated with a 7-day course of oestrogen (ethinyl-oestradiol 10 µg/day).

GnRH analogue. This long-acting agonist delivered intranasally, subcutaneously or via monthly implantation produces a state of hypogonadotrophic hypogonadism, achieving even lower levels of serum oestradiol levels than with danazol. The side-effects are those of oestradiol deprivation and bone loss occurs. If long-term therapy is contemplated, then 'addback' therapy is recommended.

Surgical

This is the only means of removing the disease.

Definitive surgery is required for the treatment of severe disease. The object of surgery is to restore normal anatomy and to remove as much endometriosis as possible. The only cure is the resection of all deposits which is increasingly being performed laparoscopically. Many surgeons use medical treatment prior to surgery to improve the resectability of the lesions. Hormone replacement therapy can be used postoperatively with a minimal risk of growth in residual endometriosis.

Presacral neurectomy. This procedure can be performed for intractable endometriotic dysmenorrhoea.

Follow-up

Medical therapy

This is usually effective in treating pain, particularly with minimal disease, but 40% of women will get a recurrence of symptoms at some time after treatment stops. Pregnancy rates of 50–75% are reported in both the groups treated and those untreated.

Surgery

The recurrence rate after adequate surgery is less than 20%. Postoperative fertility is related to the severity of the disease, with 60% conceiving after surgery for moderate disease compared to 35% for severe disease. Fertility is greatest in the first year after surgery and conception is unlikely after 2 years. After this time, assisted conception techniques should be considered.

DYSPAREUNIA

Expectations of the examiners

This is a common symptom which may be managed by general practitioners without referral to a gynaecologist. The candidate must have an understanding of the physical causes, their diagnosis and the management of this condition.

Definition

Painful or difficult intercourse. It may be divided into: (1) superficial—pain at the onset of penetration; or (2) deep—pain during or after penetration has occurred.

Interesting facts

Dyspareunia is a common symptom but many women are reluctant to talk about it. Often it must be elicited and there may be a combination of physical and psychological factors contributing to the pain. Pain due to a physical problem often leads to fear of intercourse which in turn makes intercourse more painful and this cycle may continue after the physical problem is cured. Both the physical and psychological aspects need to be addressed if the symptom is to resolve.

Table 7.1 Causes of superficial dyspareunia.

Vulva	Vulvitis 　Atrophic 　Infective(candida, herpes, HPV) Bartholinitis Dystrophy Neoplasm
Vagina	Vaginismus Vaginitis 　Atrophic 　Infective (as for vulva) Anatomical 　Vaginal atresia 　Imperforate hymen Contracture 　Atrophy 　Postsurgery 　Postradiotherapy
Urethra	Urethritis Urethral caruncle Urethral diverticulum

Pathophysiology

Superficial dyspareunia may be caused by any of the conditions listed in Table 7.1.

Any pelvic pathology may lead to deep dyspareunia but the common causes are:

1. PID
2. Endometriosis
3. Ectopic pregnancy
4. Chronic pelvic pain syndrome (see below)
5. Ovarian neoplasm, e.g. bleed into cyst.

Uterine prolapse and retroversion are commonly listed as causes but are unlikely to result in significant dyspareunia except where the uterus is involved in other pathology, e.g. endometriosis.

Assessment

History

The onset and relationship of the pain to the woman's life events and menstrual cycle are important. The menstrual, contraceptive and obstetric history should be obtained in detail and a full sexual history taken. It is important to assess the woman's attitude to sex and the family history of attitudes to pain and sex. Acute dyspareunia suggests an organic cause, while chronic superficial dyspareunia is more suggestive of psychosexual dysfunction.

Examination

A very careful pelvic examination should be performed to exclude physical causes. The woman's attitude to the examination may reflect her underlying attitude to her sexuality (or a physical problem).

Investigations

Vaginal and endocervical swabs should be taken if indicated. Deep dyspareunia usually requires laparoscopy to make a diagnosis if a cause is not apparent on examination.

Treatment

Superficial

If the cause is organic, this is usually apparent on examination and should be appropriately treated. Vaginismus plus other psychosexual dysfunction is usually treated with vaginal dilators combined with psychosexual counselling. This should be undertaken by a person with experience in this field.

Deep dyspareunia

Any organic cause should be treated appropriately. Unexplained or untreatable disease (e.g. due to previous surgery) may be improved by limiting penetration through the use of alternative positions during intercourse.

Follow-up

The treatment of physical disease causing superficial dyspareunia is usually successful provided that the woman has a supportive sexual partner. The outcome of psychosexual treatment is variable but pure vaginismus can be effectively cured. The results of treatment of deep dyspareunia depend on the underlying cause. If no cause is found then it may become a chronic problem.

PELVIC PAIN

Expectations of the examiners

Pelvic pain is a common gynaecological problem and the candidate must understand how to approach the problem, exclude organic disease and deal effectively with the psychological aspects of this symptom.

Definition

Pain is localized to the pelvis but it may include lower abdominal and lower back pain.

Interesting facts

Twenty-five per cent of women referred to gynaecology outpatients complain of pelvic pain. The non-gynaecological causes include bowel (e.g. irritable bowel syndrome (IBS), appendicitis, diverticulitis) or urinary tract disease (e.g. UTI, ureteric calculus) and rarely spinal disease. In 30% of patients with pelvic pain no cause can be found at laparoscopy and these patients are characterized as having chronic pelvic pain (syndrome). Malignant gynaecological tumours may present with lower abdominal or pelvic discomfort. Significant pain is usually a late feature of advanced gynaecological malignancy.

Pathophysiology

All nerves from the pelvic organs ascend to the T10–L1 spinal segments but the pain is poorly localized and may be referred to the appropriate dermatome. The cause of the pain is unclear—acute distension of the fallopian tubes or ovaries causes pain (e.g. ectopic pregnancy) but chronic slow swelling may be asymptomatic (e.g. dermoid cyst). Venous congestion of the pelvis causing pain is a controversial issue and unresolved at present. Venous congestion is often striking in acute pelvic inflammatory disease, although whether this is the source of the pain is unknown. Dysmenorrhoea is caused by prostaglandin-induced myometrial contractions and anything that stimulates uterine contractions will cause pain (e.g. labour, incomplete abortion).

Assessment

History

A full history is fundamental in dealing with pelvic pain adequately and the pain should be defined as accurately as possible:

1. Site and radiation of pain
2. Character of pain (sharp, dull)
3. Duration and nature of onset
4. Periodicity of pain (constant, intermittent)
5. Severity of pain (e.g. effect on sleep, work, leisure)
6. Bowel patterns, abdominal bloating
7. Relationship to menstruation, food, movement, coitus, defaecation, micturition, posture
8. Any alleviating factors and effect of analgesics.

A full sexual history and a detailed social history focusing on stressful life events and current circumstances must be taken. While taking the history, an assessment of the woman's psychological status including mood and level of anxiety should be made.

Examination

A careful general and abdominal examination must be performed. If the pain is well localized, an organic cause is more likely. Similarly, abdominal guarding and rebound are unlikely to be elicited without underlying pathology. Pain of a gynaecological cause is usually most severe suprapubically. After speculum examination has been performed to exclude abnormality, a bimanual examination should be undertaken.

Investigations

Obvious gynaecological or non-gynaecological disease should be managed appropriately. Often the diagnosis is unclear and the only investigation of value in the absence of clinical findings is a laparoscopy. Fifty per cent of women with chronic pelvic pain and a normal pelvic examination will have laparoscopic abnormalities but, conversely, only 15% of women with an abnormal pelvic examination will not have an abnormality on laparoscopy.

Treatment

The treatment of any chronic pain disorder begins in the history taking with the establishment of rapport between the woman and her examining doctor. In 30% of women with chronic pain, no abnormality can be detected and the pain may well be due to IBS or 'psychosomatic'. Treatment should combine support, an attempt to increase the woman's awareness of how her pain is affected by stress or emotions, and analgesia. Initially aspirin or paracetamol should be used or a prostaglandin synthetase inhibitor if dysmenorrhoea is a component. Once a physical abnormality has been excluded (by physical examination and laparoscopy) the therapeutic approach can shift to the perspective of how the woman is going to deal with the pain and still function in her normal life. Trained psychological support may also be beneficial when the woman has accepted that no physical cause can be found.

Many of these women have been demonstrated to have abnormal pelvic venograms. Whether this venodilatation is a cause of, or an association with, pelvic pain is unproven. Research into this phenomenon continues in subspecialty clinics which also provide a well-organized and effective psychological support service.

In women with chronic pelvic pain cognitive behavioural therapeutic approaches are often successful. Women who have admitted past or current sexual abuse require expert counselling and psychological support.

Follow-up

Women with pelvic pain need to be followed for 1–2 years, as a large proportion will have recurrent pain. This is a difficult management problem, particularly in those women who have had surgery for their pelvic pain (often including abdominal hysterectomy ± bilateral salpingo-oophorectomy). The corollary to this is that surgery should be avoided in the absence of obvious pathology.

8. Infertility

M. Chapman

Expectations of the examiners

The candidate will be expected to have an organized approach to the investigation and management of the infertile couple. A basic understanding of reproductive endocrinology is necessary but the more complex aspects including detailed knowledge of sophisticated drug regimens are not essential.

Definition

Infertility can be defined as the failure to conceive after a period of 12 months of unprotected intercourse. The time period is arbitrary but relates to natural rates of conception, i.e. 80% of couples will be pregnant after 12 cycles.

During the second year of attempted conception 50% of those remaining will conceive spontaneously. Subsequently the chances of conception are in the order of 50% in the following 4 years. Any treatment for infertility must improve that background rate of conception.

The differentiation of infertility into primary (no previous pregnancies) and secondary (previous pregnancies) is useful in that the incidence of causes for each are different, e.g. secondary infertility is more likely to be due to tubal damage. Male factors are more likely in primary infertility.

Pathophysiology

The three major causes of infertility are:

1. Semen quality—40%
2. Ovulatory disorders—30%
3. Tubal problems—30%.

Unexp - 30%
Sperm - 25%
Ovary - 20%
Tubal - 15%
Other - 10%

Other causes include:

1. In the male
   a. Impotence
   b. Retrograde ejaculation
   c. Antisperm antibodies

64

2. In the female
    a. Cervical factor (including antisperm antibodies)
    b. Severe endometriosis.

The diagnosis of unexplained infertility is reached after exclusion of the above causes.

Assessment

A detailed history from both partners can suggest the underlying problem(s). An assessment of the couple's general health and of their current life stresses, e.g. occupation, family problems, etc., is useful to provide a background to the problem. Regularity of sexual intercourse and timing and any associated problems need to be explored with both partners. Infertility itself may contribute substantial psychological pressure and impair the ability to conceive.

Male

In the male, causes for poor semen quality should be sought:

1. Infections, e.g. mumps as an adult, gonococcal infection leading to blocked vasa deferentia
2. Operations, e.g. inguinal herniorrhaphy, orchidopexy
3. Drugs, e.g. antimitotic agents, β blockers, alcohol (in excess), nicotine.

Information about previous pregnancies should be obtained from each partner separately. Examination should be performed to assess that the genitalia are normal. The size and consistency of the testicles should be noted as well as the presence of vasa deferentia and varicocele.

Female

In the female the history is aimed at providing evidence of ovulation. Signs and symptoms suggesting ovulation include:

1. Regular cycles
2. Mid-cycle pain (mittelschmerz)
3. Changes in vaginal discharge
4. Premenstrual symptoms, e.g. breast tenderness
5. Primary spasmodic dysmenorrhoea.

The reproductive history should be documented in detail. Factors suggesting tubal disease should be sought, i.e. pelvic inflammatory disease, previous pelvic or abdominal surgery, intrauterine device usage, chronic lower abdominal pain and secondary dysmenorrhoea. Full physical assessment including pelvic examination should be performed.

Investigations

Male

Semen analysis. Instruction for collection should include 3 days' abstinence from ejaculation and rapid transport to the laboratory (< 1 hour) of a specimen obtained by masturbation.

Normal parameters (WHO criteria)

1. Volume: 2–5 ml
2. Concentration: > 20 million/ml
3. Motility: > 50%
4. Normal forms: > 50%

Specimens with subnormal parameters should be repeated in 4–6 weeks before final assessment of quality is made.

Diagnostic categories

1. Normal (as above)
2. Azoospermia (no spermatozoa seen)
3. Oligospermia (concentration < 20 million/ml)
   a. Severe
   b. Moderate
   c. Mild.
4. Asthenospermia (decreased motility).

Further investigations: LH, FSH, testosterone.

Impaired semen quality is predominantly due to spermatogenic failure of unknown cause. The importance of varicoceles in male subfertility is controversial.

Postcoital test. This test involves aspiration of a sample of cervical mucus around the time of ovulation within 6 hours of intercourse. A positive test, i.e. motile sperm in the cervical mucus, excludes a cervical problem and confirms vaginal intercourse has occurred. A negative test can be caused by many factors other than mucus hostility, e.g. poor timing and infection, and therefore its value is limited.

Female

Ovulation

Temperature charts. The basal body temperature chart has a limited role but is worth recording for a maximum of two cycles to:

1. Define cycle length
2. Determine frequency of intercourse

3. Check biphasic pattern indicating ovulation (correlation with biochemical parameters of ovulation: 70–80%).

Serum progesterone. This is taken 7 days prior to the menses, e.g. day 21 of a 28-day cycle or day 25 of a 32-day cycle. Serial measurements should be taken if the cycle is irregular. Values greater than 30 nmol/l indicate ovulation.

Other methods of assessment. These include ultrasound monitoring, direct visualization of a corpus luteum at laparoscopy, and monitoring of serum LH levels to time ovulation.

Tubal patency

Hysterosalpingogram (HSG). HSG demonstrates intrauterine and tubal anatomy and patency but it provides little information about problems elsewhere in the pelvis, e.g. adhesions. It is an outpatient procedure but generally causes discomfort or pain. There is a small risk of introducing or reactivating infection.

Laparoscopy and dye instillation. This procedure demonstrates pelvic anatomy and pathology, e.g. adhesions, endometriosis, ovarian disease and tubal patency. It is an inpatient procedure requiring general anaesthesia, with an operative mortality of 1 : 16 000. The correlation of HSG and laparoscopy findings is 70–80% and therefore it may be necessary to perform both investigations. Most women have a laparoscopy and dye instillation initially, followed by an HSG if indicated. Hysteroscopy at the time of laparoscopy can show intrauterine pathology, such as adhesions, polyps, or fibroids.

Rubella status. This should be checked prior to commencing treatment. Non-immune patients must be vaccinated and advized to avoid pregnancy for 3 months.

Treatment

Male

The outlook for azoospermia and oligospermia has been poor. Cold showers, loose underwear, varicocele ligation and hormonal strategies (except in hypopituitarism) have not been shown to be of any significant benefit. Recently developed micromanipulation techniques (Intracytoplasmic Sperm Injection — ICSI) in conjunction with In Vitro Fertilization (IVF) have been successful in severe cases offering new hope in this group. Mild and moderate oligospermia may improve spontaneously and pregnancies do occur. Semen preparation (e.g. Percoll) can significantly improve the chances of conception with assisted repoduction techniques in this group. Artificial insemination with donor semen is successful in 50–60% of cases (for 12 cycles) but is only acceptable to 60% of suitable couples.

Female

Ovulatory problems (see 'Amenorrhoea'). The use of ovulation induction techniques has substantially improved the chances of conception to almost normal rates. The first line of treatment is clomiphene citrate, initially 50 mg from days 2 to 6 of the menstrual cycle. Clomiphene increases FSH production by acting as an antioestrogen at the pituitary level. Serum progesterone levels should be checked to confirm ovulation. The use of other ovulation induction agents (gonadotrophins, LHRH analogues) is only appropriate in specialist units. The complications of ovulation induction agents include hyperstimulation and multiple pregnancy.

Tubal problems. The overall success rate of tubal surgery is 20–30%. In specialized centres, success rates in selected cases can be up to 50%.

In vitro fertilization. IVF produces a 'take home baby' rate of 15–20%. The procedure is used in cases of infertility due to tubal disease. It involves the induction of ovulation and collection of multiple ova (either by laparoscope or ultrasound guided needle aspiration) followed by extracorporeal fertilization. Embryos are replaced into the uterine cavity transcervically after 48 hours.

Unexplained infertility. This is an increasingly diagnosed situation. Gamete IntraFallopian Transfer (GIFT) and Intrauterine Insemination (IUI) have been shown to enhance the pregnancy rate. GIFT involves ovulation induction and oocyte collection using the laparoscope. At the time of operation the oocyte and freshly washed semen are replaced into the fallopian tube where fertilization occurs. 'Take home baby' rates of 25–30% can be expected. IUI has rates of 10–15%/cycle.

Other problems. Cervical factors and antisperm antibodies are poorly understood and difficult to treat. Spontaneous pregnancies do occur and assisted conception can be useful.

The general practitioner's role in management

The initial investigation (except for tests of tubal patency) of an infertile couple can be performed in a general practice setting. In cases of straightforward failure of ovulation, treatment by the general practitioner with clomiphene for 3–6 months is appropriate. Failure to conceive within this period necessitates specialist referral.

SUMMARY

Infertility is a common problem affecting 1 : 6 couples wishing to conceive. History is important and investigation should be structured to produce a diagnosis in a short time. Referral to specialist centres is mandatory if pregnancy is not achieved relatively quickly, as the psychological effects of infertility can aggravate the problem.

9. Congenital abnormalities of the female genital tract

J. Rymer

Expectations of the examiners

A detailed knowledge of the abnormalities is not required but the candidate is expected to know the complications that they may produce.

Definition

An anomaly of the female genital tract that is present at birth.

Interesting facts

Women with congenital abnormalities of the uterus often have renal tract anomalies. The cause of congenital abnormalities of the genital tract is thought to be of polygenic aetiology rather than a single genetic cause.

Pathophysiology

The paramesonephric (Müllerian) ducts are the precursors of the fallopian tubes, uterus, and upper two-thirds of the vagina. The lower third of the vagina develops from the urogenital sinus. The paramesonephric ducts develop parallel to the mesonephric ducts from an invagination of coelomic epithelium. They progress caudally and cross the mesonephric ducts ventrally, and fuse to form a Y-shaped uterovaginal primordium which projects into the urogenital sinus. Canalization of the paramesonephric ducts begins before fusion of the ducts and proceeds craniocaudally. The vaginal septum disappears before the uterine septum. The uterine fundus then bulges cranially to form a convex dome.

The classification of the congenital uterine anomalies may be based on the embryological developmental defect:

1. Failure of development, e.g. no paramesonephric duct development or unilateral development
2. Failure of paramesonephric duct canalization
3. Failure of fusion of paramesonephric ducts
4. Failure of median septum loss

5. Failure of fundal dome development
6. Failure of fusion of paramesonephric ducts with urogenital sinus
7. Failure of transverse septum loss between paramesonephric system and urogenital sinus.

See Figure 9.1.

Assessment

The following features are associated with congenital abnormalities of the uterus:

1. Primary amenorrhoea (cryptomenorrhoea)
2. Recurrent first trimester miscarriages
3. Recurrent second trimester miscarriages
4. Preterm labour
5. Abnormal fetal presentations in late pregnancy
6. Intrauterine growth retardation
7. Incoordinate uterine action
8. Retained placenta.

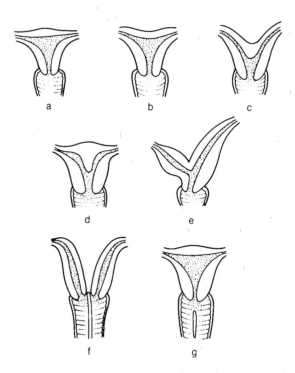

Fig. 9.1   Congenital abnormalities of the uterus and vagina.
a. Normal uterus and vagina; b. arcuate uterus; c. bicornuate uterus; d. subseptate uterus; e. rudimentary horn; f. uterus didelphys; g. normal uterus with partial vaginal septum.

As many of the above features can occur with other conditions, diagnosis is difficult. A high index of suspicion is needed and diagnostic procedures should be undertaken early.

Investigations

1. Examination under anaesthesia
   a. Probing the fundus of the uterus: this may detect an arcuate uterus
   b. Passing a dilator through the cervix: if a size 7 Hegar dilator can be passed through easily, then cervical incompetence may be present
   c. Dilatation and curettage: this procedure should detect partial septums or double systems.
   d. During a manual removal of the placenta an abnormality may be detected.
2. Hysterography: dye is injected through the cervix and X-ray pictures are taken. The uterine cavity and tubal lumina can be seen.
3. Hysteroscopy.
4. Ultrasound.
5. Laparoscopy ± dye insufflation.

Management

Each case must be dealt with individually and depends on:

1. Time of diagnosis
2. Previous obstetric history
3. Nature of the lesion
4. Mode of presentation.

Non-pregnant

1. Cervical incompetence: this condition usually occurs after previous dilatation of the cervix, however congenital cervical incompetence can occur. A cervical cerclage can be inserted prior to pregnancy, but most are performed at 14–16 weeks of pregnancy.
2. Uteroplasty: the septum is surgically excised at laparotomy. Most operations reduce the size of the uterine cavity but the fundal dome is increased and all patients must have caesarean sections in subsequent pregnancies.
3. Hysteroscopic incision of the uterine septum: under direct visualization through a hysteroscope the uterine septum is divided, either surgically or by laser. The uterus remains arcuate.

During pregnancy

1. Cervical cerclage: ideally performed at 14–16 weeks. The suture is removed at about 37 weeks. If the woman goes into spontaneous labour prior to this the suture must be removed.
2. Bed rest: the benefit has not been ascertained.
3. Intrauterine growth retardation: placentation on the septum may cause IUGR and patients must be managed appropriately.

During labour

1. Incoordinate uterine action: if inefficient uterine action results because of congenital abnormality of the uterus this should be corrected with oxytocin.
2. Malpresentations or fetal distress are dealt with appropriately.
3. Vaginal septum: this can be excised if there is delayed progress in the second stage of labour.
4. Retained placenta: as the incidence of retained placenta is increased, active management of the third stage is required (see Ch. 26).

SUMMARY

As it is so difficult to diagnose congenital abnormalities of the uterus, it is difficult to assess the various forms of treatment. In cases of recurrent first trimester miscarriages, mid-trimester miscarriages, preterm labour, and retained placentas, the index of suspicion should be high.

10. Hirsutism and virilism

M. Chapman

Expectations of the examiners

Hirsutism is a common complaint which is not usually managed particularly well. The examiners will expect a limited understanding of the physiology of androgen metabolism. Candidates should have a knowledge of basic investigations, their interpretation and subsequent management. Specialist endocrinological referral will be part of the management in severe cases.

Definition

Hirsutism can be defined as excessive hair growth outside the normal female distribution. Difficulties have arisen in differentiating 'normal' from 'abnormal'.

Virilism is defined as masculinization of the female involving one or more of the following features: clitoral hypertrophy, muscle hypertrophy, breast atrophy, hirsutism, deepening of the voice.

Interesting facts

Hirsutism is common. Depending on the stringency of the definition, more than 10% of females could be deemed to be hirsute. Only a small proportion complain.

Management of the psychological effects of hirsutism is the most important aspect of this problem. In almost all cases the underlying hormonal imbalance is benign.

Virilism is extremely rare (<1% of patients referred with hirsutism).

Pathophysiology

The physiology of the androgens is complex. There are many androgens with differing relative biological activities which are produced from a variety of sites. For example, dehydroepiandrosterone (DHEA) is produced predominantly by the adrenal gland and has a very weak biological activity when compared to testosterone. Dihydrotestosterone

(DHT), which has greater biological activity, is produced by peripheral conversion of weaker androgens.

Binding of the androgens to sex hormone binding globulin (SHBG) and albumin reduces the availability of the free steroid.

In hirsutism, various disorders of androgen metabolism can occur. Production rates of the androgens can be increased from the ovary (e.g. in polycystic ovarian disease) or the adrenal gland (e.g. in the case of a tumour) or peripheral conversion can be enhanced (e.g. in obesity or increased precursor production). SHBG may be reduced in liver disease. Finally, there may be an increased sensitivity of target organs to normal levels of testosterone (e.g. hair follicles, clitoris).

Aetiology

1. Ovarian
   a. Polycystic ovarian disease
   b. Tumour, e.g. androblastoma, teratoma
2. Adrenal
   a. Androgen secreting tumours
   b. Cushing's syndrome
   c. Congenital adrenal hyperplasia
3. Idiopathic
4. Rare causes
   a. Drugs
   b. Familial hypertrichosis
   c. Virilized intersexual disorders.

Assessment

Specific points in the history include:

Menstrual pattern

A regular menstrual cycle excludes a significant underlying hormonal disturbance. Oligo- or amenorrhoea should be investigated fully to look for polycystic ovarian disease and to exclude the rarer but potentially life-threatening hormone secreting tumours.

Racial group and family history

Hair distribution varies substantially with racial group, e.g. Scandinavian women rarely have facial hair whereas in southern Mediterranean women it is common.

Drugs

e.g. Danazol, testosterone implant.

Examination should exclude endocrine disease and signs of virilism should be noted. The severity of the hirsutism should be assessed and specific enquiry should be made about previous local treatments.

Investigations

Plasma androgens

A normal or slightly elevated testosterone level suggests a benign cause for the hirsutism. High levels are strongly suggestive of an androgen secreting tumour. Raised serum DHEA and androstenedione levels indicate an adrenal origin of the excess androgens. Raised levels of 17-hydroxyprogesterone may indicate congenital adrenal hyperplasia.

SHBG

SHBG binds testosterone and reduces the free testosterone available to stimulate receptors in the hair follicles. A low level of SHBG is associated with a raised total testosterone level and a higher concentration of free testosterone.

Gonadotrophin levels

Raised LH levels and increased LH/FSH ratios are consistent with polycystic ovarian disease.

Transvaginal ultrasound will show polycystic ovaries in more than 80% of women with hirsutism.

Other

Further investigations of specific endocrine disorders should be performed as indicated.

Treatment

Serious conditions should be excluded.

Psychological

The benign nature of the condition should be explained and continuing support may be necessary.

Local treatment

This may be the most effective management and includes:

1. Bleaching agents
2. Plucking
3. Shaving
4. Depilatory creams

5. Waxes
6. Electrolysis: this is effective and permanent but it can be painful and occasionally leave scarring.

Drugs

1. Dexamethasone: adrenal (ovarian) suppression
2. Oral contraceptives: SHBG elevation
3. Cyproterone acetate : androgen receptor inhibition
4. Spironolactone: enzyme inhibition
5. GnRH analogues: pituitary down-regulation leading to reduced ovarian production of steroids.

In general practice it is appropriate to use low-dose dexamethasone or oral contraceptives but further drug therapy should be prescribed after specialist referral.

It is important to emphasize that the pharmacological therapy of hirsutism is lengthy (12–24 months). Immediate improvement should not be expected.

SUMMARY

A detailed history and examination usually provides the diagnosis but basic investigations will confirm the presence of benign androgen excess. Reassurance can then be provided and advice about cosmetic treatment should be given. More severe cases should be managed by a gynaecologist or an endocrinologist.

11. Bleeding in early pregnancy

G. Davis

Expectations of the examiners

Bleeding in early pregnancy is common and candidates will be expected to differentiate between those patients who can be managed at home and those requiring admission, and to have a knowledge of the clinical findings which distinguish the two groups. In terms of clinical management, the important diagnostic decision is between threatened abortion and the remainder, but the terminology encourages examiners to ask about definitions.

Definitions

Abortion. Termination of pregnancy prior to 24 weeks' gestation, either spontaneous or induced.

Threatened abortion. Bleeding in early pregnancy without dilatation of the cervix or the passage of products of conception (POC).

Inevitable abortion. Bleeding in early pregnancy associated with cervical dilatation but without passage of POC. *(products of conception)*

Incomplete abortion. Bleeding in early pregnancy with cervical dilatation and the passage of POC.

Complete abortion. Bleeding in early pregnancy followed by the passage of all POC.

Missed abortion. Early pregnancy in which the fetus dies and the uterus fails to enlarge further. There may or may not be bleeding.

Septic abortion. Any abortion that becomes infected.

SPONTANEOUS ABORTION

Interesting facts

The commonly quoted incidence for abortion is 15% but is probably much higher (40–60%) when early pregnancies are included, i.e. prior to detection. These biochemical pregnancies probably present as slightly delayed periods which may be heavier than normal. Most spontaneous abortions occur prior to 12 weeks' gestation with a peak incidence at 7–8 weeks. The frequency of miscarriage increases with maternal age, smoking, and alcohol consumption.

Aetiology

1. *Fetal abnormalities.* These account for more than 50% of all spontaneous abortions and include chromosomal and developmental abnormalities. Chromosomal abnormalities (most commonly trisomy) are present in 80% of pregnancies in which a conceptus is not present (otherwise known as a blighted ovum or an afetal sac).
2. *Uterine abnormalities.* Malformation of the uterus may interfere with normal development of the pregnancy. Abnormalities may be congenital or acquired, e.g. submucous fibroids or mechanical damage from previous curettage.
3. *Systemic disease.* Most severe systemic diseases, e.g. connective tissue and renal disease, increase the rate of abortion. Any systemic infection or sustained pyrexia may cause abortion. Infections are not a common cause, but cytomegalovirus, toxoplasmosis and rubella are classically associated with an increased risk of abortion. Similarly, listeriosis and syphilis are uncommon causes of abortion in the second trimester.
4. *Drugs.* Cytotoxic drugs, particularly antimetabolites e.g. methotrexate, will cause abortion.
5. *Immunological.* There has been considerable debate on this subject and it has more relevance to, and is briefly reviewed in, the following section on recurrent abortion.
6. *Vascular.* An abnormal uterine arterial blood supply is associated with an increased risk of spontaneous abortion, possibly as a result of inadequate blood flow to the developing placenta.
7. *Psychological.* There is no convincing evidence that stress alone can cause abortion.

Assessment

History

1. Period of amenorrhoea.
2. Amount of bleeding.
3. Degree of pain.
4. Time of onset of pain in relation to bleeding (i.e. if pain precedes bleeding, ectopic pregnancy is more likely).
5. Passage of products of conception. This is very unreliable as organized clot is difficult to distinguish from products of conception.

Examination

There are five clinical findings of relevance:

1. The cardiovascular status of the patient.
2. Abdominal palpation. Although the uterus or lower abdomen may be tender, there should be no rebound tenderness and the pain is not usually unilateral. The exception is septic abortion where the whole of the lower abdomen may be tender with guarding and rebound. The diagnosis is usually obvious as the woman is febrile and toxic.
3. State of the cervix—whether it is starting to dilate.
4. Whether any products of conception are visible.
5. Uterine size should be equivalent to the expected size for the period of amenorrhoea.

Investigations

1. Ultrasound scan (USS). In the absence of confirmed POC or cervical dilatation, an USS is the definitive investigation in the management of abortion. If an intrauterine pregnancy is present, 45% will abort spontaneously; however, if a fetal heart is detected by ultrasound 95–98% of these women will continue the pregnancy. A pelvic ultrasound can reliably detect a live intrauterine pregnancy after 6 weeks' gestation and a transvaginal scan between 5 and 6 weeks.
2. FBC. To assess blood loss and serve as a baseline.
3. Blood group and save. If bleeding is significant, blood may need to be crossmatched and transfused. Rhesus status must be known prior to discharge from hospital and the appropriate action taken.
4. Septic abortions will require blood cultures and endocervical swabs. Further investigations will be required if the woman is septicaemic.

Treatment

Threatened abortion

The conventional management is bed rest and abstinence from intercourse. Progesterone supplementation has also been used. There is no evidence that any of these measures affect the outcome of the pregnancy. Hospital admission is not necessary but may be appropriate in selected cases.

Incomplete, inevitable, missed abortion

All require admission to hospital and evacuation of the uterus. Any products visible in the os at the initial examination should be removed with a pair of sponge-holding forceps. Failure to do so can allow the patient to go into 'cervical shock', i.e. cardiogenic shock thought to be related to vagal stimulation as a result of cervical dilatation. Ergometrine 0.5 mg i.m. may be useful in reducing blood loss and raising the blood pressure.

Septic abortion

The treatment of septic abortion is based on the principles of resuscitation, adequate antibiotic coverage and evacuation of the uterus when the patient's condition permits. In practice this usually means 12–24 hours of preoperative intravenous antibiotics, a broad-spectrum agent (such as a cephalosporin) and metronidazole, and gentamicin if the patient is septicaemic.

Evacuation of the uterus

This is usually performed with suction and completed with gentle curettage to ensure the uterus is empty. Particular care is necessary in septic abortion because of the increased risk of uterine perforation.

Complications

1. Immediate
   a. Haemorrhage
   b. Infection
   c. Uterine perforation
2. Delayed
   a. Infertility
   b. Asherman's syndrome—complete or partial loss of the endometrium due to excessive curettage
   c. Cervical incompetence—whether this occurs after spontaneous abortion is debatable.

Follow-up

Anti-D-immunoglobulin should be given to rhesus-negative women. Suppression of lactation is not usually necessary before 20 weeks. Prior to discharge the causes and prognosis should be discussed with the woman (and partner if possible). After abortion in the first pregnancy the chance of abortion in the next pregnancy is about 15–20% and slightly higher, 25–30%, after the first two pregnancies abort. The emotional reaction to abortion is variable and some women require full bereavement counselling. The Miscarriage Association is a patient-organized support group which many women find helpful (contact: Clayton Hospital, North Gate, Wakefield, West Yorkshire). Avoidance of pregnancy for at least 6 and preferably 12 months may be recommended for psychological reasons, but each couple must be dealt with on an individual basis.

RECURRENT MISCARRIAGE/RECURRENT PREGNANCY LOSS

Definition

Loss of three or more pregnancies at less than 24 weeks' gestation with no more than one living child from the current partnership.

Interesting facts

The incidence of recurrent miscarriage (RM) is quoted as 2–5% of those couples who have conceived. The mean gestational age of miscarriages in women with RM tends to be greater than in sporadic miscarriage. If the couple have had a live child the incidence of RM is halved. The likelihood of a successful pregnancy following three consecutive miscarriages is about 60–65%.

Aetiology

The aetiology of RM can be different according to the gestation at which the pregnancy losses occurred. The majority occur in the first trimester.

First trimester loss

Polycystic ovary syndrome. Fifty-six per cent of women with RM have been found to have polycystic ovaries on ultrasound scan. An association with a raised luteinizing hormone (LH) concentration has been found, although the mechanism whereby this abnormality may cause RM is not understood. It is thought that this raised LH may cause the oocyte to mature too early so affecting the 'quality' of the embryo but there is no evidence to prove this.

Autoimmune disease. The most important association with RM is with antiphospholipid antibodies and up to 30% of women with first trimester RM have been found to carry these antibodies. These are detected by measuring anticardiolipin antibodies (ACA) and lupus anticoagulant (LA). The latter test is called the Russell viper's venom test and has to be performed on a fresh specimen of blood (within 2 hours of venepuncture). If this test is positive the patient is at increased risk of thrombosis in pregnancy and should probably avoid the oral contraceptive pill. ACA are associated with the development of systemic lupus erythematosus (SLE), although the majority of women with RM who are ACA positive are asymptomatic. It is thought that these antibodies are a marker for poor trophoblastic implantation and may be associated with a poor obstetric history, e.g. neonatal death, IUGR as well as miscarriages in both the first and second trimesters. Other autoimmune diseases such as rheumatoid arthritis do not seem to be associated with an increased risk of RM.

Chromosomal. The majority of the embryos of women with RM are chromosomally normal. Approximately 4–5% of couples with RM are found to have a structural chromosomal abnormality, most commonly a balanced translocation.

Endocrine. Diabetes mellitus and hypo/hyperthyroidism have been thought to be associated with an increased risk of miscarriage. There is no evidence that established diabetes increases the risk of miscarriage but thyroid disease has been found to be an association in 1–2% of women with RM.

Immunological. It has previously been thought that the genetic dissimilarity between the parents might trigger the production of a 'blocking factor' by the mother which prevents the embryo being 'rejected' by the maternal immune system. Based on this theory women were tested for antipaternal cytotoxic antibodies and about 50% of women with RM were found to be negative. They were then 'immunized' with their partners' leucocytes in order to develop these antibodies. While an initial study showed a significant improvement in outcome, a large multicentre trial did not confirm these findings. The treatment has been abandoned in the majority of centres particularly as there is a risk of transmitting HIV and hepatitis B and C. There is no scientific evidence to support this original theory. More recently, special HLA antibodies (HLA-G) on the surface of the embryo have been found which are not recognized by the maternal immune system. It seems likely, therefore, that it is the embryo which carries the 'mask' to prevent its rejection rather than an 'anti-immune' response by the mother.

Second trimester loss

Cervical incompetence. True cervical incompetence is rare. The classic history is of painless loss of one or more pregnancies after 16 weeks. It is not usually preceded by spontaneous rupture of the membranes or infection. It is usually associated with a past history of trauma to the cervix particularly second trimester therapeutic abortions performed under general anaesthesia with forced cervical dilatation to over 10 mm. Another association is following a cone biopsy. Incompetence is very rare after a loop excision or laser ablation but may occur after a knife cone biopsy which tends to remove a longer core from the cervix. The diagnosis should be made by performing a hysterosalpingogram which will show ballooning of the internal os as the dye is introduced. It can be diagnosed by transvaginal ultrasound at 12–14 weeks' gestation.

Uterine abnormalities. These affect 2–3% of women with RM. The commonest abnormality is a bicornuate/unicornuate uterus. An association with RM can only be made if the septum dividing the two halves of the uterus reaches more than half-way down the cavity. The miscarriages tend to get later each time as the ability of the uterine muscle to hypertrophy improves with each successive pregnancy. If the placental site is on the septum, then trophoblastic implantation may be impaired and cause a loss earlier in pregnancy. Our knowledge of the causes of RM is sadly deficient and much research needs to be done to identify the processes by which miscarriage can occur.

Assessment

History of pregnancy loss

1. How many losses?
2. What gestation?
3. Was a beating fetal heart seen prior to the loss or was the sac empty?
4. Were the losses preceded by bleeding and/or pain?
5. Were they all with the same partner?
6. How many living children/other obstetric history?
7. Ease of conception.
8. Menstrual cycle length.

Medical/surgical history

1. History of systemic disease
2. Previous surgery to cervix
3. Family history of miscarriage.

Examination

1. General for endocrine/SLE in particular
2. Pelvic examination (rarely positive).

Investigations

1. Days 5–8 of cycle: LH, FSH, testosterone, TFTs (PCOS).
2. Rubella (important to vaccinate prior to conception if non-immune).
3. Anticardiolipin antibodies, lupus anticoagulant (APS, SLE).
4. Chromosomes of both partners.
5. Ultrasound scan (PCOS, uterine abnormality).
6. Haemoglobinopathy screen of both partners if from West Africa or of Mediterranean/Asian origin (α thalassaemia, sickle cell disease).
7. Hysterosalpingogram (cervical incompetence, uterine abnormality).

Treatment

All groups require psychological support and regular ultrasound scans to confirm that all is going well or to pick up another miscarriage at the earliest possible opportunity. This has been shown to be as effective as any other treatment offered. There are no conclusive data to show that progesterone supplementation improves the outcome of pregnancy.

PCOS

1. Down-regulation with gonadotrophin releasing hormone (GnRH) agonists followed by ovulation induction with gonadotrophins has not been shown to improve the outcome.
2. Human chorionic gonadotrophin (hCG) 5000 i.u. twice weekly: one small study has suggested that hCG from the time of diagnosis of pregnancy to 14 weeks' gestation significantly improves the outcome in women who are oligomenorrhoeic (cycle length greater than 35 days) but there are no data for women with PCOS who have regular cycles. There is, therefore, not enough evidence to support the use of hCG in women with PCOS as an association for RM except in the context of a randomized controlled trial.

Autoimmune disease (ACA±LA positive)

A recent randomized trial suggests that the use of aspirin 75 mg/day and heparin 5000 i.u./day during pregnancy is associated with a significantly better outcome of pregnancy than aspirin alone which is significantly better than placebo. This should be administered by appropriately trained specialist units.

Chromosomal

These couples should be referred to a geneticist for counselling.

Immunological

There is no evidence that immunotherapy improves pregnancy and since there is a risk of hepatitis B and C and HIV transmission it should be actively discouraged.

Cervical incompetence

Cervical cerclage is indicated for women shown to have a shortened cervix or where the internal os is open/opens under pressure during hysterosalpingography. The Shirodkar suture which entailed an incision in the cervix to push the bladder up and place the suture around the cervical–isthmic junction has been replaced by the McDonald suture. This is a simpler technique which encircles the cervix with a four-bite suture as high up the cervix as possible from a vaginal approach. The suture is removed at 37 weeks. In women who miscarry despite this technique, a transabdominal approach has been used to place a stitch around the cervix with good results. The women all have a caesarean section leaving the stitch in place until the woman decides to not have any more children.

THERAPEUTIC ABORTION

Definition

Medical termination of pregnancy prior to 24 weeks' gestation.

Features

Since the 1967 Abortion Act, termination of pregnancy is possible in England and Wales providing it is carried out (in a licensed place) by a registered medical practitioner and two registered medical practitioners have signed the appropriate consent form (Certificate A). The grounds for abortion under the Act are:

A. The continuance of the pregnancy would involve risk to the life of the pregnant woman greater than if the pregnancy were terminated.
B. The termination is necessary to prevent grave permanent injury to the physical or mental health of the pregnant woman.
C. The pregnancy has NOT exceeded its 24th week and that the continuance of the pregnancy would involve risk, greater than if the pregnancy were terminated, of injury to the physical or mental health of the pregnant woman.
D. The pregnancy has NOT exceeded its 24th week and that the continuance of the pregnancy would involve risk, greater than if the pregnancy were terminated, of injury to the physical or mental health of any existing child(ren) of the family of the pregnant woman.
E. There is substantial risk that if the child were born it would suffer from such physical or mental abnormalities as to be seriously handicapped.

The vast majority of therapeutic abortions are carried out on the basis of the second reason—risk to the physical or mental health of the pregnant woman. In 1994, abortions constituted 20% of total births and abortions, i.e. about one in five pregnancies were terminated.

The rate of legal terminations in 1992–94 was approximately 12.3/1000 women aged 14–49. Most NHS hospitals provide a termination service and there are a number of private clinics and private gynaecologists who also provide this service.

Assessment

Assuming that the practitioner follows the woman's (and partner's, if present) wishes, three pieces of information are required:

1. Is she pregnant and, if so, what is the gestation?
2. Does the woman definitely want an abortion?
3. Is she fit for an anaesthetic?

Abortion services should provide counselling so that the woman's commitment can be adequately assessed and she can have the opportunity to discuss her decision in a supportive environment. As most women are referred by their general practitioner, they should have discussed it with him/her and the doctor referring should sign the medical consent form which the woman can bring with her.

History

1. Pregnancy
   a. Period of amenorrhoea
   b. Menstrual cycle
   c. Previous contraception
   d. Symptoms of pregnancy
2. Past medical and obstetric history.

Examination

1. Physical examination
2. Uterine size.

Investigations

1. Ultrasound scan if <8 or >14 weeks' gestation to confirm gestation
2. FBC
3. Blood group and antibody screen.

Methods

Most terminations of pregnancy in England and Wales are carried out under general anaesthesia but in other countries local anaesthesia is used up to 12 weeks' gestation. This has the advantage of avoiding the risks of general anaesthesia and reducing blood loss, but requires greater involvement by both staff and patients.

Prior to 12 weeks

Suction aspiration. Used routinely up to 12 weeks' gestation. The cervix is dilated and a semirigid plastic suction catheter is inserted into the uterus. Most operators check that evacuation is complete with sponge forceps and *gentle* curettage.

RU486. The progesterone antagonist, RU486, in association with a prostaglandin pessary is 99% effective in termination of pregnancy prior to 8 weeks' gestation without recourse to operation. Provided that antiabortion opinion allows its general introduction, it represents the biggest single advance in the field since the 1967 Act.

After 12 weeks

Dilatation and evacuation. After 12 weeks' gestation, instrumental destruction of the pregnancy and removal of the pieces is employed, often in conjunction with suction aspiration to reduce the uterine volume. A bolus of 5–10 i.u. of syntocinon is often given intravenously during or after the procedure. This method is commonly used up to 16 weeks' gestation and by a few operators up to 20–22 weeks.

Prostaglandins (PGs) are used for second trimester terminations, usually after 16 weeks. They may be administered as repeated, frequent vaginal pessaries, infused extra-amniotically into the uterine cavity, or given as an intra-amniotic bolus injection. PG by any route, but particularly if inadvertently given intravenously, may cause systemic side-effects of nausea, vomiting, sweating, bronchospasm, or diarrhoea. Usually these symptoms are not prominent but resuscitation equipment and adrenaline must be readily available.

PGs are used for most late terminations but the terminations may be prolonged (12–48 hours) and require considerable analgesia. Often a syntocinon infusion is added to accelerate the onset of labour (despite the relative insensitivity of the uterus to oxytocin until the third trimester).

Hysterotomy is very rarely used in modern practice. The major reason for avoiding its use is the risk of rupture of the uterine scar in subsequent pregnancy.

Complications

The risk of complications is directly related to the experience of the operator and the gestation of the pregnancy.

1. Immediate
   a. General anaesthesia
   b. Uterine perforation—usually this is minor and the woman can simply be observed overnight in hospital, but any evidence of continuing bleeding necessitates laparoscopy or laparotomy and closure of the uterine defect
   c. Incomplete evacuation leading to haemorrhage or infection.
2. Delayed
   a. Infertility due to postoperative infection

b. Asherman's syndrome (see above)
c. Cervical incompetence (see above)
d. Psychological—the response is very variable but can be prolonged and significant. Future subfertility is often attributed (both correctly and incorrectly) to previous termination of pregnancy.

Follow-up

In practice, very few centres follow up their patients despite the frequency of emotional difficulties most women experience after termination of pregnancy. In those that attempt to, attendance by the women postoperatively is sporadic.

EXTRAUTERINE PREGNANCY

Definition

Implantation of a pregnancy outside the uterine cavity, the majority in the fallopian tube (95%).

Interesting facts

In the 1982–84 Maternal Mortality report for England and Wales, ectopic pregnancy was the sixth commonest cause of maternal mortality (10 cases). The initial diagnosis is incorrect in 25–50% of cases. Its incidence (1 in 200 pregnancies) has doubled in the past 20 years and varies in different groups, e.g. 1 in 30 pregnancies in the West Indies and in 2–3% of pregnancies resulting from assisted conception.

The diagnosis is usually made late and delay between admission and operation is common. The classic symptoms of ectopic pregnancy are abdominal pain, amenorrhoea, and irregular vaginal bleeding. The diagnostic problem is that these symptoms are also associated with spontaneous miscarriage and pelvic inflammatory disease, the two commonest alternative diagnoses. Shock is present in 15–25% of cases. It is unclear how many would or do resolve spontaneously.

Predisposing factors

Pelvic inflammatory disease (PID). Histological evidence for previous pelvic infection can be found in 30–50% of ectopic gestations. Evidence suggests that previous infection increases the risk of ectopic pregnancy about 10 times. It is widely believed that the recent increase in ectopic pregnancy is related to the current epidemic of PID.

Tubal surgery. Any form of surgery to the tubes including sterilization increases the ratio of ectopic to intrauterine pregnancy.

Previous tubal pregnancy. The risk of subsequent pregnancy implanting ectopically is increased 20-fold even if salpingectomy has been performed. This is presumably because the predisposing pathology (i.e. tubal damage) is bilateral.

Infertility. Pregnancy in subfertile women, whether after induction of ovulation or assisted conception techniques (IVF or GIFT), is more likely to implant ectopically. In many cases this is due to pre-existing tubal disease.

Intrauterine devices. The overall incidence of ectopic pregnancy in IUD users is lower than normal. However, if pregnancy occurs, the ratio of ectopic to intrauterine pregnancies is 1:20.

Progestins. The low dose progestogen-only pills have a similar effect to IUDs in that they increase the ectopic to intrauterine pregnancy ratio while not affecting, or slightly reducing, the overall incidence of ectopic pregnancy. However, the addition of progestin to an inert IUD (Progestasert) appears to increase the incidence of ectopic pregnancy threefold over non-contraceptive users. The reasons for this are unclear.

Assessment

The most important aid to diagnosis is a high level of suspicion—all women in the reproductive age group who present with one or any combination of the symptoms, i.e. abdominal pain, vaginal bleeding, and amenorrhoea, should be assumed to have an ectopic pregnancy until proven otherwise.

History

1. Pain
   a. *Usually* unilateral but may be bilateral
   b. Usually starts prior to the bleeding
   c. May radiate to the shoulder tip
2. Bleeding
   a. Classically dark red and described as 'prune juice'
   b. Usually not as heavy as in spontaneous miscarriage
   c. May pass a decidual cast, mimicking products of conception
3. Amenorrhoea: *absent* in 25% of cases.

Examination

1. Cardiovascular status—may be shocked.
2. Abdomen—unilateral tenderness usually with rebound but may present with a rigid abdomen if massive blood loss.
3. Uterus enlarged, cervical excitation is usually present and a mass may be palpable, although in half of these the ectopic pregnancy will be on the opposite side.

Investigations

In the collapsed, shocked patient, no investigations are required prior to surgery. In less obvious cases the following investigations are necessary.

Pregnancy test

Sensitive tests for hCG will be positive in > 95% of ectopic pregnancies.

Ultrasound scan

If an intrauterine pregnancy is detected the diagnosis of ectopic pregnancy can virtually be excluded. The coexistence of intrauterine and ectopic pregnancies is rare (1 in 30 000) except in assisted conception. The problem arises in pregnancies at 4–6 weeks' gestation where the sac is not visible. The use of transvaginal ultrasound allows earlier detection of an intrauterine pregnancy and should be the preferred option to transabdominal pelvic ultrasound.

Laparoscopy

All women who present with pain and bleeding, a positive pregnancy test or raised serum hCG and no intrauterine pregnancy on ultrasound should have an urgent laparoscopy. Where the diagnosis is uncertain (hCG <1500, no intrauterine pregnancy), the woman should be kept in hospital and the serum hCG repeated after 48 hours. In a viable intrauterine pregnancy the hCG doubles in 48 hours and therefore a slowly rising or static hCG is indicative of an ectopic or non-viable pregnancy and other causes of pelvic pain. In these circumstances laparoscopy and uterine curettage are indicated. Undiagnosed unilateral pain (without a positive pregnancy test or raised serum hCG) which does not resolve within 24–48 hours should also be investigated by laparoscopy to exclude ectopic pregnancy and other causes of pelvic pain.

Other investigations

1. FBC
2. Cross match.

Treatment

Resuscitation

An i.v. line and resuscitation should be initiated, en route to theatre in severe cases.

Surgery

Every attempt should be made to conserve the tube. The operation of choice is controversial, ranging from salpingectomy to linear salpingotomy—opening the tube lengthwise along its antimesenteric border over the implantation site. Progressively more of the surgery for ectopic pregnancies is performed laparoscopically — usually salpingostomy or injection of methotrexate into the gestational sac. In pregnancies treated laparoscopically the serum hCG should be followed postoperatively to ensure that it falls appropriately as the persistence of trophoblast is more common. There is no evidence that removal of the ovary on the same side affects the prognosis for future fertility in any way.

Surgery for extratubal pregnancies (e.g. ovarian or intra-abdominal pregnancies) should achieve a balance between removing the pregnancy and damaging the site of implantation. Haemostasis is often a major problem.

Prognosis

1. Immediate postoperative complications are uncommon. Occasionally if the pregnancy is 'milked out' of the fimbrial end, residual trophoblast may continue to grow, requiring further surgery. Routine postoperative management and follow-up should be undertaken.
2. Future pregnancy: only one-third of women wishing to have a further pregnancy will succeed in having a child and 10% will have a further ectopic pregnancy. The chances of intrauterine pregnancy depend on the extent of tubal damage pre- and postoperatively. The impact of laparoscopic management of ectopic pregnancy on these figures is not known.
3. Undiagnosed ectopic pregnancy may result in tubal abortion into the peritoneal cavity with subsequent reabsorption of the products or, rarely, abdominal implantation. Chronic bleeding from an ectopic pregnancy can lead to a pelvic haematocele — a pelvic haematoma surrounded by inflammatory change and adhesions.

HYDATIDIFORM MOLE

Definition

A benign tumour of trophoblast.

Features

The incidence in the UK is lower (1 in 2000 pregnancies) than in South East Asia (1 in 200 pregnancies). The aetiology is unknown and there are two types which are genetically and clinically dissimilar: complete (classical) in which no fetus is present; and partial where a fetus (or fetal material) is present. Complete moles are rare. The cells contain 46 chromosomes of *paternal* origin and they may lead to choriocarcinoma.

Partial moles are more common; they have 69 chromosomes (triploid) of which the additional haploid set are again paternal in origin and probably do not give rise to choriocarcinoma. A mole may become 'invasive' and penetrate the uterus and/or metastasize, particularly to the lungs. This is distinct from choriocarcinoma which is a malignant tumour of trophoblast.

Pathology

Complete mole

There is a triad of microscopic features:

1. Hyperplasia of both syncytiotrophoblast and cytotrophoblast
2. Villous oedema forming multiple small collections of fluid 'cisterns'
3. Absence of fetus.

Partial mole

The placenta shows *focal* hyperplasia which is usually confined to the syncytiotrophoblast, and focal villous swelling with cistern formation. The fetus usually dies early and the only remnants may be the presence of erythrocytes in placental vessels. The diagnosis may be difficult as villi are often swollen in aborted tissue so the diagnosis rests with the pathologist. Where a fetus is present, multiple congenital abnormalities are evident, consistent with the triploid state.

Assessment

Moles usually present with irregular vaginal bleeding in pregnancy. The massive production of hCG may lead to exaggerated symptoms of pregnancy.

History

1. Amenorrhoea
2. Bleeding
3. Hyperemesis (25–30%)
4. Passage of grape-like vesicles
5. Rarely, metastatic spread: haemoptysis, pleuritic pain.

Examination

1. Pre-eclampsia may develop early (15–20%)

2. Uterus is usually larger than dates (55%), but may be smaller (15–20%)
3. Fetal heart is usually absent
4. Theca lutein cysts may be palpable (10–20%).

Investigations

1. Ultrasound: scanning reveals a typical 'snow storm' appearance in the uterus. A fetus is not usually identified
2. hCG is usually significantly elevated
3. Chest X-ray to exclude pulmonary metastasis.

Treatment

Suction evacuation

This may need to be repeated if bleeding persists or hCG levels are still elevated 6 weeks after initial evacuation. This will cure 90% of patients. The risk of perforation is increased.

Extra-amniotic prostaglandin infusion

This procedure is used if the uterus is thought to be too large for surgical evacuation.

Hysterectomy

Hysterectomy may be performed in older women as they have a greater risk of developing choriocarcinoma.

Follow-up

All patients with molar pregnancy should be registered at a centre for trophoblastic disease. Meticulous follow-up of all women with molar pregnancies is essential. Estimations of hCG should be performed 3 weeks postevacuation and then fortnightly until negative. They should then be assessed monthly for 2 years. Any rise or plateau in the hCG levels requires chemotherapy as outlined below under choriocarcinoma. These cases (10% of total) usually become evident between 3 and 6 weeks after evacuation.

Prognosis

The mortality from trophoblastic disease is 6–8 women per year in the UK. The incidence of hydatidiform mole in a subsequent pregnancy is 1 in 120. Pregnancy is contraindicated for 1 year and oral contraception is not recommended. In subsequent pregnancies, women are asked to attend early for exclusion of molar pregnancy by ultrasound and a hCG should be performed 3 weeks after delivery.

CHORIOCARCINOMA

Definition

Malignant tumour of trophoblast.

Interesting facts

This may follow normal or molar pregnancy but choriocarcinoma is a thousand-fold more common after molar pregnancy, i.e. a woman presenting with choriocarcinoma has an equal chance of the preceding pregnancy being normal or molar. One in 30 moles become choriocarcinoma and it is vastly more common in South East Asia.

Local extension is frequent and metastatic spread is usually vascular to the lungs (70%) or brain.

Treatment

1. Methotrexate and folinic acid plus evacuation of the uterus or hysterectomy.
2. Resistant or high-risk cases require combination chemotherapy.
3. Invasive mole and choriocarcinoma are treated similarly, the treatment depending more on risk factors such as age and degree of spread than histology.
4. Follow-up of hCG levels is required similar to that in molar pregnancy.

Prognosis

Remission can be expected in all women except the few with metastases other than pulmonary. Pregnancy after choriocarcinoma is possible after 2 years free of disease and is managed in a similar way to pregnancy following other trophoblastic disease.

12. Benign conditions of the female genital tract

A. Rodin

Interesting facts

Benign lesions of the female genital tract are common and they may be congenital or acquired. Occasionally, they are manifestations of systemic disease.

THE VULVA

Abnormal appearance of the external genitalia at birth may represent an intersex state; further discussion of intersex is beyond the scope of this book. Clitoromegaly may occur in certain virilizing conditions (see Ch. 8).

PRURITUS VULVAE

Vulval irritation can occur at any age and it may be an extremely distressing symptom. It is most commonly caused by *Candida albicans* infection (Table 12.1).

Table 12.1 Causes of pruritus vulvae.

Local causes
    Infection
        Candida albicans
        Herpes genitalis
        Genital warts
        Other sexually transmitted diseases
        Threadworms, pubic lice, scabies
    Atrophic vulvitis
    Vulval dystrophies
    Tumours

General causes
    Skin diseases, e.g. eczema, psoriasis
    Medical conditions, e.g. diabetes mellitus, hypothyroidism, liver disease, chronic renal failure, Crohn's disease, polycythaemia
    Drug reactions
    Psychogenic

Management of this complaint is aimed at identifying the cause and then treating appropriately. A history is taken and a physical examination is performed to look for generalized causes of pruritus. The vulva is inspected and a gentle speculum examination is performed and microbiological swabs are taken prior to digital examination. Glycosuria should be excluded and blood tests should be performed as clinically indicated. Skin biopsies should be taken if epithelial changes are suspected.

CHRONIC EPITHELIAL DYSTROPHIES OF THE VULVA

The chronic vulval dystrophies are of unknown aetiology and mainly occur in postmenopausal women. They are classified according to their histological appearance.

Classification of vulval dystrophies

1. Hyperplastic dystrophy
   a. Without atypia
   b. With atypia
2. Hypoplastic dystrophy
3. Mixed dystrophy
   a. Without atypia
   b. With atypia.

Pruritus vulvae is the commonest symptom and on examination the vulva appears atrophic and white plaques (leukoplakia) may be present. Fusion of the labia may occur with stenosis of the introitus. The changes do not extend into the vagina. The diagnosis is confirmed by histological examination of skin biopsies.

In hypoplastic dystrophy (lichen sclerosus et atrophicus) there is thinning of the epidermis with hyperkeratosis and chronic inflammation in the dermis. Hyperplastic dystrophy is characterized by thickening and hyperplasia of the epidermis. Leukoplakia describes thickening and whitening of the skin and is seen in several conditions. Malignant change may occur in dystrophy associated with the presence of nuclear atypia.

Treatment

Topical

1. Corticosteroid cream—hyperplastic
2. Testosterone cream ⎫ hypoplastic
3. Oestrogen cream ⎭

Local

1. Laser
2. Cryosurgery.

Surgery

Vulvectomy is usually reserved for cases in which there is nuclear atypia but may be used to provide palliation in cases where there is intractable pruritus vulvae.

VULVAL LUMPS AND SWELLINGS

Lumps and swellings of the vulva are common and in the majority of cases they are benign. Any skin condition may affect the vulva. (See Table 12.2.)

Bartholin's gland swellings

The Bartholin's glands are paired structures which lie deep to the posterior ends of the labia minora posteriorly. The duct on each side opens between the labium minus and the hymen and is about 0.5 cm long. Normally the gland cannot be palpated. Obstruction of the duct results in accumulation of secretions and cyst formation. Women present with a painless vulval swelling. A Bartholin's abscess is painful and women present with a tender, red and sometimes fluctuant lump. Treatment of both cysts and abscesses is by marsupialization. This involves making an elliptical incision into the roof of the cyst, draining the cavity and suturing the cyst wall to the skin to allow continuing drainage. Excision of the Bartholin's gland is rarely performed.

Urethral caruncle

This term is applied to any reddened area involving the posterior margin of the urethral orifice and is thought to be due to prolapse of the posterior urethral wall. Caruncles are often symptomless and are usually found in postmenopausal women. They occasionally cause bleeding and

---

Table 12.2   Causes of swellings of the vulva.

General causes
    Sebaceous cyst
    Haematoma
    Varicose veins
    Benign tumours, e.g. lipoma, papilloma, fibroma, hidradenoma
    Malignant tumour: primary/secondary

Specific causes
    Bartholin's gland: cyst/abscess
    Urethral caruncle
    Endometriosis
    Carcinoma of the vulva
    Inguinal hernia
    Hydrocele of Canal of Nuck

dyspareunia. Treatment with topical oestrogen cream is usually effective but sometimes surgical excision is necessary.

Causes of vulval ulceration

See 'Sexually transmitted infections in women (Ch. 39).

VAGINA

VAGINAL SEPTUM

See 'Congenital abnormalities of the female genital tract' (Ch. 9).

VAGINITIS

See 'Sexually transmitted infections in women (Ch. 39).

VAGINAL CYSTS

These are usually remnants of the lower portion of the mesonephric (Wolffian) duct and they occur anterolaterally in the vagina. They are usually asymptomatic and require no treatment.

THE CERVIX

The vaginal portion of the cervix is covered by stratified squamous epithelium and the endocervical canal is lined by columnar epithelium. Before puberty, the squamocolumnar junction is in the endocervical canal. During adolescence, the ovarian hormones cause eversion of the lower part of the cervical canal so that columnar epithelium appears on the ectocervix. The columnar epithelium is exposed to the acid environment of the vagina and columnar epithelium is replaced by stratified squamous epithelium (squamous metaplasia). If the process of squamous metaplasia results in the obstruction of cervical glands, retention cysts may form which are known as nabothian follicles.

CERVICAL ECTROPION

Eversion of the lower cervical canal occurs during adolescence, during pregnancy and while taking the combined oral contraceptive pill and the characteristic appearance of the cervix in these circumstances is known as cervical ectropion. The florid appearance of the cervix in these situations gives rise to the term 'erosion', however this term is a misnomer and should be avoided.

Ectropion may also result from cervical tears sustained during childbirth. Cervical ectropion is usually asymptomatic, but occasionally causes excessive vaginal discharge or postcoital bleeding. A cervical smear should be taken. Treatment is rarely necessary but women with persistent symptoms can be treated with cryocautery as an outpatient procedure .

CERVICITIS

Chronic cervicitis is a non-specific condition which is difficult to define. It is a common clinical diagnosis which is rarely confirmed by bacteriology.

CERVICAL POLYPS

These develop from the endocervix and protrude from the external os into the vagina. They are covered by columnar epithelium which often undergoes squamous metaplasia. They are usually asymptomatic, but the dependent part of the polyp may ulcerate causing intermenstrual and postcoital bleeding. They may also cause an increase in vaginal discharge. Cervical polyps are rarely malignant.

Cervical polyps should be avulsed and sent for histological examination. Their base should be cauterized to prevent regrowth and an endometrial biopsy should be taken at the same time to exclude other causes of irregular vaginal bleeding.

THE BODY OF THE UTERUS

POLYPS

Various types of polyps form in the cavity of the uterus including:

1. Endometrial polyps (adenomatous)
2. Fibroid polyps
3. Placental polyps.

Endometrial polyps are the most common and may be multiple in premenopausal women but are usually single in postmenopausal women. Occasionally they extrude through the cervix causing dysmenorrhoea. They may be symptomless but usually present with abnormal vaginal bleeding. Menorrhagia and intermenstrual bleeding may occur and in the older woman there may be postmenopausal bleeding. If the polyp has passed through the cervix there may be postcoital bleeding. Ideally, endometrial polyps should be removed under direct vision using a hysteroscopic resectoscope. The polypoid tissue must be sent for histological examination to exclude malignancy.

UTERINE FIBROIDS

Fibroids or leiomyomata are the commonest tumours of the female genital tract and are present in at least 20% of women over the age of 30 years. Their aetiology is unknown but their growth is oestrogen dependent and they regress after the menopause. Fibroids are associated with nulliparity in white women and they are more prevalent in Afro-Caribbean women.

Fibroids are mainly derived from smooth muscle but also contain some fibrous tissue elements. They form well-defined tumours with a false capsule and may be found in various sites: intramural fibroids lie within the uterine wall, subserous fibroids project from the peritoneal surface of the uterus, and submucous fibroids encroach on the uterine cavity, sometimes distorting it and increasing its surface area. Subserous fibroids may become pedunculated and a submucous fibroid may become extruded to form a fibroid polyp. Only 2% of fibroids arise in the cervix.

Fibroids are usually multiple and vary in size from seedlings to large tumours. They may undergo various types of degenerative changes:

Hyaline degeneration. This is the commonest change and it occurs as the fibroid outgrows its blood supply. Areas liquefy and cysts form.

Calcification. This occurs in postmenopausal women.

Infection. Subserous or pedunculated fibroids may become infected by spread from adjacent structures. Ascending infection may complicate submucous fibroids.

Red degeneration. This occurs during pregnancy when the blood supply is insufficient to support growth of the fibroid; the cut section of the fibroid appears red.

Malignant change (leiomyosarcoma) is rare (< 0.5% of fibroids) and may be suspected when there is rapid or painful enlargement of fibroids.

Assessment

The majority of fibroids are asymptomatic and are detected at routine pelvic examination. The commonest symptom is menorrhagia which is particularly associated with submucous fibroids. Some women present with abdominal distension and others complain of pressure symptoms such as increased frequency of micturition and stress incontinence. Pain is an unusual feature but occasionally fibroids present as an acute abdomen following torsion of a pedunculated fibroid or haemorrhage into a large fibroid. Fibroids do not cause infertility unless they are obstructing the cornua of the uterus.

Pelvic examination reveals an enlarged and often irregular uterus which may be palpable per abdomen. The main differential diagnosis is from ovarian tumours where the uterus should be detected separately from the pelvic mass. The presence of ascites is highly suggestive of ovarian pathology. In practice, it may be difficult to distinguish between the two clinically.

Investigations

Ultrasonography may be useful to distinguish between uterine and ovarian pathology. Abnormal vaginal bleeding should not be assumed to be due to fibroids and other pathology should be excluded. A cervical smear should be performed and the patient should have an endometrial biopsy.

Blood tests may reveal iron deficiency anaemia but large fibroids are rarely associated with polycythaemia (due to erythropoietin production).

Treatment

Conservative management

Conservative management is appropriate in the following situations:

1. Uterus smaller than 16 weeks' gestation
2. Asymptomatic
3. During pregnancy
4. Menopause approaching
5. Fertility required.

Medical treatment of fibroids using GnRH analogues has produced disappointing results. Fibroids regress during treatment but rapidly regrow when therapy is discontinued. Duration of treatment is limited by bone loss due to oestrogen deficiency.

Surgery

Surgery is indicated in the following situations:

1. Fibroids causing symptoms
2. Uterus >16 weeks' size
3. Rapid growth in fibroids
4. Recurrent miscarriage/fibroid-related complications in previous pregnancy (see below)
5. Diagnosis uncertain.

Hysterectomy is the definitive procedure. Myomectomy can be technically difficult and regrowth of fibroids after this procedure is common. Myomectomy should be reserved for women who wish to retain fertility and for those who decline hysterectomy. Submucous fibroids can be resected hysteroscopically. Pedunculated and subserous fibroids can be removed laparoscopically.

Fibroids in pregnancy

Fibroids may be detected for the first time in pregnancy. They may cause the uterus to feel large for dates. They do not usually influence the outcome of the pregnancy but they may be associated with some complications:

1. Recurrent miscarriage: submucous fibroids distort the uterine cavity and may be associated with repeated early pregnancy loss.
2. Pain: red degeneration may occur in large fibroids causing pain and localized uterine tenderness; torsion of a pedunculated fibroid may occur.
3. Malpresentations/abnormal lie.
4. Obstructed labour (rare).
5. Postpartum haemorrhage.

Surgical treatment of fibroids is not undertaken during pregnancy, except in the rare situation when a pedunculated fibroid undergoes torsion. Red degeneration is treated with rest and analgesia.

THE OVARIES

70%

Functional cysts of the ovaries are common and they usually cause no symptoms. Follicular cysts are rarely >5 cm in diameter and are usually diagnosed by ultrasound in women with anovulatory cycles and those receiving fertility treatment. Corpus luteal cysts are associated with short periods of secondary amenorrhoea followed by heavier than usual bleeding. Multiple theca lutein cysts are characteristically associated with trophoblastic disease and hyperstimulation associated with fertility treatment. Functional cysts usually resolve spontaneously and should be followed up by ultrasonography. Persistent cysts should be removed laparoscopically and examined histologically.

ENDOMETRIOSIS   *Dermoid Cyst - 5%*

See 'Endometriosis, dyspareunia and pelvic pain' (Ch. 7).

OVARIAN NEOPLASMS

See 'Gynaecological oncology' (Ch. 13).

13. Gynaecological oncology

A. Hollingworth

Expectations of the examiners

Candidates are expected to understand the natural history of the common gynaecological malignancies, to know their mode of presentation and the principles of their management. An appreciation of the role of screening will be important for the general practitioner.

Screening

The criteria for introducing a screening test were formulated by Wilson and Jungner and, of the 10 listed, at least seven need to be fulfilled before a test should be introduced. The criteria are as follows:

1. The condition sought should be an important health problem.
2. There should be an accepted treatment for patients with recognized disease.
3. Facilities for diagnosis and treament should be available.
4. There should be a recognizable latent or early symptomatic stage.
5. There should be a suitable test or examination.
6. The test should be acceptable to the population.
7. The natural history of the condition, including development from latent to declared disease, should be adequately understood.
8. There should be an agreed policy on whom to treat as patients.
9. The cost of case-finding (including diagnosis and treatment of patients diagnosed) should be economically balanced in relation to possible expenditure on medical care as a whole.
10. Case-finding should be a continuing process and not a 'once and for all' project.

Screening for the different types of gynaecological malignancy will be discussed where appropriate.

THE VULVA
VULVAL INTRAEPITHELIAL NEOPLASIA

The incidence of vulval intraepithelial neoplasia (VIN), though difficult to assess, appears to be on the increase. It is a premalignant lesion although its malignant potential for transformation to vulval cancer is not as great as CIN (cevical intraepithelial neoplasia) to cervical cancer.

The average age of presentation is 38 years. In premenopausal women <50 years, the disease may be multicentric and multifocal and coexist with CIN. The disease is usually a single focus in postmenopausal women (>50 years). The most common site is the labia minora.

Predisposing features include:

1. Coincidental CIN
2. Previous genital tract infections, e.g. warts, herpes simplex, gonorrhoea, trichomonas vaginalis
3. History of immunosuppression.

Women may present with the following symptoms:

1. Local discomfort
2. Superficial dyspareunia
3. Pruritus
4. Local red spot
5. White lesion
6. Asymptomatic (noted at time of colposcopy).

If there is a suspicious lesion then a biopsy must be taken.

Histological appearance

VIN1   The epidermis is thickened and nuclear atypia is confined to the lower third of the epithelium.
VIN2   Marked nuclear atypia in the lower half of the epithelium.
VIN3   Carcinoma in situ, marked nuclear atypia extending through the full thickness of the epithelium.

Treatment

Treatment depends on the site and size of the lesion(s), as well as the age and general condition of the patient. Follow-up is essential as recurrences do occur.

1. Local destruction
   a. Laser vaporization
   b. Cryotherapy
   c. 5-FU cream
2. Excision methods
   a. Wide local excision
   b. Simple vulvectomy
   c. Skinning vulvectomy with skin grafting.

CARCINOMA OF THE VULVA

Vulval carcinoma accounts for about 4% of all genital tract tumours.

Incidence

In 1988, 1125 new cases of vulval carcinoma were reported in England and Wales (OPCS). The number of deaths from this disease was 512 in 1992.

Age

Most tumours occur in the 65–70 year age group, though there is an increasing number of cases in younger women with multifocal premalignant changes in the lower genital tract.

Geography

There is no obvious geographical distribution.

Predisposing factors

A history of vulval irritation may be a predisposing factor. In younger women, there may be some relationship to HPV. VIN may progress to invasive disease. Any woman with a history of lichen sclerosus should be reviewed regularly as she is also at risk.

Staging

I Lesion confined to the vulva, maximum diameter 2 cm. No suspicious groin nodes.

II Lesion confined to the vulva, diameter >2 cm. No suspicious groin nodes.

III Lesion extends beyond the vulva with no suspicious nodes *or* lesion confined to the vulva with suspicious nodes.

IV Lesion of any size with obviously positive nodes *or* lesion involving rectum, bladder, urethra or bone *or* all cases with pelvic or distant spread.

Microscopic appearance

The majority of tumours are squamous in origin (85%). The rare types include melanomas, basal cell carcinomas, sarcomas, and adenocarcinomas of the Bartholin's gland. The spread is slow with local tissue infiltration, before metastasizing to the inguinal and femoral nodes. There may be spread to the contralateral lymph nodes. Pelvic node spread is late and carries a poor prognosis.

Symptoms

The majority of women present with irritation or pruritus, a mass or an ulcer. Other symptoms may include vulval pain, bleeding, or discharge. Most tumours are ulcerative, though some may be exophytic. Death is usually due to infection, general debility, or haemorrhage. The majority of lesions occur on the labia (70%).

Prognosis

Stage	5-year survival rate
I	70%
II	50%
III	30%
IV	10–15%

Management

The preoperative investigations of patients with vulval carcinoma will reflect the age and general medical condition of the patient. All patients need an examination under anaesthesia (EUA), with a full thickness biopsy and fine needle aspiration of any suspicious nodes.

Surgical

In the case of small lesions (Stage I), a wide local excision or simple vulvectomy may be the most appropriate treatment with regular follow-up. Otherwise, the treatment of choice is radical vulvectomy with bilateral groin node dissection.

Radiotherapy

This treatment is reserved for local recurrence or nodal disease as it is usually poorly tolerated by the patient.

Chemotherapy

In some centres, mitomycin C and 5-FU have been used in conjunction with radiotherapy to good effect in large tumours.

THE CERVIX

CERVICAL INTRAEPITHELIAL NEOPLASIA (CIN)

Cervical premalignant disease (CIN 1–3) and invasive disease are thought to be part of a continuum:

CIN1 → CIN2 → CIN3 → Microinvasion → Frank invasion

The further the disease progresses to the right along this continuum, the less likely it is to regress. The evidence for these statements is that the epidemiological features of CIN and invasive disease are similar and also that progression studies have demonstrated the progression of CIN1 to CIN3, and CIN3 to invasive carcinoma.

The transformation zone

The cervix is lined by two types of epithelium, stratified squamous and columnar epithelium. The latter is one cell thick and is translucent, which accounts for its red appearance (ectropion) on visualization with the naked eye. In the prepubertal stage, the squamocolumnar junction (SCJ) is within the endocervical canal. As a result of growth of the cervix at the time of puberty, there is eversion of the columnar epithelium. The columnar epithelium may be stimulated to undergo metaplastic change to squamous epithelium. This area is known as the transformation zone (TZ) which, described simply, is the area where one type of epithelium (columnar) has transformed to another type (squamous). This metaplastic epithelium is susceptible to external agents (see 'Predisposing factors', 'Cancer of the cervix', below) and may become *dys*plastic (abnormal epithelium).

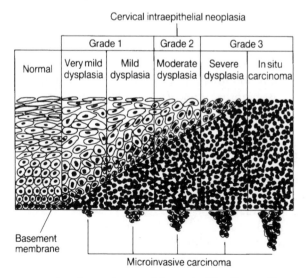

Fig. 13.1   Precursors to invasive carcinoma of the cervix. The diagram illustrates abnormal changes in the cervical epithelium in CIN1–3. Microinvasion is shown as crossing the basement membrane.

Pathology

CIN is divided into three grades, in each case the basement membrane is intact. (Figure 13.1 shows the abnormal changes seen in CIN1–3.)

CIN1   Nuclear atypia confined to the basal third of the epithelium.
CIN2   Nuclear atypia present in the lower two-thirds of the epithelium.
CIN3   Nuclear abnormalities occur throughout the full thickness of the epithelium.

Screening

Screening for premalignant disease of the cervix is by cytology. Cells are collected from the squamocolumnar junction by means of an Ayre's spatula, and are spread onto a glass slide and fixed with alcohol. The slide undergoes an automated staining process. The slides are screened for *dys*karyotic (abnormal nuclei) cells. The nucleocytoplasmic ratio is altered in abnormal cells, ranging from mild to moderate to severe changes. In the latter, there is hardly any cytoplasm surrounding an enlarged nucleus.

Current guidelines suggest regular 3-yearly screening for women between the ages of 20 and 60 years. Referral for colposcopy is advised if the cytology report shows moderate dyskaryosis or worse, or if the woman has had two mildly dyskaryotic smears 6 months apart.

Colposcopy

Colposcopy is an aid to diagnosis. The cervix is visualized through a colposcope and 5% acetic acid is used to bathe the cervix. In abnormal epithelium there is a relative excess of nuclear material (protein) and a relative lack of cytoplasm (glycogen). As a result, the epithelium appears white and may show a mosaic pattern or punctation. Aqueous iodine solution may also be used, this is taken up by normal glycogenated epithelium. In an abnormal epithelium, the area is iodine negative. The affected area is biopsied and the histology of that sample gives the diagnosis.

Treatment

1. Local ablative techniques — this will treat the whole of the TZ
    a. Laser vaporization
    b. 'Cold' coagulation
    c. Diathermy
    d. Cryocautery, which should only be used in HPV or CIN1
2. Excision techniques
    a. Laser cone biopsy
    b. Large loop excision of the TZ
    c. Cold knife, i.e. surgical under GA

d. Hysterectomy depending on other possible indications.

The lesion must fulfil the following criteria before local ablative techniques can be undertaken:
1. The whole lesion must be visible
2. There must be no suspicion of invasion.

Adequate follow-up is important with regular cytology, usually following local guidelines. Ideally a cytobrush smear should be taken to ensure that cells from either side of the SCJ have been sampled.

CARCINOMA OF THE CERVIX

The majority of these tumours are squamous in type (90–95%), adenocarcinoma accounts for 4–8%, the remainder are rarer tumours including sarcomas, lymphomas, and melanomas.

Incidence

In 1988, 4467 new cases of cervical cancer were reported (OPCS), making cervix the second commonest genital tract tumour (after ovarian cancer) in England and Wales. In 1992, there were 1647 deaths from the disease.

Age

The median age for cervical cancer is 52 years. There has been an increase in the number of younger women (20–35 years) developing the disease and the prognosis is worse in this age group.

Geography

On a worldwide basis, cervical cancer is the second commonest malignancy in women after breast cancer. It is much more common in the developing than the developed world.

Predisposing factors

1. Sexual activity is a key event in the development of cervical cancer, especially an early age of first intercourse. Other factors are the number of sexual partners and a 'high risk' male partner with many previous sexual contacts.
2. There is no definite association with the oral contraceptive pill, though sexual mores may be affected by its availability and use.

3. Smoking affects the local immunity of the cervix, making it more sensitive to oncogenic change.
4. Human papillomavirus (HPV) is the current contender for aetiological agent in cervical cancer. There are over 60 types of HPV, and HPV 16, 18 and 33 have been associated with CIN and cancer.

In the past, herpes simplex 2 virus was thought to be linked with cervical cancer though this is no longer the case.

Staging

0   CIN
I   Carcinoma confined to the cervix:
    Ia   microinvasive disease, depth of invasion <3 mm
    Ib   all other cases.
II Carcinoma extends beyond the cervix but not to the pelvic side wall; it may involve the upper two-thirds of the vagina:
    IIa no obvious parametrial involvement
    IIb obvious parametrial involvement.
III Carcinoma extends to the pelvic side wall.
IV Carcinoma extends beyond the true pelvis, or involves the bladder or rectum.

Microscopic appearance

The majority (90–95%) of tumours are squamous carcinomas with the cells being described as keratinizing, large cell non-keratinizing, or small cell non-keratinizing. Most of the remaining tumours are adenocarcinomas. The method of spread of cervical tumours is direct invasion and lymphatic permeation, which dictates the methods of treatment.

Symptoms

Invasive disease may be initially asymptomatic and if not detected at the time of routine cytology, will present with intermenstrual, postcoital or postmenopausal bleeding, plus or minus offensive discharge. Pain is usually a sign of advanced disease.

Prognosis

In terms of 5-year survival rate:

Stage I   up to 90% when microinvasive disease is included
Stage II   55%
Stage III   30–35%
Stage IV   <10%

Management

All patients with cervical carcinoma need a preoperative full blood count and an IVU or other assessment of the renal tract. An examination under anaesthetic is important for accurate staging to determine treatment modality and a biopsy is necessary. A CT scan may be done for assessment of lymphatic spread.

Surgery

1. The treatment of microinvasive disease is controversial but most authorities would suggest that cone biopsy can be used for microinvasive disease if the depth of invasion is <3 mm and there is no lymphatic involvement.
2. Radical hysterectomy with a cuff of vagina, the parametrium and pelvic node dissection plus or minus conservation of the ovaries is the treatment of choice for Stages Ib and IIa.

Radiotherapy

Stages Ib and IIa if the patient is not suitable for surgery.
   Treatment for Stages IIb onwards.

Chemotherapy

This may be used for palliation. HRT may be used in women who have had radiotherapy.
   Regular follow-up is essential, most recurrences will occur within the first 2 years of treatment.

CARCINOMA OF THE BODY OF THE UTERUS

The majority of tumours of the uterus are adenocarcinomas of the endometrium. Sarcomas account for up to 4% of all uterine tumours. Screening for endometrial carcinoma is not a practical proposition. However, any woman presenting with postmenopausal bleeding or discharge, or abnormal bleeding after the age of 40 years, needs investigation. This may include endometrial sampling, hysteroscopy, and dilatation and curettage.

Incidence

In 1988, 3789 new cases were reported in England and Wales (OPCS). In 1992, there were 913 deaths due to endometrial cancer. These figures placed uterine cancer third in frequency of genital tract tumours after ovary and cervix.

Age

80% of cases occur in postmenopausal women, with a median age of 60 years. Less than 5% of cases occur before the age of 40 years.

Geography

In the USA and parts of Australia, endometrial cancer is the most common genital tract malignancy.

Predisposing factors

Endometrial carcinoma is oestrogen dependent, so a history of unopposed oestrogen administration or, less commonly, oestrogen secreting tumours of the ovary may be significant.

Obesity is a risk factor as androgens are converted to oestrogens in the peripheral fat leading to an increase in the serum oestrogen concentration.

Other associations include nulliparity, late menopause, history of diabetes or previous pelvic radiotherapy for cervical cancer.

Staging

I Carcinoma confined to the body of the uterus:
   Ia confined to the endometrium.
   Ib confined to the uterine body with invasion of less than half the myometrium.
   Ic confined to the uterine body with invasion of more than half the myometrium.
II Carcinoma involving the body of the uterus and the cervix but not extending beyond the uterus.
III Carcinoma extending beyond the uterus but not beyond the true pelvis.
IV Carcinoma extending outside the true pelvis or involving the mucosa of the bladder or rectum.

Microscopic appearance

Most of the endometrial tumours are adenocarcinomas and are graded according to differentiation. Grade 1 is well differentiated, grade 2 moderately differentiated and grade 3 poorly differentiated.

These tumours spread locally to the cervix, via the fallopian tubes to the ovaries or invade the myometrium. There is also lymphatic spread to the pelvic and para-aortic nodes.

Symptoms

In postmenopausal women, carcinoma of the uterus usually presents early with vaginal bleeding or discharge. The disease in pre- or perimenopausal women usually presents with irregular vaginal bleeding.

Prognosis

Stage	5-year survival rate
I	72%
II	56%
III	32%
IV	10%

Management

The majority of tumours (90%) will present at Stage I or II. Depth of invasion of the tumour is the most important predictive index of the disease, with the most likely place of recurrence being the vault.

Surgery

Total abdominal hysterectomy with bilateral salpingo-oophorectomy is undertaken once the diagnosis has been made.

Radiotherapy

1. As an adjunct following surgery to prevent vault recurrence.
2. Radical radiotherapy in women who are unsuitable for surgery.
3. Palliation in advanced cases.

Chemotherapy

Progestogens have been used for recurrent disease or to reduce bleeding prior to surgery. Cytotoxic agents are used for disseminated or recurrent disease.
   Regular follow-up is essential.

CARCINOMA OF THE OVARY

Ovarian carcinoma is the commonest gynaecological tumour in England and Wales, and usually presents in more advanced stages because of its lack of specific symptoms. As a result the outlook in terms of survival remains poor.

Incidence

In 1988, 5174 new cases of ovarian cancer were reported, in 1992 there were 3880 deaths (OPCS).

Age

The incidence increases with advancing age of the woman.

Geography

More common in the developed world than in the developing world.

Predisposing factors

1. Continuous ovulation may be important, i.e. nulliparity, early menarche, and late menopause. The combined OCP is thought to be protective. There is evidence that ovulation induction agents may also increase the risk of ovarian cancer.
2. Other possible risk factors include talc and the mumps virus.
3. In a small number of cases (2%), there is a family predisposition.

Staging

This is done at the time of laparotomy.
I   Tumour confined to the ovaries:
    Ia   confined to one ovary, capsule intact and no ascites
    Ib   confined to both ovaries, capsule intact and no ascites
    Ic   confined to one or both ovaries with ascites or positive peritoneal washings.
II   Tumour involving one or both ovaries with pelvic extension:
    IIa spread to the uterus and/or tubes
    IIb spread to other pelvic tissues
    IIc IIa or IIb with ascites or positive peritoneal washings.
III Tumour involving one or both ovaries with intraperitoneal spread outside the pelvis or tumour limited to the pelvis with extension to the small bowel or omentum.
IV   Tumour involving one or both ovaries with distant spread, i.e. extra-abdominal.

Microscopic appearance

Ovarian cancer spreads directly to involve the pelvic peritoneum, and is carried upwards to cover the peritoneal surfaces of the diaphragm, liver, bowel, and omentum. Lymphatic and blood-borne spread occurs in the later stages of the disease. Differentiation of the tumours ranges from well differentiated through moderate to poorly differentiated. Some tumours are reported as borderline in that they have histological features of malignancy but no stromal invasion.

It is important to remember that ovarian tumours may be primary or secondary.
1. Primary types
   a. Epithelial tumours (85%), adenocarcinomas which includes serous, mucinous, endometrioid and clear cell
   b. Germ cell tumours (2%)
   c. Sex cord tumours (6%)
   d. Miscellaneous including sarcomas and lymphomas
2. Secondary types account for about 6% of cases and the most common primary sites include breast, stomach, colon and lung.

Symptoms

The majority of patients (70%) present in the late stages of the disease. Most of the symptoms are vague and include abdominal discomfort, increasing girth, pressure symptoms, urinary frequency, weight loss and very occasionally menstrual problems. When a patient presents, in addition to abdominal examination, it is important to palpate the supraclavicular region for lymph nodes, to examine the chest, breasts, and perform both rectal and vaginal examinations.

Prognosis

Stage	5-year survival rates (approx.)
I	70–75%
II	45%
III	20%
IV	5%

Management

Routine preoperative bloods tests should be done. The serum CA 125 level is a useful tumour marker in about 80% of cases and may be used to assess the response to treatment. Ultrasound or CT scan of the abdomen and pelvis may be useful but the final tissue diagnosis and staging will be by laparotomy.

Surgery

Staging laparotomy — peritoneal washings, total abdominal hysterectomy, bilateral salpingo-oophorectomy plus omentectomy, and as much debulking as possible. This may not be appropriate in Stage Ia if fertility is a consideration.

Radiotherapy

This may be used for remaining disease, though it is ineffective if the bulk is large and its role in treatment is controversial. It may be useful for palliation to reduce symptoms from tumour bulk or metastasis.

Chemotherapy

Adjuvant combination chemotherapy has largely taken the place of radiotherapy. The combination is usually an alkylating agent (cyclophosphamide) and a platinum compound for the epithelial tumours. Cisplatinum, etoposide and bleomycin can be used for germ cell tumours.
    Regular follow-up is important.

Screening

The difficulty in screening for ovarian cancer arises from not knowing its natural history. Tests that have been used include pelvic examinations, serum CA 125 levels and diagnostic ultrasound. The sensitivity of these tests is poor and they do not convey any prognostic value. These tests are useful if the patients are involved in trials or in the small percentage of women with a family history of ovarian cancer.

14. The menopause and hormone replacement therapy

A. Rodin and J. Rymer

Expectations of the examiners

The candidate is expected to understand the basic physiology of the menopause. A knowledge of the long-term effects of the menopause is required and a detailed understanding of the management of women on hormone replacement therapy is needed.

THE MENOPAUSE

Definition

The menopause is defined as the cessation of menstruation and it marks the end of a woman's reproductive potential. It is a retrospective diagnosis usually made after 12 months of amenorrhoea.

Interesting facts

The average age of the menopause in the UK is 51 years. Interest in menopause-related problems has grown due to the increase in mean female life expectancy, which is now 82 years (in the UK).

The average woman spends 38% of her life after the menopause and in the UK postmenopausal women number more than 9 000 000 and comprise 18% of the total population. The short- and long-term problems associated with the menopause cause significant morbidity and mortality and have important economic implications. Women who do not suffer the 'acute' symptoms of the menopause remain at risk of long-term complications.

Physiology

The menopause is the result of ovarian failure and it is preceded by a transition phase known as the climacteric which is of variable duration. The climacteric is characterized by increasing resistance of the ovarian follicles to stimulation by the gonadotrophins. Total oestrogen output by the ovaries declines and therefore gonadotrophin levels increase.

117

Anovulation becomes more frequent and as a result progesterone deficiency occurs; this may lead to prolonged or irregular vaginal bleeding. These changes commence 10–15 years before the menopause and some women complain of symptoms of oestrogen deficiency during the climacteric. The menopause may occur prematurely (<40 years) and it may follow surgery (bilateral oophorectomy) or radiotherapy.

Prior to the menopause, the main oestrogen is 17β-oestradiol which is secreted by the ovaries. This is converted to oestrone which has one-tenth the potency of 17β-oestradiol, and then to oestriol. In the postmenopausal woman, ovarian 17β-oestradiol production ceases and oestrone becomes the primary oestrogen. The major source of oestrone after the menopause is the peripheral conversion in adipose tissue of androstenedione which is produced by the adrenal cortex (70%) and the ovary (30%). After the menopause, the ovary continues to secrete androgens, mainly testosterone and androstenedione. FSH and LH levels plateau 2–3 years after the menopause and begin to decline after 5–10 years.

The effects of oestrogen deficiency

Oestrogen deficiency is responsible for the characteristic features of the menopausal syndrome. Most systems are affected but the manifestations vary between individuals. Vasomotor instability affects 75% of women and 25% are severely affected. Hot flushes and night sweats may continue for more than 5 years in 25% of women. Flushes can be socially disabling and may interfere with daily activities while night sweats result in interrupted sleep and progressive fatigue. The mechanism of menopausal vasomotor instability is uncertain but a hypothalamic mechanism has been suggested.

Atrophy occurs in all oestrogen-sensitive tissues, notably the urogenital tract, breasts and skin. In the vagina, there is flattening and thinning of the epithelium which may result in atrophic vaginitis. Loss of glycogen from the epithelial cells leads to the disappearance of the lactic acid-forming Döderlein's bacilli and, as a consequence, the vagina becomes alkaline. The bladder and urethra, which are lined by transitional epithelium, undergo similar changes to the vagina. The supporting structures of the genital tract lose tone and prolapse may become apparent. Breasts become atrophic with a reduction in adipose tissue and lobules.

The psychological effects of the menopause may be the direct result of oestrogen deficiency on the central nervous system or they may be precipitated by distressing physical symptoms or life events.

The long-term consequences of the menopause are:

Osteoporosis. Postmenopausal osteoporosis is a major health care problem. The important fracture sites are the vertebrae and the femoral neck. Twenty-five per cent of women over 60 will suffer vertebral crush fractures. The incidence of fractured neck of femur is increasing, although the reasons for this trend are unclear. Twenty per cent of women who suffer

Table 14.1 Common presenting symptoms of the menopause.

Physical	Psychological
Hot flushes	Depression
Night sweats	Anxiety/panic attacks
Exhaustion	Irritability
Joint pains	Lethargy
Dysuria	Poor memory
Vaginal dryness	Poor concentration
Dyspareunia	Decreased libido

this type of fracture die from complications and many of those that survive never return to full mobility.

Following the menopause, bone mineral is lost from the skeleton at an accelerated rate for about 5 years and then becomes more gradual. Women who have an early menopause or who have had amenorrhoea (either weight or exercise related) during their potential reproductive years are at greater risk of osteoporosis in later life .

Other risk factors include being Caucasian and having a positive family history.

Cardiovascular disease. Premenopausal women have a lower risk of cardiovascular disease compared to men of the same age group. This effect is partly due to the influence of oestrogen on the lipid profile (raises HDL-cholesterol and lowers LDL-cholesterol). Oestrogen also acts as an arterial vasodilator increasing blood flow to the myocardium and central nervous system. Following the menopause the protective effect of oestrogen is lost and the prevalence of cardiovascular disease in men and women is similar.

Assessment

The diagnosis is usually straightforward and is based on the history. Common presenting symptoms are listed in Table 14.1.

It is important to elicit how the symptoms are interfering with everyday activities and relationships. Diagnosis may be less obvious in women who have premature ovarian failure and in women who have undergone hysterectomy with conservation of the ovaries. A medical history should exclude contraindications to hormone replacement therapy. Smoking should be discouraged. General physical examination should include breast examination and height, weight and blood pressure should be recorded. Pelvic examination should include a cervical smear if indicated.

Investigations

Blood tests are rarely helpful but in cases where the diagnosis is in doubt, measure serum gonadotrophins and/or oestradiol. Oestradiol <70 pmol/l and FSH/LH >15 i.u./l are found in menopausal women. Endometrial biopsy is not performed as a routine but it is mandatory in women with postmenopausal bleeding or irregular bleeding. Mammography should be offered to women over 50 years.

Non-invasive methods are now available for the measurement of bone density in the spine and femoral neck. Dual energy X-ray absorptiometry is the most popular but dual photon absorptiometry and CT scanning may also be used. Ultrasound is currently being assessed as a diagnostic tool.

Treatment

Non-hormonal preparations have been used to treat menopausal symptoms but they are generally ineffective and provide no protection from the long-term effects of the menopause. Hormone replacement therapy (HRT) is the most appropriate treatment for women with menopause-related problems. The decision to commence HRT should be made after full discussion with the patient.

Indications for HRT include:

1. Menopause-related symptoms
2. Early menopause
3. Prevention of osteoporosis
4. Cardiovascular protection.

Contraindications to oestrogen replacement therapy are:

1. Carcinoma of the breast
2. Carcinoma of the endometrium
3. Liver disease (porphyria, active hepatitis).

Hypertension is not a contraindication to therapy but blood pressure should be stabilized before HRT is commenced. Women with a history of thromboembolic disease can be given HRT but it is often advisable to refer women with a complicated medical history to the local menopause clinic.

When considering HRT in women who have had carcinoma of the breast or endometrium, careful discussion should centre on quality of life issues. Each case should be individualized and if a woman is prepared to accept the theoretical risk of disease recurrence by taking HRT, then it is her right to choose for her quality of life.

Oestrogen therapy

'Natural' oestrogens (17β-oestradiol, oestradiol valerate, conjugated equine oestrogens) are commonly used. Tibolone is a synthetic steroid which has oestrogenic, progestogenic and some androgenic activity. Ethinyloestradiol and other synthetic oestrogens which are found in combined oral contraceptive preparations are avoided because of their effects on coagulation. Oestrogen should be given continuously and may be administered orally or parenterally. The pharmacodynamics and biochemical effects of exogenous oestrogens can vary markedly with the route of administration. Oral therapy is the most widely used. Oestrogen delivered by this route first passes through the liver. This has several effects:

1. Hepatic metabolism removes a large proportion of a given dose.
2. Oestrogen may influence the synthesis of various hepatic products and this may have beneficial or adverse effects; oral oestrogen favourably alters the HDL/LDL ratio by elevating plasma HDL-cholesterol; oral therapy may increase renin substrate production and a parenteral route of administration may be more appropriate in hypertensives; similarly antithrombin III production may be depressed, and parenteral administration may be advisable in women with clotting disorders.
3. Concurrent drug therapy (e.g. with anticonvulsants) may result in induction of hepatic enzymes leading to rapid inactivation of oestrogen.

The parenteral route avoids the first pass effect and is particularly suitable for hypertensives and women with a history of thromboembolic disease. It is a convenient method following hysterectomy. Subcutaneous implants of oestradiol (50 mg) are inserted under local anaesthesia into the anterior abdominal wall or buttock. Testosterone (50 or 100 mg) may be added to improve libido and energy levels. The procedure is repeated every 6 months. Vaginal administration of oestrogen creams results in blood levels comparable to those seen after oral therapy and endometrial hyperplasia may occur with long-term use. Oestrogen can now be administered transdermally via skin patches which are convenient and effective.

Progestogen therapy

Prolonged administration of oestrogens to postmenopausal women is associated with an increase in incidence of endometrial carcinoma. This risk can be avoided by adding a progestogen for 12 days each calendar month. Side-effects can be reduced by using the minimum dose of progestogen.

Unwanted effects of progestogen are:

1. Withdrawal bleeding which occurs in 90% of women
2. 'Premenstrual' symptoms
3. Alterations in the lipid profile which may counteract the favourable effect of oestrogen.

Tibolone therapy

Tibolone is a synthetic steroid with oestrogenic, progestogenic and androgenic activity. It does not cause endometrial proliferation and it obviates the need for withdrawal bleeds.

Approaches to treatment

For the purposes of treatment, women can be classified into two groups: those who have a uterus; and those who have previously undergone hysterectomy. Women should be fully counselled before starting treatment and they should be warned about common side-effects.

Women with a uterus. The regimen used must not cause endometrial proliferation. There are three main options:

1. Continuous oestrogen + cyclical progestogen 12/28 days. The majority of women will have withdrawal bleeds on this regimen.
2. Continuous oestrogen + continuous progestogen. The majority of users will be amenorrhoeic but some bleed irregularly, particularly in the first 6 months.
3. Tibolone. As with continuous combined therapy, irregular bleeding may occur within the first few months, but usually less than with continuous combined.
4. Insertion of intrauterine system (IUS). A progestogen-containing IUD is inserted and oestrogen can be administered orally or parenterally. The local progestogen release induces an atrophic endometrium.

Women without a uterus. These women can be given continuous oestrogen either orally or parenterally.

Follow-up of women on HRT

Women should be reviewed 3 months after treatment is commenced. Symptoms should be discussed and enquiries should be made about the pattern of vaginal bleeding (in those with a uterus). Weight and blood pressure should be recorded at each visit. Subsequently, women should be reviewed every 6 months. Smears should be taken as necessary and annual breast examination should be performed. Mammography can be repeated every 2–3 years. Unscheduled vaginal bleeding must be investigated promptly with an endometrial biopsy and transvaginal ultrasound scan.

There is no consensus about the optimum duration of hormone replacement therapy. To obtain significant protection from osteoporotic fractures, a minimum course of 5 years' treatment is recommended.

Advantages of HRT

1. Relief from menopausal symptoms.
2. Prevention of bone demineralization; oestrogen therapy halts bone loss and protects against osteoporotic fractures. It is most effective if it is commenced shortly after the menopause to avoid the period of accelerated bone loss associated with ovarian failure. The minimum bone-sparing dosages of oestradiol valerate and conjugated oestrogens are 2 mg and 0.625 mg respectively. Epidemiological evidence

suggests that treatment for 5 years is associated with a 50% reduction in hip fractures.

3. Oestrogen replacement therapy protects against cardiovascular disease and strokes. Most studies suggest a 30–50% risk reduction with HRT use.

4. Recent evidence suggests that hormone replacement therapy may decrease the incidence of Alzheimer's disease and delay the onset by about 5 years.

HRT and cancer

Concerns about the link between HRT and cancer seem to be largely unfounded. The addition of cyclical progestagens or oestrogen replacement therapy reduces the risk of endometrial cancer to below that in an untreated population. There is no association between HRT and carcinoma of the cervix and ovary. Epidemiological evidence about the effect of HRT on the incidence of carcinoma of the breast is unclear. There does not appear to be an increased risk of breast cancer in the first 10 years of HRT but some studies suggest a small increase in risk with more prolonged use.

SUMMARY

The average woman spends more than one-third of her life after the menopause. The long-term sequelae of the menopause have important medical implications. The benefits of HRT in improving menopausal symptoms, preventing osteoporosis and reducing the incidence of cardiovascular disease are well recognized.

15. The premenstrual syndrome

A. Rodin

Expectations of the examiners

The candidate should have a basic understanding of the premenstrual syndrome and the management of women with this condition.

Definition

Distressing physical and psychological symptoms which occur during the premenstrual phase of the menstrual/ovarian cycle and regress at the onset of menstruation.

Interesting facts

The premenstrual syndrome (PMS) was first described by Frank in 1931. He reported a small group of women with tension, depression and irritability occurring 7–10 days before menstruation and relieved by the onset of 'the menstrual flow'. This condition remains poorly understood. Estimates of the prevalence of PMS in the general population vary from 5% to 95%.

Pathophysiology

The aetiology of PMS is unknown. It is likely that PMS is not a homogeneous condition but it is due to a combination of physical, psychological, genetic and environmental factors. A variety of mechanisms have been proposed in PMS but they remain unproven. Popular hypotheses include progesterone deficiency, fluid retention, vitamin deficiency, hypoglycaemia or defective prostaglandin metabolism. The link between PMS and cyclical ovarian activity is certain and the condition characteristically commences after pregnancy or discontinuation of the combined contraceptive pill with the resumption of ovarian activity.

Assessment

Diagnosis is based on the history. Symptoms are many and varied and any body system may be involved. Patterns of symptoms vary between women

Table 15.1 Symptoms of premenstrual syndrome.

Physical	Psychological
Breast discomfort	Irritability
Bloating	Anxiety
Weight gain	Tension
Acne	Depression
Headache	Insomnia
Pelvic pain	Change in libido
Change in bowel habit	Poor concentration

and the severity of symptoms may vary from cycle to cycle. Common symptoms are listed in Table 15.1.

In addition, there may be behavioural changes and pre-existing medical conditions such as epilepsy, asthma or herpes may be exacerbated. If the history is suggestive of PMS, confirmatory evidence can be obtained by prospectively assessing symptoms over three cycles. Various methods have been used ranging from self-grading of severity of symptoms to the use of visual analogue scales. Blood tests are of no value in the diagnosis of PMS.

Treatment

A variety of approaches have been used and these are summarized in Table 15.2.

The placebo response in PMS may exceed 90% and consequently it is difficult to prove the effectiveness of any active treatment. The choice of first-line treatment will be influenced by the severity of symptoms. In mild cases, vitamin B6 or γ-linolenic acid may be helpful. The combined contraceptive pill or dydrogesterone 10 mg b.d. on days 12–26 of the cycle can be prescribed for moderately affected women.

In severe cases, inhibition of the ovarian cycle is the approach of choice. This can be achieved by using subcutaneous oestradiol implants combined with cyclical oral progestogen to prevent the development of endometrial hyperplasia. LHRH analogues are extremely effective but because of the suppression of ovarian oestrogen production they are not appropriate for long-term use, unless 'addback' therapy is instituted.

If single symptoms predominate, it may be preferable to try a therapy aimed at alleviating that specific complaint; for example, bromocriptine for breast pain and diuretics for bloating. Counselling or psychotherapy may be beneficial in women with PMS.

SUMMARY

PMS is associated with cyclical ovarian activity and does not occur before puberty, during pregnancy or after the menopause. Most women

Table 15.2 Treatments used in premenstrual syndrome.

Drug treatment
  Hormonal
    Progesterone
    Combined pill
    LHRH analogues
    Oestradiol implants
    Danazol
  Non-hormonal
    Diuretics
    Vitamins B6, A, E,
    Bromocriptine
    Prostaglandin synthetase inhibitors
    Psychoactive drugs
    γ-Linolenic acid

Psychological
  Psychotherapy
  Hypnosis

Other
  Diet
  Acupuncture
  Bilateral oophorectomy
  Radiation menopause

experience adverse symptoms prior to menstruation. The aetiology of PMS is unknown and treatments are non-specific. In severe cases, ovarian suppression is the treatment of choice.

16. Urinary incontinence

J. Rymer

Expectations of the examiners

The candidate will be expected to have a basic knowledge of the physiology of micturition, and the various types of incontinence. In particular, the candidate should be able to distinguish between stress and urge incontinence, and manage appropriately. In the clinical examination the candidate could be asked to demonstrate stress incontinence as described below.

Definition

Incontinence is defined as the involuntary loss of urine which is a social and hygienic problem and is objectively demonstrable.

Causes

Whenever the intravesical pressure is greater than the intraurethral pressure loss of urine will occur.

The three commonest causes of incontinence are: genuine stress incontinence, detrusor instability and overflow incontinence. Although urinary fistulas are a rare cause in the UK, they are a common cause in third world countries.

STRESS INCONTINENCE

Definition

Involuntary loss of urine coinciding with a rise in intra-abdominal pressure (e.g. laughing, coughing, jumping).

Pathophysiology

Control of micturition depends on two main factors:

1. A competent sphincter mechanism able to resist the changes in intra-abdominal pressure.

2. The capacity to inhibit a bladder contraction until it is convenient to micturate.

Urine leakage occurs when the intravesical pressure exceeds the maximum urethral pressure. Most commonly the urethral 'occlusive forces' have been diminished by childbirth trauma, surgical damage and/or menopausal atrophy, and this deficiency is aggravated by descent of the proximal third of the urethra below the level of the pelvic floor (Fig. 16.1). In addition, a chronically raised intra-abdominal pressure such as in chronic bronchitis or obesity will aggravate the condition.

Assessment

History

History is important to determine whether this is pure stress incontinence or whether an element of urgency is present. A full obstetric and gynaecological history must be obtained especially concerning previous incontinence and repair procedures. Chronic constipation, chronic bronchitis, smoking and diuretics are associated with stress incontinence and should be specifically asked about. Classically the incontinence occurs synchronously with the rise in intra-abdominal pressure. Most patients find incontinence a social and hygienic problem.

Examination

General and abdominal examination should be performed. To assess the stress incontinence, the patient should be examined in the Sims' position with a full bladder. The labia are parted, noting any excoriation, and the patient is asked to cough, and loss of urine and vaginal wall descent are

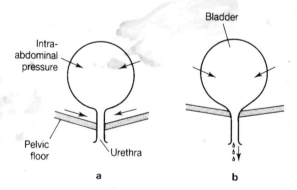

a   b

Fig. 16.1 Stress incontinence. a, Normally an increase in intra-abdominal pressure will be transmitted to the bladder and to the urethra, thus maintaining continence. b, If there is an alteration in the position of the bladder neck and most of the urethra is below the pelvic floor, then an increase in intra-abdominal pressure will increase the intravesical pressure but not the urethral pressure, so that urine will be lost.

noted. A Sims' speculum is inserted along the posterior vaginal wall and the anterior wall is observed again with coughing. Descent of the cervix is observed and traction may be applied using a sponge forceps on the anterior lip of the cervix. The speculum is gradually withdrawn noting any laxity of the posterior vaginal wall. A bimanual examination should be performed. The value of Bonney's test (elevation of the bladder neck) at the time of examination is debatable.

Investigations

MSU should be performed to exclude a urinary tract infection.

Urodynamic investigation. This should be performed in all cases to exclude voiding difficulties and detrusor instability. Operations to correct genuine stress incontinence may aggravate detrusor instability.

Treatment

Local causes should be treated appropriately, e.g. infection.

Conservative therapy is predominantly used for women with mild genuine stress incontinence or in women who have not completed their family.

Pelvic floor exercises (± interferential therapy ± faradism) may be helpful, ideally under the guidance of a physiotherapist, and vaginal cones may be a useful adjunct.

Surgery is the mainstay of treatment and there are various options. Suprapubic operations are more effective for curing stress incontinence. The choice of operation depends on the degree of uterovaginal descent, and the general health of the patient.

1. *Colposuspension.* This is an abdominal procedure in which sutures are placed periurethrally, and lateral to the bladder neck, from above, and then sutured to the iliopectineal ligament (Burch), or the periosteum overlying the symphysis pubis (Marshall–Marchetti–Krantz).
2. *Anterior colporrhaphy.* This is a vaginal procedure where the anterior wall of the vagina is elevated and any excess tissue is removed. It is a good operation to repair a cystocele but has a high failure rate for genuine stress incontinence.
3. *Sling procedures.* These can be performed abdominally or vaginally, using synthetic material, or fascia lata to elevate the urethra. The sling is then attached to the rectus sheath. They have a high success rate but high complication rate, e.g. long-term voiding difficulties.
4. *Stamey procedures.* A long needle is inserted abdominally and a suture is placed either side of the bladder neck to elevate it. The suture is secured to the rectus sheath. These procedures are reserved for elderly patients or repeat procedures.

5. *Injectables*. GAX collagen or macroplastique are injected paraurethrally to build up bulk around the sphincter.
6. *Artificial sphincter*. Complex operations which are considered an end stage operation.

Ring pessaries. If there is associated uterovaginal prolapse, these can be used in cases not fit for anaesthetic.

Summary

Genuine stress incontinence is a common problem which may be socially embarrassing and unhygienic. A careful history and examination is essential to make the correct diagnosis. Urodynamic investigations must be performed to enable an accurate diagnosis. Conservative treatment can be helpful but the definitive treatment is surgery, with the Burch colposuspension being the operation of choice.

URGE INCONTINENCE

Definition

Involuntary loss of urine caused by uninhibited detrusor contractions.

Interesting facts

Detrusor instability more commonly produces the classic triad of symptoms, namely, urgency, frequency, and nocturia (passing urine at night). Whether or not the patient leaks will depend on the integrity of the urethral sphincter mechanism. Urge incontinence may be precipitated by a urinary tract infection or gynaecological surgery.

Pathophysiology

In this condition the urethra functions normally but the bladder contracts in an uninhibited fashion, and if the intravesical pressure exceeds the urethral pressure, incontinence results.

Aetiology

1. Idiopathic
2. Secondary to an upper motor neurone lesion
3. Secondary to previous incontinence operations.

Assessment

History

History involves determining the severity of the following symptoms: frequency, urgency, and nocturia.

Examination

Examination is usually uninformative, but should include a full neurological examination.

Investigations

1. Urine microscopy and culture.
2. Urodynamics: a normal bladder can be filled to at least 500 ml with an intravesical pressure rise of less than 10 cm of water. Normally, detrusor activity is suppressed with posture changes, sudden rises in intra-abdominal pressure and rapid filling. Cystometry measures intravesical pressure during bladder filling.
3. Detrusor instability is confirmed by a sensation of discomfort or a detrusor contraction (pressure rise >15 cm water) during filling, coughing or standing.

Treatment

Bladder drill

This requires patient motivation for success. The aim is to progressively increase the interval between episodes of micturition. The usual interval should be determined, and the patient should then be instructed to pass urine at this frequency even if she has no desire to void. Once she has accomplished this, with no accidents, she should increase the time in 15-minute increments. This may take a few days, but once this is achieved, increase again, and again, until 3 hours is achieved. Essentially the bladder is 'retrained'. Ideally this should be done as an inpatient with biofeedback, but few units have these facilities. Fluid restriction and frequency volume charts may be useful.

Drug therapy

Anticholinergic agents are the mainstay of treatment. They have the side-effect of causing a dry mouth and blurred vision.

1. Propanthelene: anticholinergic; effective for diurnal frequency.
2. Oxybutynin: anticholinergic and direct smooth muscle relaxant effect; good for all symptoms of detrusor instability.
3. Imipramine: anticholinergic and central nervous system effect; good for nocturia and nocturnal enuresis.
4. Desmopressin: antidiuretic hormone analogue; prevents the patient producing urine at night, which is when it is taken; good for nocturia and nocturnal enuresis.
5. HRT: good for patients with irritative bladder symptoms especially in conjunction with other medication.

Surgery

Clam cystoplasty — this procedure results in long-term voiding problems and is reserved for intractable detrusor instability.

Summary

Detrusor instability produces the symptoms of urinary urgency, frequency, and nocturia. Cystometry is essential to confirm the diagnosis, and bladder drill is the treatment of choice. One must be cautious with drug therapy as urinary retention can be precipitated.

OVERFLOW INCONTINENCE

Definition

Frequent involuntary loss of small volumes of urine, usually precipitated by changes in posture. The urinary stream is slow with hesitancy, and after micturition, there may be a sensation of incomplete emptying.

Pathophysiology

May be caused by obstruction to bladder outflow or bladder atony. Urine leakage occurs when the intravesical pressure exceeds the maximum urethral pressure in the absence of detrusor activity. Frequency may occur due to decreased functional capacity.

Aetiology

Detrusor hypotonia

1. Lower motor neurone lesions (e.g. diabetes)
2. Drugs with anticholinergic side-effects
3. Secondary to pain (e.g. herpes), which pushes the patient into retention and then overdistends the bladder and results in detrusor damage.

Outflow obstruction

1. Pelvic mass
2. Uterovaginal prolapse
3. Inflammation
4. Constipation
5. Incontinence surgery.

Assessment

History will provide the symptoms as above, and it may have been precipitated by a recent event.

Examination may reveal a palpable mass. The passage of a urethral catheter will reveal a large residual urine.

Investigations

1. MSU.
2. Cystometry will reveal a large residual urine with a delayed first sensation, and enlarged bladder capacity. In detrusor hypotonia the voiding pressure will be reduced whereas in obstruction it will be raised. With time the detrusor compensates so that all patients may present with a reduced voiding pressure and a reduced peak flow rate regardless of cause.

Treatment

1. If drug ingestion is causing the problem, the drug regimen must be altered.
2. Urine infection should be treated.
3. Treat constipation.
4. Get the patient to double void.
5. If detrusor hypotonia is the problem then try cholinergic agents such as bethanechol.
6. If outflow obstruction is the cause then treat the cause (e.g. pelvic mass). If it is due to urethral stenosis then perform a urethrotomy.
7. In failed cases teach clean intermittent self-catheterization.
8. Some patients who are not dextrous may require a long-term in-dwelling catheter.

Summary

Overflow incontinence can be due to either detrusor hypotonia or outflow obstruction. The two may present in a similar manner but require different treatments.

TRUE INCONTINENCE

Definition

Continuous urine leakage most commonly due to a fistulous track between the vagina and either the ureter, bladder, or urethra.

Interesting facts

Congenital abnormalities are rare, e.g. ureteric ectopy which presents in infancy.

A very low urethrovaginal fistula can cause intermittent incontinence.

Aetiology

1. Prolonged labour
2. Carcinoma
3. Surgery
4. Radiotherapy.

Assessment

History of urine continuously draining from the vagina. Examination is best performed in the Sims' position, with a Sims' speculum. Colouring the urine, and placing tampons in the vagina, may aid location of the fistulous track.

Investigations

A micturating cystourethrogram, and/or an IVP may help location.

Treatment

1. Wait—some fistulae will heal spontaneously if given enough time with continuous bladder drainage.
2. Surgery.

FUNCTIONAL INCONTINENCE

Definition

Patient complains of intermittent or continuous incontinence but all investigations reveal no evidence of abnormality. Reassurance is helpful, and referral to a psychiatrist may be indicated.

17. Uterovaginal prolapse

A. Rodin

Expectations of the examiners

The candidate is expected to have a basic understanding of the support structures of the female genital tract. The candidate should be aware of the clinical features of different types of prolapse and should be competent in the appropriate examination. Management options should be clearly understood but details of surgical repair techniques are not required.

Definition

Uterovaginal prolapse is defined as descent of a pelvic organ or structure into and sometimes outside the vagina.

Interesting facts

Uterovaginal prolapse is a common gynaecological problem which accounts for a large proportion of major gynaecological surgery. It is caused by a failure of the support structures of the genital tract.

Causes of uterovaginal prolapse

1. Congenital (rare) e.g. connective tissue disorder
2. Acquired (common).

Parity

Childbirth is the principal risk factor for uterovaginal prolapse. Many factors contribute but surprisingly little is known about which components of pregnancy and labour are implicated in the causation of prolapse. The considerable weight of the pregnant uterus may play a part and, in addition, the effects of prolonged labour, pushing before full dilatation, and genital tract trauma may be of importance. Multiparity increases the risk of subsequent prolapse.

Raised intra-abdominal pressure

Conditions which result in chronic elevation of intra-abdominal pressure may cause or aggravate prolapse:

1. Chronic cough
2. Chronic constipation
3. Intra-abdominal masses
4. Heavy lifting.

Prolapse commonly becomes clinically apparent after the menopause. Oestrogen deficiency results in atrophy of the vaginal skin and laxity of the uterine supports leading to prolapse which was initiated by childbirth many years before.

The support structures of the female genital tract

The main supports of the uterus and the upper vagina are the cardinal ligaments (transverse cervical ligaments) and the uterosacral ligaments. These are formed from condensations of the endopelvic fascia. The cardinal ligament fans out from the lateral cervix and upper vagina to reach the lateral walls of the pelvis. The uterosacral ligaments pass posteriorly, lateral to the rectum and upwards to insert onto the sacrum. Anteriorly, the fascia runs from the cervix and under the bladder to reach the pubic symphysis (the pubocervical ligament). The round ligament does not have a support function.

The pelvic floor is the other important support for the female genital tract. It comprises the levator ani muscles which each have three components: ischiococcygeus, iliococcygeus, and pubococcygeus. It is thought that damage to the levator ani in childbirth may be one of the major events predisposing to later prolapse.

Types of prolapse (Fig. 17.1)

Prolapse of the anterior vaginal wall and bladder is known as a cystocele. This may be accompanied by prolapse of the urethra or urethrocele.

Prolapse of the rectum and posterior vaginal wall is known as a rectocele.

An enterocele is a hernia of the pouch of Douglas through the posterior vaginal fornix. There is a peritoneal sac which may contain small intestine. Enterocele is usually associated with uterine prolapse but may occur in isolation or after hysterectomy. It is a recognized complication of colposuspension procedures.

Uterine prolapse

Uterine prolapse is usually associated with anterior and posterior vaginal wall prolapse. There is descent of the cervix and uterine body into the vagina. Three stages of uterine prolapse are recognized:

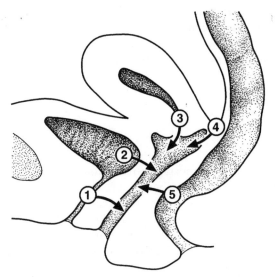

Fig. 17.1   Types of prolapse in the female reproductive system: 1, urethrocele; 2, cystocele; 3, uterine prolapse; 4, enterocele; 5, rectocele.

1.   First degree in which there is descent of the cervix but it does not reach the vaginal introitus.
2.   Second degree in which the cervix reaches the introitus.
3.   Third degree prolapse or procidentia in which the cervix and body of the uterus lie outside the introitus.

Vault prolapse

Vault prolapse is an inversion of the vaginal vault that can occur after hysterectomy.

Clinical features

Prolapse is often asymptomatic and may be detected at routine screening. It commonly presents as a vaginal swelling which may cause discomfort. The swelling is often worse at the end of the day and may disappear when the patient is recumbent. The patient may be aware of a dragging sensation in the pelvis.

Cystocele is sometimes associated with urinary symptoms. Stress incontinence may occur but is not necessarily associated with a cystocele (see Ch. 16). Incomplete voiding may leave an increased volume of residual urine in the bladder increasing the chances of urinary tract infections.

Rectocele may be associated with difficulty in defaecation. Patients may sometimes need to reduce the posterior wall prolapse digitally before the rectum can be emptied. Enterocele may present with small bowel obstruction secondary to incarceration. This is a very rare complication.

Procidentia may be associated with decubitus ulceration of the cervix. Rarely, bilateral ureteric obstruction occurs and chronic renal failure has been reported.

Assessment

History

From the history it is important to ascertain the degree to which the prolapse is causing interference with daily activities and impairing quality of life. Specific questions must be asked about urinary and bowel symptoms. Postmenopasual women must be asked about vaginal bleeding and premenopausal women must be questioned about menstrual disorders. If surgical repair is being considered it is essential to record whether the woman is sexually active.

Further questions must be asked about chronic conditions which may aggravate prolapse, e.g. chest disease and smoking. The success of surgical repair in these women may be prejudiced. Record the patient's occupation and social circumstances, as work involving heavy lifting is unsuitable after surgical repair.

Examination

General physical examination. To assess whether the patient is fit for anaesthesia and to exclude conditions which may aggravate prolapse, e.g. chest disease, abdominal masses. (A thorough abdominal examination must always be performed prior to a pelvic examination.)

Pelvic examination. Ask the patient to turn to the left lateral position for examination with a Sims' speculum. Separate the patient's buttocks with assistance if necessary. Ask the patient to cough. Insert the blade of the Sims' speculum along the posterior vaginal wall and retract to display the anterior vaginal wall. Ask the patient to cough again to assess the degree of prolapse of the anterior vaginal wall and note any stress incontinence (remember the patient's bladder may be empty and she may have stress incontinence but it may not be demonstrable). Support the anterior vaginal wall with a sponge forceps and ask the patient to cough again while continuing to support the anterior vaginal wall with the sponge forceps. One can then observe for cervical descent. The patient is asked to bear down again and the speculum is then removed slowly. While anterior vaginal wall support is maintained the top of the vaginal vault and the posterior vaginal wall can then be visualized sequentially to detect the presence of an enterocele or a rectocele respectively. A bimanual examination should then follow.

When discussing the examination findings anterior and posterior wall prolapse is usually described as 'mild, moderate or severe'. These descriptions are highly subjective.

Management

Treatment is not indicated when prolapse is found at routine examination and is asymptomatic.

General measures which should be considered include weight reduction, stopping smoking, and hormone replacement therapy. Aggravating conditions, e.g. chest infections, should be treated when possible before definitive treatment.

Surgery is the mainstay of treatment for uterovaginal prolapse. In some women conservative measures may be more appropriate.

Conservative management

1. Indications
   a. patient's choice
   b. unfit for surgery
   c. temporary problem, e.g. in pregnancy
2. Methods
   a. pelvic floor exercises (only suitable for minor degrees of prolapse)
   b. pessaries.

Many devices have been used. The ring pessary is now in common use. It is inserted to occupy the posterior fornix and the lower part of the anterior vaginal wall, and works by putting redundant vaginal skin on stretch. Use of this pessary is effective for anterior vaginal and uterovaginal prolapse but less effective for posterior wall prolapse. It should be changed every 6 months and may cause erosion of the skin of the vaginal walls.

Surgical repair

The choice of repair procedure will be influenced by the preference of the gynaecologist. These are guidelines:

Cystocele/urethrocele. Anterior colporrhaphy ± bladder neck support.
Rectocele. Posterior colporrhaphy.
Enterocele. Hernia sac identified and opened. Contents reduced and neck tied. Sac excised. Combined with posterior repair. Sacrocolpopexy. Sacrospinous fixation.
Uterovaginal prolapse. Vaginal hysterectomy ± repair.

The Manchester (Fothergill) repair is occasionally used. This involves amputation of the cervix, approximating the cardinal ligaments in front of the cervical stump, anterior and posterior colporrhaphies. The uterus is conserved and reproductive potential is retained in younger women.

SUMMARY

Uterovaginal prolapse is common in postmenopausal women and is usually caused by childbirth. Symptoms may be influenced by the type of prolapse present. Surgical repair is usually the treatment of choice.

18. Minimally invasive surgery

B. J. Auld

Expectations of the examiners

Whilst a detailed knowledge of this kind of surgery is not required, some general understanding of these new procedures is expected. One should be able to give a basic explanation of the techniques involved and some indication of the pattern of recovery and the expected outcome. As with any new form of treatment an appreciation of the potential risks and benefits is of value especially while these techniques become established.

Definition

In gynaecology, minimally invasive surgery encompasses the range of therapeutic procedures which can be performed under hysteroscopic or laparoscopic guidance. In both instances the use of minimally invasive techniques is to avoid laparotomy. It is recognized that postoperative pain, complications and recovery time are related to the size and position of the initial surgical incision.

Interesting facts

It is now considered that up to 80% of all classic gynaecological operations can be carried out endoscopically. Recent technological advances have facilitated the rapid growth in minimally invasive surgery.

HYSTEROSCOPIC MINIMALLY INVASIVE SURGERY

Technique of hysteroscopy

Hysteroscopy allows inspection of the uterine cavity via the cervix and CO_2 gas or fluid is used to distend the uterine cavity. Diagnostic hysteroscopy is performed with a narrow diameter scope (2–7 mm) which often permits insertion without dilatation of the cervix thus avoiding general anaesthesia. Operative hysteroscopy including endometrial resection utilizes wider diameter instruments (10 mm) and is usually performed under general anaesthesia.

Contraindications and complications

Contraindications to hysteroscopy are pregnancy and the presence of acute pelvic infection. Uterine perforation is a complication which may follow any form of instrumentation but in operative hysteroscopy carries a greater risk of damage to intra-abdominal viscera or blood vessels. Less serious complications are: pelvic infection, excessive absorption of fluid distension media, and anaesthetic complications.

Operative hysteroscopy

Hysteroscopic surgery is indicated for a number of conditions:

1. Uterine septum
2. Uterine synechiae (Asherman's syndrome)
3. Endocervical/endometrial polyp
4. Fibroid polyps
5. Submucous fibroids
6. Dysfunctional uterine bleeding
7. Retrieval of IUD.

Most of the above conditions are treated hysteroscopically using either electrocautery techniques or by laser, which in this instance is by means of the Nd : YAg laser which has the property of transmission of laser light through a fluid medium (normal saline). The main interest and practice of hysteroscopic surgery has been in the treatment of dysfunctional uterine bleeding.

Endometrial ablation/resection

Historically many techniques have been used to remove the endometrial lining of the uterus. The operation of dilatation and curettage (D&C) removes only the superficial endometrium which regenerates. Endometrial ablation/resection seeks to remove the endometrium to a depth where the basal layer is destroyed and the underlying myometrium is exposed. Total endometrial ablation should result in amenorrhoea. It was the expectation of this outcome, performed as a day case procedure and without the need to remove the uterus, that has led to the current enthusiasm for this procedure.

Hysteroscopically two techniques are favoured, transcervical resection of the endometrium (TCRE) performed with electrocautery, and laser endometrial ablation (LEA) in which the endometrium is destroyed by energy from the Nd : YAg laser. Ablation of the endometrium using a rollerball electrocautery is an alternative technique but with slightly less effective results. Another non-hysteroscopic technique is radiofrequency endometrial ablation (RaFEA) using energy derived from a radiofrequency generator to thermally destroy the endometrium when a probe is placed in the uterine cavity.

Patient selection

The success of these procedures depends on patient selection. Women under the age of 40 years are more likely to have a poor outcome, often with recurrence of their symptoms. The ideal patients are women approaching the menopause who wish to avoid hysterectomy. The uterus should be normal size and enlargement with fibroids other than submucous fibroids is also a contraindication. Symptoms of pelvic pain and dysmenorrhoea may suggest the presence of adenomyosis. In adenomyosis the pockets of intramyometrial endometrium allow regeneration of the endometrium and thus recurrence of symptoms. These patients are therefore not suitable. All patients with menstrual irregularities should have the endometrium sampled prior to the procedure to exclude pathology. Finally, these patients should have completed their family.

Pretreatment for endometrial ablation

Suppression of the endometrium improves the outcome but if surgery is to be carried out on unprepared patients it is more effective in the postmenstrual phase when the endometrium is thinnest. Regimens for endometrial suppression are:

1. Medroxyyprogesterone acetate 30–50 mg daily for 6 weeks
2. Danazol 600 mg daily for 6 weeks
3. GnRH analogue (goserelin implant 3.5 mg) 1 month before surgery.

Pregnancy and sterilization

Most women will be sterile following the procedure, but sterility cannot be guaranteed and occasional pregnancies have been reported. Of greater concern is the risk that pregnancy may establish ectopically in the fallopian tube particularly in its intramural segment. For this reason laparoscopic sterilization should be considered at the time of the endometrial ablation/resection.

Complications of endometrial ablation/resection

A perforation rate in the order of 1.3% is quoted but only a very few of these are associated with major trauma involving damage to great vessels, bowel, and ureter. Emergency hysterectomy is only rarely required. Other serious complications occur at a rate of about 0.2% and include water intoxication, pulmonary oedema, and haemorrhage requiring blood transfusion. A minor complication is prolonged vaginal bleeding and discharge associated with postoperative infection.

Results

The outcome of endometrial ablation resection can be assessed in terms of whether there is total amenorrhoea, a reduction in menstrual flow and return of cycle regularity or no change or even a deterioration in menstrual symptoms. One long-term outcome measure is the number of women who will subsequently require a hysterectomy for recurrent symptoms. Table 18.1 compares these outcomes for TCRE and LEA.The results for RaFEA are said to be of the same order as electrocautery techniques.

Conclusions

Overall the outcomes of endometrial ablation/resection have not proved as encouraging in the treatment of dysfunctional bleeding as had first been expected but it remains a useful treatment option. Currently an unanswered worry hangs over this technique regarding the presentation of malignancy in women who have had this operation, although the risk is very small. If the use of ablative techniques delays or masks the presentation of endometrial carcinoma, allowing it to progress, then in the long term it will prove a retrograde development.

LAPAROSCOPIC MINIMALLY INVASIVE SURGERY

Gynaecologists have been using the laparoscope as a diagnostic tool for many years. The use of the laparoscope to perform more complex operative procedures has been relatively recent. General surgeons have far more rapidly assimilated the benefits of laparoscopic surgery into their practice. The range of surgical procedures open to a laparoscopic approach now covers almost all aspects of gynaecological surgery. Operations which can be performed laparoscopically are listed below:

1. Tubal sterilization
2. Assisted reproductive procedures
3. Ovarian drilling (for polycystic ovarian syndrome)
4. Adhesiolysis

Table 18.1   Comparison of the outcomes from TCRE and LEA (%)

Operation	TCRE	LEA
Totally amenorrhoeic	35	60
Improved menstruation	50	32
No improvement in menstruation	15	8
Requiring hysterectomy	16	—

5. Surgery for endometriosis
6. Uterosacral ligament transection
7. Tuboplasty, fimbrioplasty, neosalpingostomy
8. Treatment of ectopic pregnancy
9. Ovarian cystectomy
10. Salpingo-oophorectomy
11. Myomectomy
12. Hysterectomy (supracervical and total) with combined vaginal approach
13. Colposuspension and sacrocolpopexy
14. Presacral neurectomy
15. Pelvic lymphadenectomy
16. Radical hysterectomy
17. Pelvic floor repair.

Laparoscopic treatment of endometriosis

Data are accumulating to suggest that laparoscopic treatment of endometriotic deposits is more effective than medical treatment, and that a combination of both treatments may be best of all. The surgical approach avoids the side-effects of medical therapy, particularly when pregnancy is actively sought. In patients with endometriomas it is possible to remove these laparoscopically or to ablate the lining using the KTP-532 laser which is assisted by the haemosiderin pigment. Surgical treatment has resulted in pregnancy rates as high as 80%. It is also claimed to be an effective treatment for those patients who also complain of pelvic pain and dysmenorrhoea resulting from endometriosis.

Laparoscopy for tubal infertility

Laparoscopic surgery to restore normal tubal anatomy and to unblock a hydrosalpinx (neosalpingostomy) has been shown to achieve pregnancy rates of 60% when the endosalpinx of the tube is healthy.

Laparoscopic treatment of ectopic pregnancy

Advances in the use of transvaginal ultrasound and quantitative hCG testing mean that increasingly ectopic pregnancy is being diagnosed early, usually before tubal rupture has occurred. This allows a more conservative approach with preservation of the tube. The patient may be discharged from hospital the next day but requires continued follow-up of serum hCG levels. Static or rising levels indicate the presence of residual trophoblastic tissue which can be treated by systemic therapy with methotrexate and folinic acid. Subsequent intrauterine pregnancy rates are reported between 20 and 83%, with recurrent tubal pregnancies between 10 and 22%.

Laparoscopic treatment of polycystic ovarian syndrome

As an alternative to classical open wedge resection, the ovaries are now drilled ('pepperpotting') laparoscopically using either a diathermy needle or a fibre laser (KTP or Nd : YAG). These multiple holes in the ovaries destroy the androgen producing stroma which leads to a restoration, albeit temporary, of normal ovarian activity. Ovulation rates of 75% have been reported with pregnancy rates of 50–75% in women previously unresponsive to clomiphene. The effect may only last for three to six cycles however.

Laparoscopic oophorectomy and ovarian cystectomy

Ultrasound assessment of all adnexal masses is essential regardless of the age of the patient. Masses should be less than 10 cm diameter with distinct borders and have no evidence of irregular solid parts, thick septae, ascites or matted bowel loops. The serum CA125 concentration should be less than 35 i.u./ml. At laparoscopy the abdominal cavity is fully inspected for evidence of malignant disease. If concern exists about the risk of malignancy or if the contents of the cyst are toxic (dermoid cysts), ovarian tissue can be placed inside a retrieval bag and the bag closed by means of a drawstring to avoid spillage before removal. If the tissue bulk is too large to remove through a small trocar point a posterior colpotomy in the vagina will allow removal via this route. Oophorectomy is sometimes practised as an adjunct to treatment for breast cancer or to relieve pain in women with residual or entrapped ovarian syndrome.

Laparoscopic pelvic lymphadenectomy

Laparoscopic dissection of the pelvic lymph nodes in pelvic malignancy can be performed, however its role in management is still being evaluated.

Laparoscopic hysterectomy and laparoscopically assisted vaginal hysterectomy

Interesting facts

In the UK some 73 000 hysterectomies are performed annually, of which 75% are abdominal and 25% vaginal. Abdominal hysterectomy prolongs the hospital stay and the morbidity from abdominal surgery is significantly greater than vaginal surgery. The laparoscopic approach to hysterectomy offers the opportunity to convert the outcome for hysterectomy from that associated with abdominal surgery to an outcome like that of vaginal hysterectomy or even better.

Reich first described laparoscopic hysterectomy in 1989. He differentiated between two levels of laparoscopic hysterectomy. In true laparoscopic hysterectomy (LH) the laparoscopic approach is used to secure all the pedicles down to the level of the uterine arteries and below. In laparoscopically assisted vaginal hysterectomy (LAVH) the laparoscopic approach is used to secure only the upper pedicles and the uterine arteries are secured from the vaginal end.

It is now clear that most surgeons in practice rarely remove the ovaries via the vaginal route. One of the benefits of LAVH therefore is that when it is required to remove the ovaries at the time of hysterectomy then LAVH will avoid an abdominal operation. Similarly, laparoscopy may facilitate a vaginal hysterectomy when there are adhesions in the pelvis which can be dealt with laparoscopically and without which a vaginal operation would not have been possible. In addition, the risk of vault haematoma should be reduced although the evidence for this is not yet available.

Technique of laparoscopic hysterectomy

The laparoscope is inserted in the usual subumbilical position having first achieved a pneumoperitoneum with carbon dioxide. Further trocar points are inserted, either two or three, usually low down in the suprapubic area. Major vascular pedicles can be secured by the use of electrocautery, endosuturing techniques or the use of disposable endostapling devices which simultaneously insert rows of parallel haemostatic staples and divide the pedicle between these rows. Such instruments add to the costs of the operation but reduce the length of operating time.

Following the laparoscopic procedure the vaginal approach is used to secure the remaining vascular pedicles. The uterus and adnexal structures are removed through the vagina which is then repaired in the normal fashion. A final laparoscopic inspection is made to ensure haemostasis.

Classical Abdominal Semm Hysterectomy (CASH)

This form of laparoscopic hysterectomy has been devised by Semm and results in laparoscopic removal of only the supracervical part of the uterus. Subtotal hysterectomy is an operation which has largely been discarded because of the concern about leaving behind a cervical remnant with its potential for malignant change. The risk of this occurring is actually rare but to counter this problem Semm has devised a technique whereby the epithelial lining of the cervical canal is reamed out like an apple core thus removing the risk of transitional zone neoplasia.

A laparoscopic subtotal hysterectomy is then performed removing the fundus of the uterus above the level of the uterine arteries by morcellation within the abdominal cavity. The proponents of this operation argue that conserving the cervix also conserves the ligamentous supports of the vaginal vault preventing later prolapse. They also maintain that the cervix is an integral component of sexual stimulation and satisfaction for the female.

Results and complications of laparoscopic hysterectomy

The early experience of this operation suggests a long-term outcome similar to abdominal hysterectomy but with a reduced perioperative morbidity. The major advantage is in terms of shortened hospital stay (1–3 days) and shortened recovery to normal activities (21 days). Most patients are pleased with the cosmetic outcome and particularly appreciate the minimal postoperative pain they experience.

Any laparoscopic operation carries a risk of damage to internal structures. These risks reflect the skill and learning curve of the surgeon and the degree of difficulty in relation to any existing pathology encountered. Despite this the risks of laparoscopic hysterectomy remain low, probably less than 1% and usually in the form of uncontrollable haemorrhage or damage to the bowel or urinary tract. The major complication most commonly recognized is ureteric injury which usually occurs in laparoscopic hysterectomy when the uterine arteries are divided laparoscopically.

Conclusions

The main drawbacks of laparoscopic surgery are the capital costs needed to set up the necessary facilities and the considerable learning curve to acquire the skills needed to carry out these operations. The risks of complications which may be serious should encourage lengthy preoperative counselling of patients regarding the possiblity of undergoing a laparotomy.

In all these procedures the avoidance of a laparotomy incision benefits the patient by a less painful, more speedy recovery, which in turn shortens the length of hospital stay and hastens the return to normal activities. The surgical outcomes of most of these procedures are the same as their laparotomy counterparts. In theory however a potential benefit of laparoscopic surgery is the avoidance of the inevitable handling of tissues necessary at open laparotomy. Also tissue damage with instruments such as the laser and bipolar diathermy used at laparoscopy is much reduced resulting in less postoperative adhesion formation and fewer complications overall. The consequences of this are that laparotomy is no longer a justifiable approach in many instances and we must expect that laparoscopic surgery will become the normal practice for most gynaecological procedures.

DEBATE

The growth of minimally invasive surgery is leading to a fundamental change in the practice of primary health care and hospital-based services. The ability to discharge patients early from a hospital-dependent situation may lead to the use of hotel-type recovery facilities or a greater role of community care in postoperative recovery. This will have a major impact on reducing inpatient hospital costs but may shift this burden onto the resources of community-based services.

19. Prepregnancy counselling and prenatal diagnosis

G. Davis

PREPREGNANCY COUNSELLING

Expectations of the examiners

Candidates will be expected to know the range of disorders in which prepregnancy care is of benefit and the principles of management of the common conditions.

Definition

Prepregnancy counselling is the discussion and investigation of medical conditions either past or present which may influence fetal or maternal health in future pregnancies.

Interesting facts

Because of the emotional and financial cost of special care for infants or mothers with medical conditions, preventive medicine should be as widely practised as possible. Counselling is indicated in women with medical illnesses that may become complicated because of pregnancy or those who may be at risk of giving birth to an infant with a genetic or environmentally induced birth defect.

Assessment

An increasing number of women are seeking advice prior to pregnancy with questions concerning diet, smoking, alcohol, drugs, and exercise. The use of folic acid around the time of conception reduces the recurrence rate of neural tube defects (NTDs) in at-risk women. In low-risk populations prophylaxis is recommended to prevent a primary NTD. All women wishing to conceive should receive supplementation at least 6 weeks prior to conception. Smoking, alcohol, and drugs (both prescription and illicit) should be avoided. Prescription drugs should be reduced to minimal essential levels and changed to those known to be safe in early pregnancy if possible. There is no evidence that exercise adversely affects either

Table 19.1   Indications for prepregnancy counselling.

Maternal conditions
Diabetes and other metabolic endocrine disorders
Hypertension
Specific maternal infections, e.g. genital herpes, HIV
Risk of genetic disease, e.g. maternal age, family history of genetic abnormalities
Drug exposure—either prescription or illicit
Abnormal maternal nutrition, either obesity or subnormal weight
Chronic medical problems, e.g. renal disease, SLE, heart disease, epilepsy, neurological disorders

Previous obstetric history
Previous pregnancy loss, e.g. stillbirth, recurrent miscarriage
Previous preterm delivery, growth retardation
Previous infant with congenital anomaly or mental retardation
Previous adverse delivery experience

conception or development (unless excessive exercise induces anovulation and amenorrhoea).

All these questions can be answered by the general practitioner but women with more specific problems, as outlined in Table 19.1, should be referred to an obstetrician. Some of these problems can then be dealt with by the obstetrician directly, e.g. previous delivery experience, but others will require referral for further medical evaluation or genetic counselling. The obstetrician then remains the contact point for the woman, and can discuss with her the options given by the physician or geneticist. Ideally, the woman should make an informed choice either to conceive or, rarely, to avoid conception.

Follow-up

It is essential that prepregnancy counselling is followed by consultation early in the pregnancy to confirm the presence of a viable intrauterine pregnancy, to allow accurate dating of the pregnancy and to arrange for prenatal diagnostic investigations if appropriate (see following section).

PRENATAL DIAGNOSIS OF FETAL ABNORMALITIES

Expectations of the examiners

Candidates will be expected to have a knowledge of the basic methods of prenatal diagnosis and the risks of common congenital disorders. They should also be familiar with the use and interpretation of routine prenatal screening tests for congenital anomalies.

Definition

Prenatal diagnosis is the detection of fetal disease or abnormality prior to delivery.

Interesting facts

Serious congenital abnormalities now account for 20% of perinatal deaths, are present in 2% of all births, and account for 30% of all paediatric admissions to hospital. Prenatal diagnosis is required in up to 10% of all pregnancies and although it has been described as 'preventive medicine', in reality many affected fetuses are terminated thereby removing them from the perinatal mortality statistics. However, some parents prefer to know if their child is abnormal prior to delivery in order to prepare themselves adequately for the birth.

Pathophysiology

Congenital abnormalities can be divided into four groups:

1. Chromosomal abnormalities arise during gamete formation or early in embryonic cleavage. They account for 60% of spontaneous abortions. Common examples are the trisomies 21 and 18, and Turner's syndrome 45XO. The incidence of many chromosomal disorders increases with maternal age.
2. A single gene defect accounts for many autosomal recessive diseases such as inborn errors of metabolism.
3. Structural abnormalities may result from multifactorial influences but some may occur in association with chromosomal abnormalities (e.g. duodenal atresia in Down syndrome) or drugs (e.g. phocomelia with thalidomide).
4. Environmental factors causing abnormality are mostly drugs or infections. Congenital infections are uncommon but may cause developmental abnormalities, intrauterine death or neonatal illness. Infections in this category include: rubella, syphilis, listeria, cytomegalovirus, and toxoplasma.

Incidence of common congenital abnormalities

Down syndrome (trisomy 21)

Overall incidence 1 in 650 live births (LB). (See Table 19.2.)

Table 19.2 Incidence of Down syndrome.

Maternal age	Approximate risk of affected child	Risk of recurrence
20	1 in 2000	1 in 100
30	1 in 900	(irrespective of age)
35	1 in 365	
40	1 in 110	
42	1 in 70	
46	1 in 25	

Neural tube defects

The overall incidence of NTDs in the UK is difficult to determine as many affected fetuses abort or are terminated. The birth prevalence varies from 3 to 5 in 1000 total births in the north and west of the country to 2 in 1000 total births in the south and east. The recurrence rate is 1 in 30 after one affected child, rising to 1 in 5 after three affected children. The risk of a NTD in the offspring of one affected parent is 5%, and 30% if both parents are affected. Fifty per cent of affected fetuses have anencephaly (which is incompatible with life), 45%, spina bifida and 5% encephaloceles. There are varying degrees of handicap but of those born with open spina bifida, 70% will die within the first 5 years and only 10% will be free of major handicap.

Congenital heart disease

The incidence of serious congenital heart disease is 8 per 1000 live births of which 50% are major defects. The recurrence risk is 1 in 50 and there is a 5% risk of having an affected child if one parent is affected.

Cystic fibrosis

Cystic fibrosis is inherited as a classical autosomal recessive trait with a birth prevalence of 1 per 2500. Males are sterile due to obliteration of the vas deferens but females can reproduce. The risk of an affected woman having an affected child is 1–2%.

Antenatal screening

Ninety per cent of congenital anomalies will arise in women who do not have any risk factors and screening is therefore important. Routine screening tests are:

1. Ultrasound at 18–20 weeks
2. Serum screening for Down syndrome at 14–20 weeks
3. Testing for sickle cell disease in Afro-Caribbean women
4. Haemoglobin electrophoresis to detect thalassaemia in Mediterranean or Asian women
5. Testing for rubella immunity.

Routine anomaly scan

This is performed at 18–20 weeks to confirm gestation and to exclude major fetal structural abnormalities. The fetus is carefully scanned with particular attention to the head, spine, four chamber view of the heart, kidneys, bowel, presence of a bladder, and moving limbs of normal length.

Ninety per cent of NTDs (the commonest structural abnormality) will be detected in this manner and it is rare to miss a major NTD.

Maternal serum α-fetoprotein (AFP) levels

Serum AFP is raised in a large number of conditions, including NTDs, twin pregnancy, abdominal wall defects in the fetus, fetal death, and fetal hydrops. Levels also rise as pregnancy progresses, therefore an accurate knowledge of gestation is essential for correct interpretation. Low levels of maternal AFP have been shown to be associated with chromosomal abnormalities in the fetus. Many units have abandoned serum AFP screening and use the detailed ultrasound scan to detect NTDs.

Biochemical screening for Down syndrome

In this test the values for AFP, hCG and unconjugated oestriol in the blood in combination with maternal age are used in an algorithm to produce a risk estimate for Down syndrome. If the risk is higher than the risk of Down syndrome for a woman aged 35, then amniocentesis for karyotyping is offered. This test relies on the empirical observation that in Down syndrome pregnancies, AFP and oestriol levels are low, while hCG levels are usually higher than average. This test should detect about 60% of babies with Down syndrome. It remains controversial because on a population basis the same number of normal babies will be lost due to complications of amniocentesis as cases of Down syndrome detected. In many centres only AFP and hCG are used, which apears to be just as efficient.

Ultrasound screening for Down syndrome

Increased nuchal thickness measured at 11–13 weeks is strongly associated with aneuploidy. The efficacy of this procedure as a screening test is currently being investigated.

Testing for sickle cell disease and thalassaemia

In women who are known to carry the trait or have the disease, haemoglobin electrophoresis is performed on their partner's blood. If the partner is a carrier and hence the fetus at risk of having the disease, then prenatal diagnosis can be performed by DNA techniques or chorionic villus sampling (CVS) or fetal blood sampling. The former technique is preferable as it can be performed earlier in gestation.

Rubella immunity

Most women should be immune to rubella through the nationwide immunization of teenage girls, and now of children. Non-immune women are identified and managed appropriately.

Table 19.3 Women at risk of having a fetus with congenital abnormality.

History
    Previous abnormal child/fetus
    Family history of abnormality
    Maternal age >35

Current pregnancy
    Maternal diabetes (4 × risk)
    Abnormal maternal AFP
    Exposure to teratogens—drugs, radiation
    Suspicious findings on routine ultrasound scan
    Breech presentation (4 × risk)
    Oligohydramnios
    Polyhydramnios
    Severe symmetrical growth retardation
    Twin pregnancy (2 × risk)
    Contact with or suspicion of maternal infection with known teratogenic
    pathogen, e.g. rubella, CMV

Identification of risk groups

Women at risk of having a fetus with congenital abnormality are outlined in Table 19.3 and should be referred early in pregnancy for prenatal diagnosis.

Investigations

Methods

Ultrasound scan. This is used to detect structural abnormalities in the central nervous system, gastrointestinal tract, urinary system, skeleton, and heart. In addition, cleft lip and palate can be detected if a specific search is made. Routine ultrasound screening for structural abnormalities is performed at 18–20 weeks, which is a compromise between performing the procedure earlier (so that safer termination of pregnancy may be carried out) and later (when the structural details become more obvious).

Amniocentesis. Removal of liquor for the culture of desquamated fetal fibroblasts permits karyotyping and the detection of enzyme defects. This is now performed under ultrasound guidance. It takes 2–3 weeks for the cells to proliferate sufficiently for investigation and culture is unsuccessful in <1.0% of cases. It is ideally performed between 15 and 18 weeks when sufficient liquor is available. Amniocentesis at earlier gestations, particularly 10–13 weeks, appears to carry a higher risk of miscarriage. The risk of pregnancy loss after the procedure is 1% over the background loss rate for that period of gestation.

Chorionic villus sampling (CVS). CVS involves aspirating placental tissue under ultrasound guidance either transcervically or transabdominally with a needle. Karyotyping and other investigations can usually be performed immediately on placental tissue, significantly reducing the delay between the procedure and result. It is also carried out earlier in pregnancy

(10–13 weeks), permitting earlier and safer termination if necessary. Fetal loss secondary to the procedure is reported to be 2% but probably improves as the operator gains experience.

Cordocentesis. Ultrasound-guided sampling from the umbilical cord permits the direct assessment of the fetal blood, e.g. rapid karyotyping, acid-base status, haemoglobinopathies, electrolytes, and pathogens, and is possible after 18 weeks' gestation. Because of the invasive nature of this technique, its use is restricted to at-risk fetuses, e.g. severe growth retardation, suspected congenital infection, and structural cardiac abnormality, and it is now used routinely for intrauterine transfusions of fetuses with haemolytic disease. Rates of fetal loss are approximiately 3% but figures for the procedure risk are difficult to obtain because of the high-risk group in which the procedure is used.

Fetoscopy. An alternative method for sampling fetal blood or tissue is to do so under direct vision using a fine laparoscope. Fetal losses from this procedure are reported to be about 5% but the technique has been largely superseded by cordocentesis.

Laboratory investigations

Chromosome analysis. Nuclei are either stained immediately (chorionic villus biopsy, cordocentesis) or the cells are cultured and then the nuclei are stained. Duplication of chromosomes and gross rearrangements (e.g. translocations) are then detectable. The commonest chromosomal abnormalities which survive until term are the trisomies (21, 18, 13) and Turner's syndrome (45XO).

Enzyme defects. These are now usually detected by molecular biological techniques identifying the altered gene, but previously they were detected by direct assay in chorionic villi or occasionally by incubation of fetal cells with a specific substrate. It is only possible where the fetus is known to be at risk of an inborn error of metabolism, i.e. where the parents have had an affected infant previously or screening has revealed the parents to be carriers.

Tests on fetal blood. Rapid karyotyping, FBC, platelet count, and a number of other haematological parameters may be measured directly on fetal blood, e.g. factor VIII to detect haemophilia A and β globin to detect thalassaemia. These latter methods are largely being replaced by analysis (see below). Recently, fetal blood sampling to assess acid-base status and electrolytes has become more common in high-risk pregnancies. This is currently only of value after fetal viability (24 weeks' gestation) and is used to assist in the management of severely compromised fetuses.

DNA analysis. Using these methods, abnormal genes are detected in two ways, either directly or indirectly (linkage studies). Direct detection is possible where the specific mutation has been identified, e.g sickle cell disease or cystic fibrosis. Indirect detection relies on the fact that most

Table 19.4   Conditions for which probes are available.

X-linked recessive
   Duchenne muscular dystrophy
   Fragile X syndrome
   Haemophilia A and B

Autosomal recessive
   Cystic fibrosis
   Phenylketonuria
   Sickle cell anaemia
   Thalassaemia

Autosomal dominant
   Huntington's chorea
   Neurofibromatosis

chromosomes have differences in the DNA sequence of homologous (same number, e.g. 21) chromosomes which do not cause genetic disease (polymorphism). If a mutation is close to a *detectable* polymorphic change, then the mutation and the polymorphic change will usually travel together in any recombination of genetic material that occurs. In this way, the detectable polymorphic marker can be used to determine whether the fetus has the affected gene.

Some of the more common conditions for which gene probes are now available are listed in Table 19.4.

Management of at-risk couples

Irrespective of whether at-risk couples opt for termination of pregnancy or not, genetic counselling is of value. General practitioners and obstetricians should be familiar with the risks and preliminary management of the conditions for which women are routinely screened in antenatal clinics. For at-risk couples, most practitioners will need to involve a medical geneticist, although the management principles are the same.

These principles include:

1. Knowledge of which couples are at risk from their history or clinical features. It is important that the diagnosis of the affected member(s) of the family is accurate before proceeding further
2. The natural history of the disease
3. The range of its clinical manifestations
4. Possibility of treatment, and risks of treatment
5. Accuracy of treatment and prognosis
6. Possibility of detecting carriers
7. Psychological implications
8. Likelihood of recurrence and management in subsequent pregnancy.

It is important that information, which is often quite complex, is presented to the parents in a way which they can understand. Although it is impossible to present information in an unbiased manner, this should be the goal. Genetic counselling has been shown to fail to educate at-risk couples adequately in 40% of cases, so repeated counselling is usually necessary. Other attendants involved in their care should avoid confusing the situation if they are not fully conversant with the disorder. Couples will often experience grief which must be dealt with before information can be passed on. Most couples then regard the problem in terms of how it will affect their relationship, their immediate family, and their financial status.

Follow-up

The need for close follow-up of affected pregnancies is self-evident. If an affected child is delivered, then ongoing paediatric care is usually necessary and the couple then need to return for reinforcement of the information on outcome of the affected child and recurrence risk in future children. Couples that have opted for termination of pregnancy attend for the results of the post-mortem (if possible) and to discuss again the possibility of, and management in, subsequent pregnancy.

20. Antenatal care

G. Davis

Expectations of the examiners

The routine management of pregnancy and the assessment of obstetric risk are fundamental to the appropriate care of obstetric patients and the examiners will therefore expect candidates to have a comprehensive grasp of all aspects.

Definition

'A planned programme of observation, education, and medical management of pregnant women directed toward making pregnancy and delivery a safe and satisfying experience.' *American College of Obstetricians and Gynaecologists*.

Interesting facts

The major objective of antenatal care is to reduce perinatal and maternal morbidity and mortality. Whether this objective is best achieved by the manner in which antenatal care is currently practised is debatable. At least 80% of pregnant women would deliver healthy babies without any antenatal care and very few of the measures used routinely have been properly evaluated.

The objectives of antenatal care are:

1. To predict problems on the basis of the medical, social and obstetric history and physical examination of the women.
2. To prevent, or reduce, the severity of problems by prophylactic measures.
3. To detect and treat conditions which have harmful effects on the mother or fetus.
4. To provide education, information and reassurance for the pregnant woman and her partner.

The current approach to routine antenatal care ideally involves:

1. Prepregnancy counselling (see Ch. 19)
2. Booking visit

3. Routine antenatal visits
4. Antenatal education classes
5. Inpatient care if required.

BOOKING VISIT

Assessment

The booking visit is the most important visit in most women's antenatal care. At this visit, risk factors are assessed and future antenatal care and place of delivery decided. Pregnant women are usually seen by a midwife initially and a history taken, special investigations performed or ordered, information on maternity benefits and antenatal education classes given and a date made for a further appointment. At the next visit the woman sees a member of the medical staff, by which time results of initial investigations are available to assist in further decisions. This process may also be completed at a single visit.

Timing

Ideally the woman should be seen as early as possible to confirm pregnancy and to deal with any early problems, e.g. chorionic villus sampling at 10–12 weeks. At the latest, the woman should be seen at 16–18 weeks' gestation to allow biochemical screening tests for Down syndrome, assessment of gestational age and exclusion of structural anomalies by ultrasound, and amniocentesis if necessary.

History

The booking history should include:

1. Identification details
2. Social history
3. Menstrual/contraceptive history
4. Past obstetric history
5. Medical conditions
6. Factors associated with genetic risk
7. General condition.

Identification details. These should include the woman's full name, address, next of kin, and race. In addition, her general practitioner's name, address and whether he or she wishes to undertake shared care should be recorded.

Social history. Details of the woman's occupation, marital status and social circumstances should be noted. It should include her attitude to the pregnancy and that of her partner. Her partner's race, occupation and support should be recorded. Details of housing are important as these may need to be changed during pregnancy and eligibility for benefits assessed.

A full drug history should be obtained including prescribed and illicit drugs, alcohol, and tobacco. All women should be encouraged to give up the latter three and prescribed medications may need to be modified in pregnancy.

Menstrual/contraceptive history. The date (and degree of certainty) of the last menstrual period (LMP) must be established and the regularity and length of the menstrual cycle. If the LMP was abnormal the last normal menstrual period should be recorded and any subsequent bleeding. If the woman was using the combined oral contraceptive then it should be determined whether the LMP was a withdrawal bleed. In some cases, such as pregnancy after a period of amenorrhoea or after previous pregnancy, no menstrual history is available. Previous duration and treatment of infertility should be noted.

If an intrauterine device is still present (and the strings are visible on examination) this should be removed to reduce the possibility of later septic miscarriages. As in all women of reproductive age who present with amenorrhoea, ectopic pregnancy should be excluded.

Past obstetric history. This is the most important part of the history in terms of identifying risk factors in the current pregnancy. Details of all previous pregnancies including abortions, terminations of pregnancy and ectopic pregnancies should be recorded. The gestations of previous pregnancies, complications and details of delivery and postnatal complications should be noted. The paternity of all previous pregnancies should also be determined. Previous stillbirth or intrauterine growth retardation is an indication for increased monitoring of fetal well-being in the third trimester. A history of recurrent, painless mid-trimester abortion suggests cervical incompetence which may require a cervical suture. A previous baby delivered spontaneously and prematurely is the best predictor of preterm delivery in the current pregnancy. If a previous baby was delivered by caesarean section, the indications for operation, type of procedure and woman's attitude to the operation must be carefully determined to assess whether a trial of labour is suitable. This may require communication with a previous hospital. Any problems in the third stage of labour will necessitate the presence of an obstetrician at subsequent deliveries. A previous baby with a congenital abnormality or other neonatal problems may be an indication for prenatal diagnosis.

Medical conditions. Any medical condition in the woman should be noted. A brief series of direct questions to exclude major disease should include:

1. Diabetes mellitus (pregnancy induced or otherwise)
2. Epilepsy
3. Thromboembolic disease
4. Anaemia

5. Chest diseases
6. Tuberculosis
7. Hypertension
8. Cardiac disease (congenital or acquired)
9. Renal disease
10. Endocrine disease (thyroid, adrenal)
11. Sexually transmitted disease
12. Rubella.

All of these conditions affect, or are affected by, pregnancy to a greater or lesser extent.

Previous operations, particularly those with relevance to the pregnancy, e.g. previous cone biopsy (risk of cervical incompetence) or bladder surgery (risk of weakening repair) should be recorded. Any psychiatric history increases the risk of postpartum psychiatric problems and should be specifically elicited as many women wish to avoid discussing this. Any allergies should be prominently recorded in the hospital notes and any record the woman keeps.

All women should be asked the date and result of their last cervical smear and this should be repeated if it has not been done in the previous 3 years or was previously abnormal.

Genetic risk. Individuals at increased risk of fetal abnormality include:

1. Maternal age greater than 35 years—risk of chromosomal abnormality
2. Afro-Caribbean women—risk of sickle cell disease
3. Mediterranean or Asian women—risk of thalassaemia
4. Ashkenazi Jews—risk of Tay–Sachs disease
5. Previous child with abnormality
6. Family history of fetal abnormality, inherited diseases, e.g. haemophilia.

Prenatal diagnosis should be discussed with all these women and appropriate action taken (see Ch. 19).

General condition. The woman should be asked if she has any complaints currently including vaginal bleeding or discharge, vomiting or concern over the pregnancy. Any questions the woman has about antenatal care or her health should be answered at this stage.

Examination

The woman should be weighed and her height and blood pressure measured. The cardiovascular and respiratory systems are examined and the breasts checked for masses or inverted nipples. Abdominal examination is performed to confirm the presence of a pelvic mass (after 12 weeks' gestation) or later in pregnancy, fetal growth, presentation and lie.

The fundus reaches the umbilicus at 20–24 weeks' gestation and the xiphisternum at 36–38 weeks. The presence of the fetal heart is confirmed with a Pinard fetal stethoscope (after 28 weeks' gestation) or a sonicaid (after 12–14 weeks). The lie is readily determined after 28–30 weeks.

Pelvic examination confirms gestation, excludes pelvic pathology and permits a cervical smear to be taken. However, unless a cervical smear is required, the value of a routine pelvic examination is debatable in a setting where routine ultrasound is performed.

Investigations

Blood tests

The blood tests routinely performed at booking are:

1. FBC
2. Blood group and antibody screen
3. Serology for hepatitis B, syphilis, rubella
4. HIV and triple test screening are usually offered.

Also in at-risk groups:

1. Sickle test
2. Haemoglobin electrophoresis.

The most common form of anaemia detected is due to iron deficiency. The lower limit of normal in pregnancy is reduced because of the haemodilution that occurs (10.5 or 11 g/dl). If the hepatitis serology is positive (HBsAg), then further testing for HBeAg and HBsAb is carried out. Routine testing for syphilis usually includes VDRL and TPHA and if positive, testing for current infection is carried out. Rubella immunity is assessed by screening for IgG unless there has been a possible recent contact, in which case the IgM levels are measured and repeated in 2 weeks to look for a rise in titre (indicating recent infection). If the IgG is negative and there is no prenatal infection, vaccination is performed after delivery.

Maternal serum α-fetoprotein (AFP)

This is measured at 16–18 weeks and if it is more than 2.5 times the mean for gestation, further testing is required to exclude neural tube defects or other abnormality. Many units have discarded serum AFP testing (see Ch. 19).

Triple test for Down syndrome

This is performed at 16–18 weeks and amniocentesis indicated if there is increased risk (see Ch. 19).

Routine ultrasound scan

In most units this is carried out at 18–20 weeks for the following reasons:

1. Accurate assessment of gestation—even in those women with certain dates, ultrasound has been demonstrated to be more accurate. It is also important for interpretation of maternal serum AFP levels and triple test for Down syndrome.
2. Detection of multiple pregnancy.
3. Detection of congenital abnormalities in the fetus.
4. Baseline for further scans if necessary later in the pregnancy.
5. Determination of the placental site. Although the placental site can usually be detected accurately at this gestation, many units do not routinely rescan those women with a low-lying placenta because the vast majority will resolve as the lower segment forms at 28–34 weeks.
6. Reassurance for mother and partner.

There has never been any reliable evidence that ultrasound used as it is in the prenatal period is dangerous for the fetus (or the mother).

Assessment of risk

Many lists of risk factors have been published and a recent one is included in Appendix II. Failing to identify risk factors or to take appropriate action when they are known to be present is a common error in obstetric practice. Obstetric patients can be classified as having low, moderate or high risk and their pregnancy managed accordingly. Risk based on factors in the history is assessed at the booking visit but the development of any problems in pregnancy may necessitate a reappraisal of the degree of risk.

Type of antenatal care

For most women this will be a choice between full hospital care shared between general practitioner and hospital or total midwifery care. For low-risk patients, shared care is usually more convenient and reduces waiting times in hospital antenatal clinics. High-risk patients should usually be seen exclusively at the hospital while the care of those with moderate risk should be decided individually.

Place of delivery

Only 1% of women now deliver at home. If the woman wishes to do so, then she should be at low risk and be supervised by a registered domiciliary midwife and doctor. Ideally, these women should be seen at the hospital for a booking visit and at least one visit later in pregnancy although, in practice, some women who opt for home delivery avoid hospitals. Low-risk patients suitable for home delivery must:

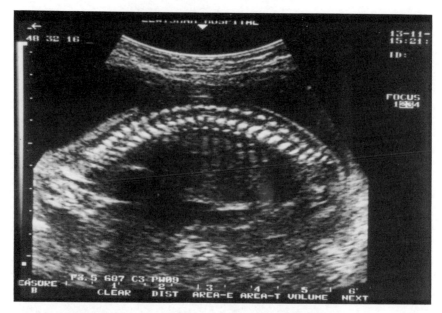

Fig. 20.1   Ultrasound scan in which the spine is seen in its entirety.

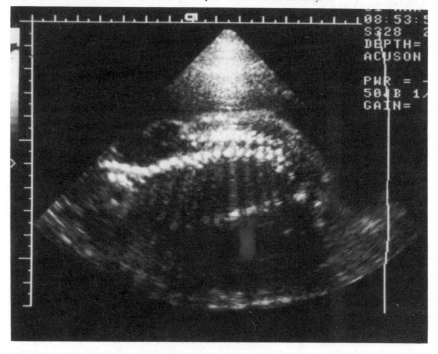

Fig. 20.2   Ultrasound scan. The defect in the spine (spina bifida) is clearly seen.

1. Be healthy women aged 19–34 years
2. Be para one or two
3. Have no major contraindications.

Major contraindications include:

1. Previous complicated obstetric/medical history
2. Major gynaecological surgery or condition (including infertility)
3. Under 152 cm in height (5 ft)
4. Gross obesity
5. Any abnormality in current pregnancy
6. Postmaturity in current pregnancy
7. Severe social problems
8. No telephone available/difficult access.

An alternative to home delivery offered in most delivery units is 'domino' (domiciliary in and out) care. Women in labour of low or moderate risk are cared for in the delivery unit by domiciliary midwives and, provided all is normal, discharged 6–12 hours after delivery. If there are any problems in labour, then care can be safely and efficiently transferred to the hospital.

SUBSEQUENT VISITS

The timing of routine antenatal visits is variable but is usually every 4 weeks until 28 weeks, fortnightly until 36 weeks and weekly thereafter. If the woman is receiving shared care then the same routine should be followed but hospital visits should be at 32 weeks, and 40 or 41 weeks.

There is wide variation between hospitals on the timing of these visits. If an abnormality is detected then the frequency of visits is increased and care may be transferred completely to the hospital.

Examination

As most antenatal visits will reveal no abnormality, it is important to avoid complacency and to maintain a high degree of alertness to potential problems. At each visit, the woman's blood pressure is measured and a urine sample tested for protein and glucose.

The blood pressure usually falls in the second trimester and should be considered abnormal if it is more than 140/90 mmHg on two separate occasions 24 hours apart, or if there is a rise of 20 mmHg or greater in the diastolic pressure.

Proteinuria may be due to contamination of the specimen by vaginal discharge. If present on a mid-stream urine early in pregnancy, it is usually due to infection or chronic renal disease and these should be investigated appropriately. Its appearance later in pregnancy suggests infection again or serious pre-eclampsia and in the presence of even mildly elevated blood pressure warrants admission for further assessment.

Glycosuria on more than one occasion is an indication for an oral glucose tolerance test to exclude maternal diabetes, although it is commonly due to the lowered renal threshold for glucose excretion in pregnancy.

Abdominal examination is performed to assess fetal growth and the symphysiofundal height may be measured. There is debate over the relative merits of the tape measure verus the hand, but candidates should be able to use a tape measure to assess fundal height whatever their clinical practice. The most important diagnostic aid is a high degree of awareness. The liquor volume is assessed and presentation checked from 32 weeks. After 36 weeks persistent breech presentation should be managed appropriately (see Ch. 29). The fetal head usually engages from 36–38 weeks in nulliparous women but in at least 40% of parous women, engagement does not occur until labour begins. An unengaged head may be due to:

1. Pelvic mass—placenta praevia, tumour
2. Large presenting diameter—hydrocephalus, malpresentation, malposition
3. Large uterus—polyhydramnios, multiple pregnancy
4. Small pelvis—cephalopelvic disproportion, abnormal pelvis.

The ease with which the head enters the pelvis can be determined by gently pressing the head into the pelvis with the woman semiseated. A pelvic examination should be performed to exclude major bony abnormality, and many obstetricians will repeat the ultrasound scan if the head remains high after 38 weeks.

Investigations

Routine screening tests have been described. The haemoglobin concentration and antibody titres in rhesus-negative women are measured at 30 and 36 weeks unless they are abnormal.

The most common causes of anaemia in pregnancy are iron deficiency and folate deficiency. These can be almost completely avoided by the administration of combined iron/folate preparations but many women find them difficult to take. Opinion on their routine use varies, but anaemia, particularly if associated with microcytosis and/or hypochromasia, should be treated with oral iron. Women should be seen weekly and compliance checked by asking the woman the colour of her stools, and measuring the haemoglobin concentration and reticulocyte count. Iron infusion is dangerous and it is better to admit the woman to ensure compliance rather than give an iron infusion.

In many centres, rhesus-negative women are routinely given anti-D immunoglobulin at 28 and 34 weeks to reduce the incidence of sensitization prior to delivery. It is now common to perform a screening test for abnormal glucose tolerance between 28 and 32 weeks. This usually comprises a 50 or 75 g oral glucose load with a blood glucose level 1 hour later. Normal values vary widely depending on the load given and the criteria adopted by the particular hospital.

Assessment of fetal growth and/or well-being

One of the major reasons for antenatal care is the detection of reduced fetal growth and yet failure to do so is common (50% undetected). The means of monitoring fetal well-being/growth are:

1. Clinical assessment at antenatal visits/symphysiofundal height
2. Fetal movements
3. Fetal heart rate recordings
4. Ultrasound assessment
5. Biophysical profile of the fetus
6. Doppler investigation of fetoplacental circulation
7. Cordocentesis.

The use of tests representing placental synthetic function, e.g. urinary oestriol, HPL, has largely been superseded by other measures. This is principally because these tests do not specifically measure fetal well-being and may be unreliable.

Clinical assessment

The importance of vigilance during routine antenatal clinics has been stressed.

Fetal movements

Every pregnant woman attending for antenatal care should be questioned regarding fetal movements over the preceding few days. A significant decrease in movements warrants further investigation, i.e. ultrasound scan and fetal heart rate recording and subsequent closer surveillance.

Most women report that their babies move less towards term and it often remains difficult to assess. It is better to be overcautious in this respect. The efficacy of fetal movement charts is debated but they probably make women more aware of fetal activity.

Ultrasound assessment

Ultrasound will only assess fetal growth if used in a serial manner.

Although a single scan may suggest growth retardation, i.e. disproportionately low overall fetal measurements (symmetrical growth retardation), or reduced abdominal circumference (asymmetrical growth retardation) or reduced liquor volume, a follow-up scan is often necessary to assess growth. The routine scan at 18–20 weeks is vital to confirm that gestation is correct.

Biophysical profile

A fetal heart rate monitor and ultrasound machine are used simultaneously to assess in the fetus:

1. Limb and body movements
2. Breathing movements
3. Tone
4. Amniotic fluid volume
5. Heart rate variability.

Each of these variables is scored to make up the profile. However, to evaluate all these parameters is time consuming, and so limb and body movement, amniotic fluid volume and fetal heart rate recordings are often assessed without the others.

Fetal heart rate recording

This gives an indication of the current status of the fetus. A normal pattern with accelerations in response to fetal movements is a good indication of normal fetal well-being. However, computerized analysis is now available to aid in interpretation.

The significance of some patterns can be difficult to interpret, particularly in very preterm fetuses. The presence of decelerations when the woman is not in labour usually indicates that immediate delivery is required.

Fetoplacental blood flow

The use of the Doppler principle to measure blood flow velocity in the uterine and umbilical arteries, together with the fetal arterial system, is helpful in the assessment of the high-risk pregnancies. Perinatal outcome has been shown to improve using these investigations. Studies in the general population on the use of Doppler as a screening test for detecting fetal compromise have shown no benefit.

Reduced, absent, or even reverse flow in the umbilical artery during diastole is an indication of increased placental resistance and therefore probably impaired fetal oxygenation. Used in conjunction with other tests it may be helpful in judging when to deliver preterm fetuses.

Cordocentesis

Rarely cordocentesis is being used to monitor the condition of the severely compromised fetus, usually in the second trimester when a karyotype is also required. The measurement of fetal arterial pH, acid-base status and oxygenation may give information about a severely compromised fetus at one time point, but unfortunately cannot give predictive information. As the risks of serial sampling are not insignificant, non-invasive assessment is preferred.

General advice in pregnancy

Pregnancy is a stressful time for both partners (and other children). Antenatal visits should provide the opportunity for women to ask about minor problems as well as ensuring that all screening tests and routine assessment is carried out. Most hospital clinics provide mothers with an easily readable information booklet, e.g. *Pregnancy Book* by the Health Education Council.

Diet

Although pregnancy increases the mother's dietary requirements, a balanced diet is sufficient to provide all the calories, protein, minerals and vitamins required. The only exception is iron. If iron is not given in pregnancy, iron stores will decline. However, provided that these were adequate initially this is not a problem. Women who are already anaemic, have depleted iron stores (grand multipara, recent pregnancy) or who have a multiple pregnancy should have combined iron and folate supplementation.

Exercise

The amount of exercise desirable in pregnancy has never been determined. It seems prudent not to begin vigorous exercise when pregnant and similarly safe to continue routine exercise as long as it is not causing serious discomfort.

Sexual activity

There is no evidence that coitus is harmful in pregnancy. Most obstetricians advise against coitus in the first trimester in women who have had recurrent miscarriages, but there is no evidence to support this view. Many women lose their inclination for sex as pregnancy advances because of their increasing awkwardness and feelings of not being attractive. Couples should be encouraged to communicate these feelings. Sexual techniques may need to be modified to avoid pressure on the uterus.

Rest and sleep

Most women are more easily fatigued in pregnancy and there is some evidence that regular resting improves fetal outcome. Resting should therefore be encouraged, particularly in women with demanding lives.

Sleep patterns tend to become less regular with more frequent waking as pregnancy continues and women may need daytime naps to catch up.

Employment

The evidence on the effect of work on pregnancy is difficult to assess. Jobs involving a lot of standing may lead to reduced fetal growth but other variables are important, such as the number of children the pregnant woman cares for at home. It seems sensible to advise each woman individually depending on her wishes, type of work, and demands of her home life.

Heavy manual labour should be avoided and pregnant women must be allowed to rest if necessary. Noxious fumes, extremes of temperature and working to exhaustion should be avoided.

Clothing

A supportive brassiere and comfortable clothes are the basic requirements. Most women find flat-heeled shoes more comfortable in later pregnancy.

Preparation for lactation

All participants in antenatal care should strongly encourage breast-feeding. In the antenatal period it is important to ensure that the woman understands the advantages of breast-feeding and the normal events in milk production after delivery.

There is no need to encourage frequent handling of the nipples to prepare them for feeding. Inverted nipples usually correct themselves during pregnancy and can be made to protrude with gentle manipulation. If these measures are unsuccessful then nipple shields are used and kept in place by the brassiere.

Antenatal education

Classes are usually available in hospital clinics. A wide range of matters need to be covered including changes in late pregnancy, when to come in to the delivery suite, choice of methods for delivery position and pain relief, what clothes the baby will need and when to buy them, how to cope with a new baby and discussion on how the baby is likely to affect the couple.

Most classes take prospective parents on a tour of the labour and postnatal wards to prepare them for delivery. Birth plans are encouraged at most hospitals but it is important to emphasize that labour and delivery can be unpredictable and that all women (and their partners) need to retain an open mind. Questioning should be encouraged and all answers should be given in terms which can be easily understood.

Follow-up

One of the most important aspects of antenatal care is that follow-up should occur so that the woman and her partner have the opportunity to discuss their labour and management. Much of this discussion occurs on the postnatal ward and with the visits of the domiciliary midwife after discharge from hospital. This information is important in ensuring that misunderstandings are corrected and negative experiences discussed.

21. Minor disorders of pregnancy

G. Davis

Expectations of the examiners

As these disorders are not usually disabling they are often treated initially by general practitioners. The examiners will therefore expect candidates to have a sound knowledge of their causes and a common sense approach to their management.

Nausea and vomiting

The majority of women experience some nausea in early pregnancy and 50% will vomit. Although classically worse in the mornings it may occur throughout the day and is often made worse by the odours associated with preparing food. If severe, multiple pregnancy and hydatidiform mole need to be excluded. Symptoms usually improve after 14–16 weeks although many women continue to experience nausea, and sometimes vomiting, more frequently than when not pregnant.

Management

In most instances, symptoms can be controlled by dietary measures. Greasy or highly spiced foods should be avoided and frequent small meals usually improve the nausea. A rearrangement of housekeeping duties may be required if the woman is responsible for these. Reassurance, practical help in coping with the symptoms and the knowledge that the problem usually improves, are important aspects of the medical care.

Admission to hospital is required if the woman is becoming dehydrated (ketones in urine), if there is significant weight loss or if the social situation is getting out of control. In hospital, fluids are given intravenously (with potassium supplementation), antiemetics are used (initially metoclopramide then prochlorperazine if this is ineffective) and no oral intake is permitted. The condition is usually improving by 24–36 hours and dry biscuits can usually be introduced by 48 hours. If there is no improvement, then intravenous alimentation may be required. Early discharge from hospital is discouraged as it is often followed by prompt readmission.

Heartburn

This is also common in pregnancy and results from gastric reflux due to relaxation of the lower oesophageal sphincter and pressure from the enlarging uterus later in pregnancy.

The condition should be treated by discouraging smoking (increases sphincter relaxation), recommending frequent, light, bland meals, avoiding a late meal, and raising the head of the bed about 20 cm. Antacid preparations, e.g. magnesium trisilicate, may also be helpful but those that are likely to cause constipation should be avoided (aluminium containing).

Constipation/bloating

It is thought that these symptoms are due to decreased bowel motility because of high levels of progesterone. Normal measures should be used to combat constipation: dietary fibre and fluid intake should increase, sugar intake should decrease and a bulk laxative, e.g. ispaghula husk, used if necessary. Bloating seems to occur independently and is difficult to treat effectively.

Haemorrhoids

These occur more frequently in pregnancy due to progesterone-induced venodilatation, obstruction of venous return from the lower body by the enlarged uterus, and increased bearing down because of constipation or at delivery.

Prolapse is best treated with ice packs and replacement if possible. Bleeding is common and a rectal examination should be performed in this instance. For mild symptoms, a soothing preparation with a mild astringent action is usually sufficient. Rarely surgical intervention may be necessary.

Epistaxis

This occurs as a result of increased peripheral vascularity. Normal first aid measures usually suffice and definitive treatment is rarely necessary.

Varicose veins

Varicosities occur mostly in the legs but also in the vulva and vagina and cause aching and tiredness. Thrombophlebitis is the commonest complication and deep venous thrombosis may also occur, although this is more common in the puerperium.

For leg varicosities, the best treatment is a combination of elevation and the use of full-length support tights. Surgical management is best reserved for at least 2–3 months postpartum when the veins will have returned to normal after pregnancy.

Backache

This is a common symptom and results from increased joint laxity in the lumbar spine and the exaggerated lordosis which occurs in pregnancy. Sacroiliac joint laxity may also cause pain. Management is conservative: rest, analgesia, and improvement in posture.

Breast soreness

This is commonest in early pregnancy as the breasts increase in size. Reassurance and symptomatic relief with a brassiere that provides adequate support are all that is needed.

Fatigue

This is a common symptom early in pregnancy when the cause is unclear, and late in pregnancy when it is due to the increased physical effort required for everyday life and often a disturbed sleep pattern. The only treatment is frequent rest and reassurance that it is normal.

Peripheral paraesthesiae

Numbness and tingling occur due to compression of peripheral nerves because of fluid retention, most commonly the median nerve (carpal tunnel syndrome). Other nerves may be affected such as the lateral cutaneous nerve of the thigh which supplies the lateral aspect of the thigh. No treatment is usually required when the cause has been explained to the patient.

Headache

This is usually a typical tension headache and is best treated by rest and mild analgesia. Migraine often improves but may deteriorate, stay the same or occur de novo, in pregnancy. The use in pregnancy of agents normally used in the treatment of migraine is not associated with adverse fetal outcome but doses should be kept to the minimum required.

Postural hypotension

This is more likely to occur in pregnancy because of venous pooling in the lower limbs (see 'Haemorrhoids' above). It is best prevented by avoiding precipitating factors: standing up quickly, hot baths, standing in hot weather.

Pruritus

Itching in pregnancy may be localized or generalized. Local causes are usually infectious (e.g. scabies, thrush). Generalized itching (pruritus gravidarum) usually begins in the third trimester and is almost always associated with some degree of biliary obstruction. Frank jaundice is rare but cholestasis of pregnancy must be distinguished from other causes of liver disease in pregnancy and non-pregnancy.

Cholestasis in pregnancy used to be considered a benign condition. However, more recent evidence suggests an increased perinatal mortality. For this reason, most obstetricians would induce labour at 36–38 weeks depending on the severity of the cholestasis. The pruritus disappears shortly after delivery but recurs in 50% of subsequent pregnancies. Treatment with skin lubrication and topical antipruritics is usually sufficient and antihistamines are of limited benefit.

Frequency of micturition

Again this is a symptom of early pregnancy when it may be due to increased renal filtration, and of late pregnancy when it is due to pressure from the enlarged uterus. There is no treatment for this symptom except delivery. Urinary tract infection is also common in pregnancy and needs to be excluded.

Insomnia

Disturbed sleep results from normal anxieties about being pregnant and later the increased size of breasts and abdomen. Sedatives should be avoided unless the woman is exhausted and should then be used for a very brief period, e.g. 2–3 nights. Relaxation exercises to relieve anxiety may be of benefit.

SUMMARY

Minor disorders of pregnancy are very common but serious conditions need to be excluded, e.g. imminent eclampsia causing headache, viral hepatitis causing pruritus. Education and reassurance together with simple, practical remedies are the basis for treatment of most of these conditions.

22. Infections in pregnancy

A. Rodin

Expectations of the examiners

An understanding of the effects on the mother and the fetus of significant infections in pregnancy is needed.

Interesting facts

Maternal infections during pregnancy are common and are usually insignificant but may result in congenital infection and handicap. The incidence of death or handicap as a result of intrauterine infection is estimated to be 0.4 in 1000 live births. The incidence of many congenital infections shows marked regional variation, e.g. toxoplasmosis is commoner in France than in the UK. In some cases, congenital infections can be prevented and/or treated. The role of ascending infection in the causation of preterm labour is currently being evaluated.

Pathogenesis

Infections may reach the fetus by four main routes:

1. Transplacental spread from the maternal bloodstream
2. Ascending infection from the genital tract after rupture of membranes
3. Infection acquired during passage of the fetus through the birth canal
4. Rarely, infection may follow invasive intra-amniotic procedures, e.g. amniocentesis and fetoscopy.

The effects on the fetus depend on the nature of the infective organism, the gestation at which infection occurs and the immune status of the mother. Following maternal infection there may be no spread to the fetus; however, it may reach the placenta and infect the fetus in utero. Fetal infection may manifest itself by abortion or stillbirth. If the pregnancy continues, the infant may be born with a variety of abnormalities (TORCH syndrome, see below) and it may develop acute neonatal illness. An infant of an infected mother who appears normal at birth may develop late effects and should be followed up.

The infectious agents causing the TORCH syndrome are:

1. Toxoplasmosis
2. Rubella
3. Cytomegalovirus
4. Herpes simplex.

These cause a mild, non-specific maternal illness and similar patterns of fetal damage. Features of the TORCH syndrome include:

1. Low birth weight
2. Microcephaly
3. Congenital heart disease
4. Eye lesions
5. Jaundice
6. Hepatosplenomegaly
7. Petechiae/purpura
8. Late effects:
   a. Visual defects
   b. Deafness
   c. Developmental delay
   d. Mental retardation.

RUBELLA

The association between maternal rubella infection in pregnancy and congenital heart disease and cataracts in the neonate was first described in 1941. Rubella is a RNA virus and is spread by droplet infection.

Maternal illness

Mild febrile illness with a macular rash and lymphadenopathy; many infections are subclinical. One infection confers a high degree of immunity and congenital infection usually follows primary maternal infection.

Fetal effects

The risk of congenital defects depends on the gestation when infection occurs: infection in the first trimester carries a high risk of major defects and infection between 12 and 16 weeks may cause sensorineural deafness. Hearing impairment is the most frequent defect associated with rubella.

Screening

All women are screened for rubella antibody (IgG) at booking. Susceptible women who develop a rash or come into contact with rubella have blood taken to check rubella IgG. If this is positive, IgM is measured to confirm recent infection.

Immunization

A live attenuated virus vaccine was introduced in 1970 and this was given to prepubertal girls and non-immune women.

Ninety-eight per cent of women in the UK attending antenatal clinics are now immune to rubella.

In 1988, the MMR vaccination (measles, mumps and rubella) was introduced and this is given to all male and female infants between 1 and 2 years of age in an attempt to eradicate rubella. Vaccination of prepubertal girls and non-immune women will continue until sufficient numbers have received MMR vaccination.

Vaccination should not be administered during pregnancy and conception within 3 months should be avoided.

CYTOMEGALOVIRUS

Cytomegalovirus (CMV) is the most common congenital infection and approximately 3 in 1000 live births are infected in England and Wales each year. CMV is a DNA virus of the herpes group and it is spread venereally by the oropharyngeal route, or by blood transfusion.

Maternal illness

CMV infection is usually symptomless, therefore diagnosis is retrospective following discovery of a congenitally infected infant. Fifty per cent of adults have antibodies to CMV. Fetal infection may follow primary maternal infection or reactivation of maternal infection.

Fetal effects

Diagnosis is made by isolation of the virus from urine or a throat swab in the first few weeks of life.

Defects may follow infection at any gestation and 10% of infected infants have significant handicaps. Sensorineural deafness is the most common sequel. Acute neonatal illness (cytomegalic inclusion disease) occurs in 5% of infected infants and is associated with a high mortality.

Screening

This is not useful because congenital infection may follow reactivation of an old infection and defects may follow exposure at any gestation. Most cases of maternal CMV infection are asymptomatic.

Immunization

Immunization is not available.

TOXOPLASMOSIS

This is an infection with the protozoon *Toxoplasma gondii*. Oocysts from this organism are found in raw meat and cat faeces. This is a rare congenital infection in the UK and approximately 1 in 100 000 live births are infected.

Maternal illness

Infection is usually subclinical and only 10% of affected women have fever and lymphadenopathy.

Fetal infection is seen only after primary infection in the mother.

Fetal effects

Congenital infection occurs in 30% of infants whose mothers seroconvert during pregnancy. The earlier the infection occurs the more severe the effect. Classical manifestations are hydrocephaly, retrochoroiditis and intracranial calcification. Stillbirth, neonatal death or severe handicap occur in 5% of these infants and late effects may occur.

Screening

Screening is not done routinely at present in the UK.

Treatment

Spiramycin is the drug of choice for treatment of the mother with primary infection. This may reduce the fetal infection rate by 60–70%. Treatment is continued until term.

HERPES SIMPLEX

Herpes simplex virus (HSV) is a DNA virus and is widespread in human populations. Most perinatal infections are caused by HSV type 2. Transplacental infection is rare and infection usually occurs during delivery.

Maternal illness

Genital ulceration follows primary infection by HSV type 2. Reactivation of infection may occur during pregnancy but rarely causes neonatal disease.

Fetal effects

There is a small risk of infection during delivery but the mortality from disseminated neurological disease is high.

Screening

Taking cervical swabs for the detection of HSV in later pregnancy is common practice, but their value is controversial. It is estimated that this method detects only 25% of women shedding virus at the time of delivery.

Management

This is controversial. In most centres, women with active genital lesions or positive viral cultures in later pregnancy are delivered by elective caesarean section. If membranes have been ruptured for 4 hours or more, the risk of infection is thought to be no greater from vaginal delivery than from caesarean section. The mortality from neonatal herpes infection has been reduced by the use of antiviral agents.

VARICELLA

Varicella (primary herpes zoster, chickenpox) is rare during pregnancy as most adults were infected during childhood.

Maternal illness

Varicella is a febrile illness with a characteristic rash and reactivation of the virus may cause shingles.

Fetal effects

Congenital varicella syndrome with characteristic limb hypoplasia and skin scarring is extremely rare.

Varicella carries a high morbidity and mortality in infants who develop a rash 5–10 days after birth. However, if the rash appears before this, the illness is benign; this is because when maternal illness occurs >7 days before delivery, maternal antibodies cross the placenta and confer passive immunity. If infection occurs after this, antibody levels are too low to be protective.

Treatment

In cases of maternal varicella at around the time of delivery, the neonate is given antivaricella zoster immune globulin.

LISTERIA

Listeriosis is caused by *Listeria monocytogenes*. This is a gram-positive bacillus which is widely distributed in the environment. It has been found in soft cheeses and prepacked foods. Listeriosis occurs in 1 in 7000 pregnancies.

Maternal effects

Non-specific febrile illness.

Fetal effects

Listeriosis is associated with spontaneous abortion, stillbirth and neonatal death.

Treatment

Ampicillin.

OTHER INFECTIONS IN PREGNANCY

Urinary tract infections

Urinary tract infections are common and range in severity from asymptomatic bacteriuria to pyelonephritis. *E. coli* is responsible for up to 90% of urinary tract infections during pregnancy. Bacteriuria (>100 000 bacteria/ml urine) may be asymptomatic and is found in 5% of women on routine screening. Acute pyelonephritis complicates up to 2% of pregnancies and is associated with an increased incidence of preterm labour. Patients are admitted to hospital and treated initially with intravenous antibiotics.

See also Chapter 39, 'Sexually transmitted infections in women'.

23. Major complications of pregnancy

PART 1
PRETERM LABOUR
A. Rodin

Expectations of the examiners

A clear understanding of this subject is essential and the candidate is expected to be able to discuss the areas of controversy in the management of this problem.

Definitions

Prematurity is defined as delivery prior to 37 completed weeks of pregnancy (WHO definition). In practical terms, most complications occur at gestations less than 34 weeks and most obstetricians would allow delivery beyond this gestation. Low birth weight infants weigh less than 2500 g at delivery and they may be preterm, growth retarded or both. Very low birth weight infants weigh less than 1500 g at delivery.

Interesting facts

Preterm labour complicates 5–10% of pregnancies and it is the major factor contributing to perinatal mortality and morbidity. Preterm delivery is responsible for 75% of all perinatal deaths and 85% of neonatal deaths not due to congenital abnormality. The diagnosis of preterm labour is difficult and up to 50% of women who complain of painful uterine contractions prior to 37 weeks do not proceed to delivery.

The survival rate of preterm infants has increased in recent years and this is mainly due to advances in neonatal care. After 32 weeks, survival is almost equivalent to those infants born at term, and in most centres, survival of infants weighing >1000 g is 70%. Preterm delivery may be associated with long-term handicap.

Pathophysiology

The mechanism of normal and preterm labour remains unknown and therefore the pathophysiology of this process remains uncertain. In about 60% of cases a cause can be identified but the remainder are idiopathic.

Causes of preterm labour

1. Maternal
    a. Pre-eclampsia
    b. Antepartum haemorrhage
    c. Chorioamnionitis
    d. Other infections, e.g. pyelonephritis
    e. Uterine abnormalities, e.g. congenital septa, cervical incompetence
    f. Polyhydramnios
2. Fetal
    a. Multiple pregnancy
    b. Intrauterine death
    c. Congenital abnormality
    d. Growth retardation.

In addition, a number of risk factors have been identified which are thought to increase the chances of preterm labour and delivery in an individual.

Risk factors for preterm labour

1. General
    a. Low socioeconomic class
    b. Multiparity
    c. Maternal age <20 years
    d. Low prepregnancy weight
    e. Smoking
2. Past obstetric factors
    a. Previous preterm labour
    b. Previous low birth weight infant
    c. Previous antepartum haemorrhage
3. Current pregnancy
    a. Threatened miscarriage
    b. Unexplained elevated AFP
    c. Antepartum haemorrhage

Attempts to devise scoring systems to predict the risk of preterm delivery have been unsuccessful and the best predictor of preterm delivery is a previous preterm delivery.

Assessment

It is essential to make an accurate diagnosis of preterm labour before any intervention is initiated. A history is taken and questions are directed at finding a cause for preterm labour. Gestational age is checked. General examination is performed and the state of the cervix is assessed noting whether membranes are ruptured or intact.

Cardiotocography is used to assess fetal condition and to confirm regular uterine activity. Ultrasound examination can be used to confirm fetal presentation, to exclude major fetal abnormalities, and to obtain an estimate of fetal weight.

The presence or absence of fetal breathing movements (FBM) has been suggested as an indicator of the outcome of preterm labour. It has been shown that in patients in preterm labour who show no FBMs over a 45-minute period, delivery in the next 48 hours is almost inevitable. The presence of FBMs indicates that the pregnancy is likely to continue.

The decision to attempt to stop preterm labour depends on a number of factors:

1. Gestational age
2. Cause of preterm labour
3. State of cervix and membranes
4. Maternal condition
5. Fetal condition
6. Local paediatric facilities.

Management

The use of tocolytics

Tocolytics act by inhibiting smooth muscle contractility. The most commonly used agents are the β sympathomimetics (salbutamol, ritodrine, etc.) which have the effect of reducing the concentration of free calcium ions within the myometrial cells and preventing contraction. These drugs have important maternal side-effects, including tachycardia and impaired glucose tolerance, and their use should be avoided in women with cardiac disease and insulin-dependent diabetes mellitus. Acute pulmonary oedema is a rare complication and is usually associated with fluid overload.

Other agents which have been used include alcohol, prostaglandin synthetase inhibitors, and calcium antagonists. Tocolytics have been shown to prolong pregnancy, however they have not yet been shown to improve perinatal mortality. They may be used in the short term to permit prenatal transfer or in the longer term to allow steroid-induced maturation of the fetal lungs. There is no evidence to support the use of oral sympathomimetics as prophylaxis for preterm labour.

The use of glucocorticoids

Antepartum administration of glucocorticoids reduces the incidence of respiratory distress syndrome (RDS) and mortality from RDS in infants between 28 and 32 weeks' gestation. (Steroids may be effective at gestations <28 weeks but evidence is lacking.) For optimum effect, delivery should take place more than 24 hours and less than 7 days after the start of treatment. A suitable regimen is betamethasone 12 mg—two doses are given intramuscularly 12 hours apart. The use of steroids in the presence of ruptured membranes is controversial because of the theoretically increased risk of intrauterine infection.

Delivery

If local neonatal intensive care facilities are inadequate, consider transfer of the patient. In utero transfer is preferred to neonatal transfer.

The mode of delivery of premature infants is controversial. Generally, infants presenting by the vertex are delivered vaginally. The routine use of forceps in these cases confers no benefit and may contribute to morbidity. Elective episiotomy is generally used. There is no consensus about the safest route of delivery for preterm infants presenting by the breech.

Prevention of preterm labour

There is much interest currently in strategies aimed at preventing preterm labour and delivery. Advice about smoking and nutrition is given routinely. Specific measures can be taken in the minority cases when there is an identifiable cause, e.g. cervical cerclage in cases of cervical incompetence. Screening techniques to identify those at risk of preterm labour are undergoing evaluation. Fetal fibronectin has been proposed as a biochemical marker for preterm delivery. This glycoprotein is found in amniotic fluid and placental tissue. Its presence in cervicovaginal secretions during the second and third trimester identifies a group of women who will deliver preterm.

PRETERM PREMATURE RUPTURE OF MEMBRANES (PPROPM)

Definition

Rupture of the membranes before the onset of labour and before completion of the 37th week of pregnancy.

Interesting facts

PPROM occurs in up to 40% of all labours.

Assessment

On admission, a history is taken and a sterile speculum examination is performed to confirm the presence of ruptured membranes. An endocervical swab is taken for microbiological examination.

Management

The risks of maternal and fetal infection must be balanced against the risks of prematurity and in the presence of group B streptococci or active genital herpes, delivery must be expedited regardless of gestation.

If gestation is 34 weeks or more, there is little to be gained by delay and labour should be induced if spontaneous contractions do not commence within a reasonable period of time. At earlier gestations, management is conservative and both mother and fetus are carefully monitored for signs of intrauterine infection:

1. Maternal pyrexia >37.2°C
2. Maternal leucocytosis
3. Uterine tenderness
4. Offensive liquor
5. Fetal tachycardia
6. Raised C reactive protein.

If contractions occur, intrauterine infection must be excluded before tocolytics and steroids are administered.

SUMMARY

Preterm delivery is a major cause of perinatal morbidity and mortality. In about 40% of cases, the cause is unknown. The use of risk factors to identify at-risk pregnancies is generally unsuccessful. The risks to the mother and fetus through continuing the pregnancy must be balanced against the risks to the fetus of preterm delivery.

PART 2
HYPERTENSIVE DISORDERS
J. Rymer

Expectations of the examiners

As pre-eclampsia is one of the commonest complications of pregnancy, the examiners will expect a thorough knowledge of all aspects of the subject. They will expect you to know how to classify 'hypertension' in pregnancy.

Definition

Hypertension may be defined as:

1. Mild—two diastolic blood pressure (DBP) recordings of 90 mmHg or more 4 hours apart or a diastolic blood pressure of 110 mmHg or more on one occasion.
2. Severe—two DBP recordings of 110 mmHg or more 4 hours apart, or DBP of 120 mmHg or more on one occasion.

Classification (WHO, RCOG)

Gestational hypertension. Hypertension after 20 weeks, during labour or the puerperium.

Pre-eclampsia. Proteinuric (>0.3 g/24 hours) hypertension after 20 weeks' gestation.

Chronic hypertension. Hypertension before 20 weeks/pre-existing.

Chronic renal disease. Proteinuric hypertension before 20 weeks.

Unclassified. No recording before 20 weeks.

PRE-ECLAMPSIA

Definition

A pregnancy-specific syndrome that is characterized by raised blood pressure with proteinuria that develops after 20 weeks' gestation and may terminate in eclampsia.

Interesting facts

Pre-eclampsia is the most important cause of IUGR in singletons with no malformations.

Cerebral haemorrhage is the major cause of maternal death in pre-eclampsia.

Pathophysiology

The aetiology is unknown, but there is thought to be an abnormality of the trophoblast or of the maternal response to the trophoblast. In normal pregnancy, sensitivity to angiotensin is lost, but in pre-eclampsia this does not occur.

High blood pressure is caused by vasoconstriction associated with decreased circulating plasma volume. The fundamental pathophysiological process affects all maternal organs with specific effects on placenta, cardiovascular, renal, clotting and nervous systems and the liver.

Assessment

Symptoms are usually absent in pre-eclampsia. However, if it is severe, the patient may complain of headache, blurred vision and epigastric pain.

On examination the woman may have high blood pressure, vasoconstriction, hyperreflexia, vomiting, tender liver, oliguria, spontaneous bleeding, bruising, and signs of raised intracranial pressure. (Oedema is a normal phenomenon of pregnancy but may be gross in pre-eclampsia.)

Investigations

FBC and platelets

As mentioned above, pre-eclamptic women have a reduced plasma volume so the haemoglobin concentration will be elevated, as will the packed cell volume. With severe disease, platelet consumption occurs, and the platelet level drops. Disseminated intravascular coagulation can develop so clotting tests must be performed.

Urea, creatinine, urate

When the renal system becomes involved there is reduced uric acid clearance, thus elevating the plasma uric acid. With worsening disease the urea and creatinine levels will also rise and renal failure may develop in severe cases.

Urine

Screening relies on dipsticks but may give false-positive results if the urine is alkaline, and false negatives if the urine is highly dilute or contains proteins other than albumin. Any positive result (+1 or more) necessitates an MSU to exclude infection. The amount of proteinuria should be determined in a 24-hour collection.

Liver function tests

In the presence of proteinuria or a reduced platelet count, liver enzymes should be measured (e.g. plasma aspartate transaminase).

Ultrasound scan

As the uteroplacental circulation is impaired the fetus is at risk. Perinatal mortality increases once proteinuria is established. IUGR is more common with early onset disease.

Management

Mild disease

Admit for 48 hours for assessment or see daily in a day assessment unit.

1. Monitor mother
   a. 4-hourly BP
   b. Full blood count and platelets, and clotting function
   c. 24-hour urine for protein estimation
   d. Serum urate, urea and creatinine
   e. Liver function tests.
2. Monitor fetus
   a. Movement chart
   b. Ultrasound scan.

If the blood pressure settles, cases of mild disease can be managed as an outpatient with daily midwife visits to check the blood pressure and the urine for protein.

Moderate disease

As for mild disease, but inpatient rather than outpatient care is advised. The place for drug treatment in pre-eclampsia is to gain control of the blood pressure to protect the cerebral vessels. It is a temporary inpatient measure as delivery is the definitive treatment. If antihypertensive medication is commenced it must be remembered that one of the major signs of worsening disease is masked.

Severe disease

Admit and deliver.
   Do baseline investigations as above including clotting studies.
   Commence antihypertensives. It is difficult to know which patients should be commenced on anticonvulsants. Hyperreflexia can be used as an indicator but is unreliable. Clonus indicates that eclampsia is imminent especially if there are more than two beats. Assess general well-being, as a woman who feels well is unlikely to have an eclamptic fit.
   The mode of delivery depends on the gestation, the presentation of the fetus, and the state of the cervix.
   After delivery the patient is still at risk of an eclamptic fit for at least 48 hours. The clotting factors and the urine output must be watched carefully. Fluid management is difficult as the patient may be oliguric and haemoconcentrated, so a central venous pressure line is advisable.
   If a clotting disorder has developed, and the platelet count is $<100 \times 10^9/1$ an epidural is contraindicated.

Antihypertensives

Labetalol. Labetalol is an α and β adrenergic blocker that causes vasodilatation, bradycardia, and reduces myometrial activity. Commence with 100 mg b.d. and increase up to 2.6 g daily.

Methyldopa. Methyldopa acts centrally, decreasing the sympathetic outflow from the brain. An initial dose of 500 mg is given and then 250 mg 6-hourly to a maximum of 750 mg 6-hourly.

Hydralazine. Hydralazine is a non-specific vasodilator that causes a reflex tachycardia, and sometimes headache. Useful for the acute reduction of blood pressure, where it can be given intravenously, e.g. 5 mg boluses given every 5 minutes titrated against the blood pressure (maximum of 20 mg).

Nifedipine. Nifedipine is a calcium channel blocker and vasodilator. It is useful for treating the acute rises in blood pressure. It is taken sublingually (10 mg) and may cause headache.

Anticonvulsants

It is difficult to identify the patients who need anticonvulsants. If there are symptoms or signs of imminent eclampsia then anticonvulsants are advisable. The purpose of anticonvulsants is to prevent fitting rather than to sedate the patient.

Magnesium sulphate is significantly more effective then phenytoin or diazepam in preventing convulsions. It is given as an i.v. infusion and the respiratory rate and patellar reflexes must be checked regularly. Reduced patellar reflexes usually precede respiratory depression. If one measures $MgSO_4$ levels the desirable levels are between 2.0 and 3.5 mmol/l, and should be checked at 1 and 4 hours and then 6-hourly.

ECLAMPSIA

This is a serious complication of pre-eclampsia because it is associated with increased maternal and fetal morbidity and mortality.

Aetiology

Fitting is a result of brain hypoxia due to ischaemia secondary to oedema and intense vasospasm.

Management

Prevention is important and most women with severe pre-eclampsia should be commenced on anticonvulsant therapy. If fits occur, basic measures are needed to establish an airway, maintain breathing and circulation. The fit should be stopped with intravenous diazepam, the blood pressure controlled, and anticonvulsants commenced. If the fetus is still in utero delivery must be expedited. Maternal sedation is needed postpartum and should be continued for at least 48 hours. Urine output, clotting and liver function tests should be closely monitored.

HELLP SYNDROME

This is an acronym for haemolysis, elevated liver enzymes and low platelets. It is a variant of pre-eclampsia affecting 4–12% of those with pre-eclampsia/eclampsia and is commoner in multigravidae. There may be acute renal failure and disseminated intravascular coagulation, and there is an increased incidence of abruption. Management is as for severe pre-eclampsia.

ESSENTIAL HYPERTENSION

In essential hypertension, the prepregnancy blood pressure is elevated and there is an absent mid-trimester drop. Essential hypertension is one of the major predisposing factors to pre-eclampsia (five times the risk). The majority of hypertensive women who do not develop pre-eclampsia can expect a normal perinatal outcome. The control of moderate chronic hypertension in early pregnancy does not lessen the eventual incidence of superimposed pre-eclampsia.

The general aims of antenatal care are to keep the blood pressure at a safe level, and to monitor maternal renal function. Growth of the fetus should be assessed regularly by serial ultrasound.

PART 3
RHESUS ISOIMMUNIZATION
A. Rodin

Expectations of the examiners

The candidate should have a knowledge of the pathophysiology of this uncommon complication, and the importance of anti-D prophylaxis should be understood.

Interesting facts

The incidence of rhesus isoimmunization has fallen dramatically since the introduction of anti-D prophylaxis in the late 1960s and rhesus disease is no longer a major cause of perinatal mortality and morbidity. The few cases that occur are mainly due to a failure of prophylaxis or to haemolytic disease occurring in the rhesus-positive mother with other maternal alloantibodies.

Pathophysiology

The rhesus gene is made up of three parts which may be C or c, D or d, and E or e, respectively. Rhesus-negative women constitute 15% of the population and they are homozygous for d. Maternal anti-D antibodies (IgG) may form when rhesus-positive fetal cells enter the circulation of a rhesus-negative mother. This commonly occurs at delivery, but fetomaternal haemorrhage may follow other complications and procedures.

Causes of fetomaternal haemorrhage

1. Spontaneous abortion
2. Termination of pregnancy
3. Ectopic pregnancy
4. Antepartum haemorrhage
5. External cephalic version
6. Amniocentesis/chorionic villus sampling
7. Delivery
8. Manual removal of placenta.

As immunization usually occurs at the end of the woman's first pregnancy, it is the second and subsequent pregnancies which are affected by haemolytic disease. If the fetus is rhesus-positive in the next pregnancy there is a rise in maternal anti-D IgG which crosses the placenta and causes haemolysis of fetal red cells. This results in anaemia and, in severe cases, hydrops fetalis.

Destruction of fetal red cells leads to a rise in unconjugated bilirubin which crosses the placenta to reach the maternal circulation and liver. Some of the unconjugated bilirubin enters the amniotic fluid where levels can be measured. After delivery, haemolysis continues and levels of unconjugated bilirubin continue to rise with a risk of kernicterus (free unconjugated bilirubin is toxic to cells of the CNS and this may be a fatal condition; surviving infants may have cerebral palsy, mental retardation, and deafness).

Assessment

Assessment of the sensitized woman is aimed at determining whether treatment is necessary and when treatment should be initiated.

Past obstetric history

Severity of disease increases in successive pregnancies and this helps to plan management of the current pregnancy.

Serology

If antibodies are detected, the partner's genotype is checked and if he is rhesus-negative further action may be unnecessary if paternity is certain. If the antibody titre exceeds 4 i.u./ml, amniocentesis is indicated.

Amniocentesis

Amniotic fluid bilirubin concentrations correlate with the severity of haemolysis. Spectrophotometry at an optical density of 450 nm produces a peak which is directly proportional to the amount of bilirubin in the liquor. Timing depends on past history and maternal antibody levels. Action-line analysis charts are used to interpret the result and plan future management.

Fetal blood sampling

Cordocentesis provides a means of directly assessing the haematological state of the fetus.

Management

At booking, screening for irregular antibodies is performed on all women. An ultrasound scan to confirm gestation is particularly important. Early referral to a regional unit is indicated for women who have had previous affected pregnancies.

In non-sensitized rhesus-negative women, screening is repeated at 28, 32, and 36 weeks. If antibodies are detected and the partner's genotype is rhesus-positive the woman is referred to a regional unit for care. Maternal antibody levels are monitored. Further management is guided by the results of amniocentesis and/or fetal blood sampling. Premature delivery may be necessary.

Treatment

1. Plasmapheresis. This has been used to reduce the maternal circulating antibody level before intraperitoneal transfusion can be performed (<20 weeks). This technique continues to be controversial.

2. Intrauterine transfusion
   a. Intraperitoneal
   b. Intravascular.

Blood tests at delivery

1. Maternal—Kleihauer test (see below)
2. Fetal—haemoglobin, blood grouping, Coombs' test, bilirubin.

Prevention of rhesus isoimmunization

The administration of anti-D IgG to the mother within 72 hours of a fetomaternal haemorrhage will prevent isoimmunization provided it is given in sufficient quantity. The size of fetomaternal transfusion can be assessed by performing a Kleihauer test. A film of maternal blood is treated with acid and maternal cells become ghosted because of the denaturation of haemoglobin; fetal haemoglobin is resistant and so fetal and maternal red cells may be distinguished. The finding of five fetal cells per 50 high power fields corresponds with a fetomaternal transfusion of 2.5 ml. 500 i.u. of anti-D IgG will neutralize 4–5 ml of fetal blood. This dose is given to all unsensitized rhesus-negative mothers delivering at >20 weeks' gestation. In pregnancies which terminate before this gestation 250 i.u. are sufficient.

Failure of prophylaxis may be due to failure to give any or sufficient anti-D. It may also follow silent immunization during the antenatal period. Antenatal administration of anti-D has been suggested to counter this.

SUMMARY

Rhesus isoimmunization is now an uncommon complication following the introduction of prophylactic anti-D IgG. Affected pregnancies should be supervised at regional centres.

PART 4
INTRAUTERINE GROWTH RETARDATION
A. Rodin

Expectations of the examiners

An understanding of the two patterns of growth retardation is needed. The candidate will be expected to know how this condition may be detected clinically and how the diagnosis is confirmed.

Definition

Intrauterine growth retardation (IUGR) is defined as fetal weight less than the tenth percentile for gestational age.

Interesting facts

Before the introduction of ultrasonography, IUGR could only be diagnosed at birth when the infant was found to be small for gestational age, although it may have been suspected antenatally on clinical grounds. The diagnosis of IUGR relies on accurate dating and this has been facilitated by the use of ultrasound in early pregnancy. Ethnic variations in birth weight must be considered. Growth-retarded infants have a higher perinatal mortality rate, a higher incidence of neonatal morbidity and long-term cognitive performance may be impaired when compared to normal sized infants.

Pathophysiology

The pathophysiology of IUGR differs according to its aetiology but there are two main mechanisms:

1. Asymmetrical growth retardation: the supply of nutrients to the fetus is inadequate to support growth and this usually results from 'placental insufficiency'. This type of IUGR usually presents in later pregnancy when fetal needs are increasing. The vital organs are protected and there is sparing of head growth initially.
2. Symmetrical growth retardation: this occurs when the growth potential of the fetus is reduced, e.g. it may be due to chromosomal abnormalities or intrauterine infection. This type of IUGR usually appears early in pregnancy.

IUGR may be associated with oligohydramnios.

Aetiology

1. Maternal
   a. Pre-eclampsia/hypertension
   b. Placental abruption
   c. Diabetes mellitus
   d. Renal disease
   e. Smoking
   f. Alcohol
   g. Infections.
2. Fetal
   a. Chromosomal abnormalities
   b. Sickle cell disease

c. Achondroplasia
d. Potter's syndrome
e. Anencephaly
f. Multiple pregnancy.

IUGR may be idiopathic. It is associated with low socioeconomic class and may recur in subsequent pregnancies.

Assessment

An ultrasound scan is performed routinely at 18–20 weeks to confirm gestation. Some women will be in a high-risk group because of pre-existing medical disease or a past history of IUGR. Fetal growth in this group should be checked by serial ultrasound scans. In others, detection of IUGR depends on a high index of clinical suspicion. Maternal weight gain is a poor indicator of fetal growth.

On examination the uterus may be small for dates and there may be oligohydramnios. Measurement of symphysiofundal height is a sensitive test for IUGR and when this is abnormal an ultrasound scan should be arranged.

The parameters used in ultrasound growth assessment are biparietal diameter (BPD) (Fig. 23.1), head circumference (HC), abdominal circumference (AC) (Fig. 23.2), and femur length (FL) (Fig. 23.3). In addition, liquor volume should be noted. In symmetrical IUGR, growth in all measured parameters is uniformly decreased. In asymmetrical IUGR (Fig. 23.4), rate of growth of the fetal abdomen is slowed while head growth remains normal. The role of Doppler flow studies in the assessment of the growth-retarded fetus is being evaluated.

Investigations

In symmetrical IUGR a TORCH screen should be performed and fetal karyotyping may be indicated.

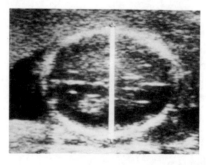

Fig. 23.1 The biparietal diameter must be measured when the head is in the occipitotransverse position, i.e. with the midline echo from the fetal brain at right angles to the ultrasound beam.

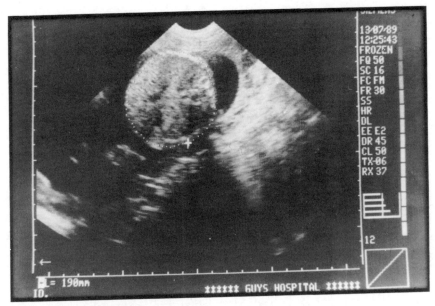

Fig. 23.2 The abdominal circumference.

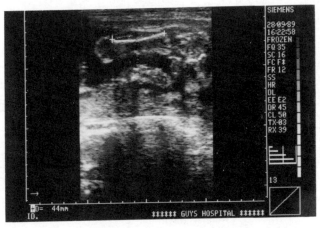

Fig. 23.3 Femur length is visualized on ultrasound scan and then measured.

Management

Once the diagnosis of IUGR has been made, hospital admission is arranged so that the condition of both mother and fetus can be monitored. History should be reviewed and a physical examination should be performed.

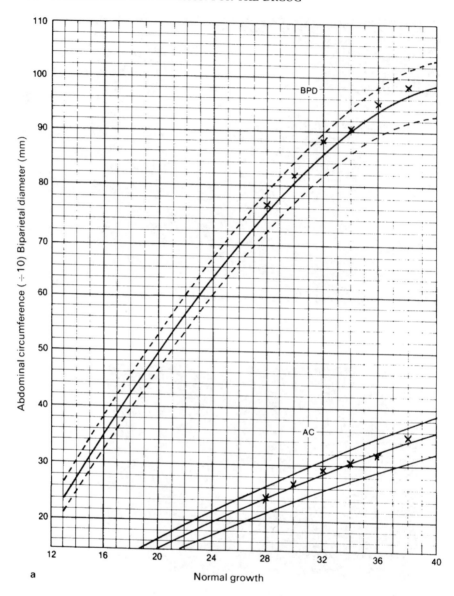

Fig. 23.4 Ultrasound measurements plotted on fetal growth charts. a, Normal growth; b, asymmetrical IUGR.

Growth scans are repeated every 2 weeks. Fetal well-being is assessed by monitoring of fetal movements and cardiotocography. Biochemical tests of placental function are no longer used routinely. In the future, Doppler flow studies and blood gas analysis of fetal blood obtained by cordocentesis may contribute to the management of these cases. Timing of delivery is usually

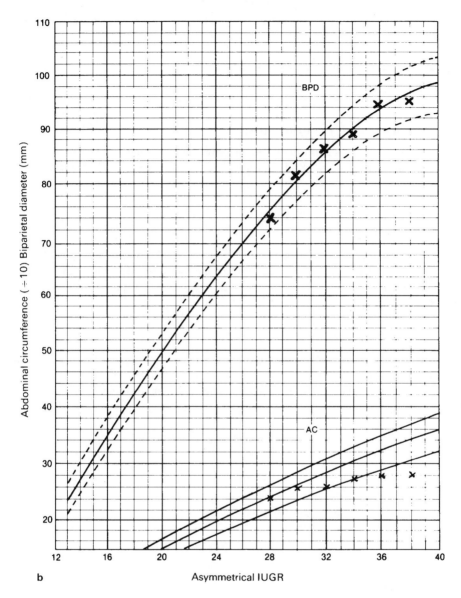

b   Asymmetrical IUGR

determined by fetal well-being. In some cases, delivery is prompted by a deterioration in maternal condition.

SUMMARY

IUGR is associated with increased perinatal morbidity and mortality. Suspected cases should be assessed by ultrasound scan. Once IUGR has been confirmed, fetal well-being should be monitored and the timing of delivery depends on fetal condition and subsequent growth.

PART 5
ANTEPARTUM HAEMORRHAGE
A. Rodin

Expectations of the examiners

The topic antepartum haemorrhage (APH) is particularly favoured by examiners and a clear understanding of the management of this condition is essential.

Definition

Bleeding from or into the genital tract after the 24th week of pregnancy and before delivery. The previous definition was after 28 weeks but as the definition of fetal viability has changed, 24 weeks is more useful.

Interesting facts

APH complicates 3% of all pregnancies and is associated with morbidity and mortality for both mother and fetus. The risk of APH rises with increasing maternal age, increasing parity, and cigarette smoking.

Causes of antepartum haemorrhage

1. Bleeding from the placenta
    a. Placental abruption
    b. Placenta praevia
    c. Bleeding from placental margin.
2. Bleeding from other sites
    a. Local causes, e.g. cervical polyp, cervical ectropion, cervical carcinoma
    b. Vasa praevia (rare)
    c. Unknown.

PLACENTAL ABRUPTION

Bleeding occurs due to separation of the placenta before delivery of the infant. This can vary in severity from a minor separation to complete placental detachment. The amount of vaginal bleeding does not correlate with the degree of placental separation and there may be total separation with no revealed bleeding.

Pathophysiology

Rupture of one or more maternal spiral arterioles occurs in the decidua basalis. The bleeding may be limited with the formation of a decidual haematoma. If bleeding continues, any or all of the following may occur:

1. Blood may track under the placenta extending the degree of placental separation and compromising the fetus.
2. Blood may dissect under the membranes to reach the cervix and vagina.
3. Blood may enter the amniotic cavity or infiltrate between the fibres of the myometrium. This causes an intense inflammatory response in the myometrium and may trigger uterine contractions. Extravasation of blood may lead to discolouration of the uterus (couvelaire uterus). Minor separation of the placental edge may occur but presentation is less dramatic than frank abruption.

Following major placental abruption there is release of thromboplastin into the maternal circulation which may trigger disseminated intravascular coagulation (DIC). Maternal death following abruption is usually associated with DIC.

Aetiology

The aetiology of placental abruption is unknown. It may occur following trauma or after sudden uterine decompression which may follow ruture of membranes in a case of polyhydramnios. Abruption is associated with low socioeconomic class, hypertension, pre-eclampsia, and previous abruption. The risk of placental abruption is increased in women who smoke during pregnancy.

Assessment

The clinical picture is determined by the extent of the abruption. Abdominal pain is the most constant feature and is usually of sudden onset. Abruption may precipitate labour. Vaginal bleeding may occur. The patient may be shocked and the uterus is tender and tense on palpation. It may be difficult to feel fetal parts and the fetal heart sounds may be absent. The differential diagnosis includes other causes of pain and bleeding in pregnancy.

Placental abruption is diagnosed clinically. Investigations are aimed at monitoring fetal and maternal well-being. Ultrasonography may reveal a retroplacental haematoma but the absence of this finding does not exclude the diagnosis of placental abruption.

Management (see also 'General management of antepartum haemorrhage' below)

When a firm diagnosis of abruption is made delivery is indicated. The diagnosis is sometimes difficult, particularly prior to 34 weeks' gestation. If the woman is in labour and there is no evidence of fetal or maternal compromise then the membranes should be ruptured, otherwise caesarean section is usually indicated.

PLACENTA PRAEVIA

The placenta is low lying in 20% of pregnancies at the end of the second trimester but the incidence falls with advancing gestation as the lower segment forms. Placenta praevia complicates approximately 0.5% of pregnancies at term, however a significant proportion deliver before this. Abruption may occur in placenta praevia.

Aetiology

The aetiology of placenta praevia is unknown but previous myometrial damage (e.g. following curettage) has been implicated. Placenta praevia is commoner in pregnancies after caesarean section and if it occurs the possibility of pathological adherence of the placenta must be anticipated. There is an association with multiple pregnancy and rhesus disease where the placental area is larger.

Assessment

Painless recurrent vaginal bleeding is the characteristic symptom of placenta praevia, however in some cases bleeding does not occur until the onset of labour. On examination, the uterus is not tender and there may be a breech presentation, abnormal lie or the presenting part may be high. These findings should raise the suspicion of placenta praevia even in the absence of vaginal bleeding. *Vaginal examination must not be performed if placenta praevia is suspected.*

Investigations

Placental localization is performed by ultrasound. This technique is usually accurate but is not infallible. There are four grades of placenta praevia:

Grade 1   Lower margin of placenta encroaches on the lower segment.
Grade 2   Lower margin of placenta reaches the internal os.
Grade 3   Placenta partially covers the internal os.
Grade 4   Placenta completely covers the internal os.

Placenta praevia is more simply classified into major and minor degrees.
A minor degree of placenta praevia is equivalent to grade 1 or 2, and a major degree corresponds with grades 3 and 4.

Management

If a low-lying placenta is detected by routine scan in early pregnancy no action is necessary, but the placental site is checked again at 32 weeks' gestation. If a major degree of placenta praevia persists the patient is admitted to hospital because of the risk of haemorrhage. Cross-matched blood is kept continuously available and ultrasound scans are repeated at 2-week intervals to monitor placental position and fetal growth.

If a major degree of placenta praevia persists at 38 weeks, delivery is by elective caesarean section. This should be performed by a senior obstetrician and general anaesthesia is advised. Women with minor degrees of placenta praevia would usually be allowed to labour spontaneously. Examination under anaesthesia is rarely indicated.

Other causes of antepartum haemorrhage

Vasa praevia is a rare condition and can occur when there is a velamentous cord insertion. The cord inserts in the membranes and the vessels course across the membranes to reach the placenta. When membranes rupture the vessels may be torn and fetal exsanguination may occur. Facilities should be available to test for fetal haemoglobin, most commonly in the form of the NaOH test.

General management of antepartum haemorrhage

Management depends primarily on the severity of the clinical situation. It is obligatory to assume that bleeding is placental in origin until proven otherwise.

Minor haemorrhage

At home
1. Refer patient to hospital
2. *Do not perform a vaginal examination.*

In hospital
1. Take a history and examine the patient
2. *Do not perform a digital vaginal examination*
3. Gentle speculum examination may be performed after the placental site is known
4. Assess fetal well-being—cardiotocography
5. Consider siting an intravenous line
6. Take blood to check haemoglobin, platelets and group and save serum
7. Admit to hospital for rest and observation
8. Arrange ultrasound scan

9. Give anti-D to rhesus-negative mothers.

It is common practice to advise women to remain in hospital for 48 hours after bleeding has stopped as there is a risk of the APH precipitating premature labour.

Major haemorrhage

At home
1. Arrange urgent admission to hospital/call obstetric flying squad
2. Insert intravenous line and commence resuscitation
3. *Do not perform a vaginal examination.*

In hospital
1. Call for assistance
2. Insert wide-bore cannula and commence intravenous infusion; two lines may be necessary
3. Request 6 units of cross-matched blood urgently
4. Send blood to check haemoglobin, platelets and clotting screen
5. Insert CVP line
6. Insert urinary catheter; monitor fluid balance
7. *Do not perform a vaginal examination*
8. If the fetus is alive, deliver by emergency caesarean section.

Complications of antepartum haemorrhage

1. Maternal/fetal death
2. Postpartum haemorrhage
3. DIC (particularly following abruption)
4. Renal failure
5. Preterm delivery.

SUMMARY

Placental abruption and placenta praevia are the important causes of antepartum haemorrhage. Assessment in hospital is essential in all cases of antepartum haemorrhage and management is determined by the clinical situation.

PART 6
MATERNAL SYSTEMIC DISORDERS
A. Rodin

Expectations of the examiners

The candidate is expected to have a knowledge of the common medical disorders which occur in pregnancy. The candidate should be able to discuss the role of the general practitioner in their management.

ANAEMIA

Interesting facts

Anaemia is one of the commonest medical complications of pregnancy.

Pathophysiology

Plasma volume increases steadily through pregnancy and reaches a plateau after 32 weeks. The magnitude of the increase is related to fetal size and the effect is exaggerated in multiple pregnancy. There is a concomitant increase in red cell mass and total haemoglobin but because of the larger rise in plasma volume, the haemoglobin concentration and PCV fall.

IRON DEFICIENCY ANAEMIA

Demands for iron increase during pregnancy due to the rise in red cell mass and fetal demands. Total iron requirement through pregnancy is 700–1400 mg with a daily requirement of 4 mg rising to 7 mg in later pregnancy. A reduction in haemoglobin concentration is a relatively late sign of iron deficiency. This is preceded by depletion in iron stores and a fall in serum iron levels.

Assessment

Iron deficiency can be detected before anaemia develops by measuring serum ferritin which gives a reflection of iron stores. Serum iron and total iron binding capacity are also useful markers.

The red cell indices suggestive of iron deficiency are reduced mean cell volume (MCV) and a reduced mean cell haemoglobin concentration (MCHC).

Management

Oral iron supplements are usually adequate for prophylaxis. Standard preparations contain between 100 and 200 mg of elemental iron often in combination with folic acid.

Treatment of established iron deficiency depends on the severity of the anaemia and the gestation. Treatment options include:

1. Oral iron supplementation
2. Parenteral iron/dextran (i.v./i.m.) } Rarely needed
3. Blood transfusion.

Adequate treatment should increase the haemoglobin concentration at the rate of 1 mg/dl/week and a reticulocyte count 2 weeks later should confirm a response to iron therapy.

MEGALOBLASTIC ANAEMIA

A deficiency in folic acid is the usual cause of this type of anaemia in pregnancy. Folate is needed for cell growth and division and requirements increase as pregnancy progresses. Folate deficiency anaemia affects 5% of pregnant women in the UK and much larger numbers in developing countries. The daily requirement of folate in pregnancy is 100 μg.

Assessment

The red cell indices show a raised MCV and macrocytes are seen on the blood film.

Management

Oral folate supplements, 5 mg daily for documented folate deficiency, are often combined with iron supplements. Prophylactic dose is 200–500 μg of folate.

SICKLE CELL ANAEMIA

Sickle cell disease is one of the most important haemoglobinopathies. It is due to a single amino acid substitution on the β chain of haemoglobin. The haemoglobin formed (HbS) is insoluble when reduced and this results in distortion of erythrocytes and subsequent blockage of small blood vessels. Sickle cell disease is common amongst black populations and in some Mediterranean groups. Heterozygotes for this abnormal gene have sickle cell trait (HbAS). Complications in pregnancy are rare. Homozygotes (HbSS) have sickle cell disease and may suffer from recurrent sickling crises. They develop a chronic haemolytic anaemia.

Assessment

Sickle cell disease and other haemoglobinopathies are detected by haemoglobin electrophoresis which should be carried out in at-risk women at booking. The partner's blood should also be tested to assess the risks of fetal disease.

Management

Women with sickle cell trait pose few special management problems. Haemoglobin electrophoresis should be performed on the baby's father to assess the risk of the infant being affected.

Women with sickle cell disease should be managed in specialist centres and further discussion is beyond the scope of this book.

CARDIAC DISEASE

Interesting facts

Less than 1% of all pregnancies in the UK are complicated by heart disease, however it remains an important cause of maternal mortality. Greater numbers of women with congenital heart disease are now reaching adulthood due to paediatric cardiac surgery and many of these women are becoming pregnant. The numbers of women with acquired (mainly rheumatic) heart disease complicating pregnancy are falling.

Pathophysiology

During normal pregnancy the cardiovascular system undergoes a number of adaptations. During the first trimester cardiac output increases by 40% due to raised stroke volume and a small increment in heart rate. Blood volume also increases by about 40% in early pregnancy and this is maintained until term. A fall in peripheral resistance occurs due to general relaxation in arterial and venous tone. An ejection systolic murmur is audible in up to 90% of normal pregnant women. At delivery, contraction of the uterus expresses about 500 ml of blood into the circulation. The normal woman can cope with these haemodynamic alterations but in a woman with heart disease they may precipitate cardiac failure.

Classification of heart disease

1. Congenital heart disease
2. Rheumatic heart disease
3. Other
   a. Cardiomyopathy
   b. Myocardial infarction.

Maternal mortality is most likely in those conditions where pulmonary blood flow cannot be increased, e.g. Eisenmenger's syndrome and primary pulmonary hypertension. Fetal outcome in patients with rheumatic heart disease and acyanotic congenital heart disease is usually good. Mothers with cyanotic congenital heart disease tend to have growth-retarded infants.

Although rheumatic heart disease is becoming rare in the UK it is the commonest form of heart disease complicating pregnancy worldwide. The most important lesion is mitral stenosis and these women are particularly likely to develop heart failure during pregnancy.

Women with artificial heart valves should receive anticoagulation through pregnancy and the puerperium.

Management

Prepregnancy

Avoidance or termination of pregnancy may be recommended in certain conditions (e.g. Eisenmenger's syndrome).

Antenatal

1. Hospital care with regular visits to obstetrician and cardiologist
2. Avoid cardiac failure
   a. Treat infections promptly
   b. Treat hypertension
   c. Avoid anaemia
3. Treat cardiac failure
4. Monitor fetal growth with serial ultrasound scans.

In labour

1. Antibiotic cover may be indicated
2. Aim for vaginal delivery
3. Adequate analgesia—epidural analgesia can be used in most cases but should be avoided in women with Eisenmenger's syndrome and hypertrophic cardiomyopathy (i.e. fixed output states)
4. Strict control of intravenous fluids
5. Short second stage
6. Do not give ergometrine.

DIABETES MELLITUS

Interesting facts

Diabetes affects about 3% of the obstetric population and before the introduction of insulin, diabetic pregnancy had a very high maternal and fetal mortality.

Pathophysiology

Hormonal changes during pregnancy have profound effects on carbohydrate metabolism. Insulin resistance develops as pregnancy advances and it is most marked in the last trimester. In normal pregnancy, increased insulin production counters the rise in insulin resistance and blood glucose levels are maintained within a narrow range. Glucose crosses the placenta freely by facilitated diffusion and maternal homeostatic mechanisms regulate fetal glucose levels in the normal situation. In the diabetic pregnancy, fetal hyperglycaemia stimulates fetal insulin production.

Glycosuria is common during normal pregnancy. This is due to an increased glomerular filtration rate and reduced tubular reabsorption of glucose.

There are three main clinical types of diabetes in pregnancy:

1. Insulin-dependent diabetes
2. Non-insulin dependent diabetes
3. Gestational diabetes.

Gestational diabetes is the term applied to women who become diabetic during pregnancy. Many will revert to normal after pregnancy, but a proportion do not.

Effects of diabetes on the pregnancy

Fetal effects

1. Increased perinatal mortality due to:
   a. Congenital abnormalities: increased risk of sacral agenesis and cardiac abnormalities due to hyperglycaemia during organogenesis
   b. Respiratory distress syndrome
   c. Birth trauma associated with macrosomia (birth weight > 4000 g)
   d. Intrauterine growth retardation
   e. Prematurity.
2. Increased neonatal morbidity
   a. Birth asphyxia/trauma
   b. Hypoglycaemia
   c. Polycythaemia
   d. Jaundice
   e. Respiratory distress syndrome.

Maternal effects

1. Pre-eclampsia: increased incidence in diabetic pregnancy
2. Polyhydramnios
3. Preterm labour.
   Good diabetic control reduces the incidence of these complications but the raised incidence of congenital abnormalities persists.

Assessment

Risk factors should be identified antenatally and these women should be offered a glucose tolerance test.

Risk factors for gestational diabetes are:

1. Glycosuria on two or more occasions
2. Maternal obesity (>20% of ideal weight)
3. Family history of diabetes in first degree relative
4. Previous congenital abnormality, neonatal death, unexplained stillbirth, macrosomic infant
5. Polyhydramnios in current pregnancy
6. Previous gestational diabetes.

Routine antenatal screening is recommended by some because about 30% of gestational diabetics have none of these risk factors.

The diagnosis of diabetes is made by the finding of a fasting blood glucose level of 8 mmol/l or more or 11 mmol/l or more after food. A fasting glucose level of <6 mmol/l excludes the diagnosis. A glucose tolerance test (GTT) with a 75 g glucose load distinguishes between diabetes, impaired glucose tolerance (IGT), and normality. The significance of IGT to the pregnancy is uncertain but some women with IGT will develop gestational diabetes later in the pregnancy.

Management

Medical management of diabetes is by diet alone or diet and insulin depending on the type of maternal diabetes. Oral hypoglycaemic agents are not used. Insulin is given at least twice daily using a mixture of short-acting and medium-acting preparations. Continuous subcutaneous insulin administration has been used with good effect.

Prepregnancy

Established diabetics should be assessed before pregnancy to achieve optimal blood glucose control before conception. Women with diabetic retinopathy and nephropathy require careful assessment.

Antenatal

1. Early booking
2. Hospital care at joint obstetric/diabetic clinic
3. Optimize blood glucose control
   a. Dietary advice
   b. Home blood glucose monitoring
   c. Regular urinalysis
   d. Regular HbA_1 and fructosamine monitoring

4. Monitor fetal well-being
   a. Check maternal serum AFP between 16 and 18 weeks
   b. Anomaly scan at 18 weeks
   c. Serial ultrasound scans to monitor fetal growth
5. Do not allow pregnancy to proceed past 40 weeks.

In labour

1. Aim for vaginal delivery
2. Continuous intravenous infusion of insulin and 5% dextrose with regular monitoring of blood glucose
3. Continuous fetal monitoring
4. Adequate analgesia.

After delivery, insulin requirements fall rapidly and careful monitoring is essential.

EPILEPSY

Interesting facts

Pregnancy does not trigger epilepsy or cause an exacerbation of pre-existing epilepsy. Untreated epileptics have an increased risk of congenital abnormalities which is poorly understood. The incidence of congenital malformations is increased two- or three-fold in infants of women on anticonvulsants. Phenytoin is associated with an increased risk of cleft lip/palate, congenital heart disease and hypoplasia of the nails and digits. Sodium valproate is associated with an increased incidence of neural tube defects.

Management

Prepregnancy

1. Check that fits are well controlled
2. Emphasize the importance of good drug compliance during pregnancy.

Antenatal

1. Continue on usual anticonvulsant at prepregnancy dose unless fits occur, then levels should be checked and the dose adjusted accordingly.
2. Women taking anticonvulsants may become folate deficient and 5 mg daily should be given throughout pregnancy.
3. Maternal serum AFP estimation at 16–18 weeks.

4. Fetal anomaly scan at 18 weeks.
5. Anticonvulsants may cause depression of vitamin K-dependent clotting factors in the mother and fetus; vitamin K should be given from 36 weeks until delivery and the neonate should be given vitamin K intramuscularly. All antiepileptic drugs are excreted in low concentrations in breast milk. Mothers taking antiepileptic drugs other than phenobarbitone should be permitted to breast-feed.

THROMBOEMBOLIC DISEASE

Interesting facts

Thromboembolic disease is an important cause of maternal mortality. The risk of thromboembolism during pregnancy and the puerperium is six times higher than in the non-pregnant state.

Pathophysiology

Pregnancy is accompanied by changes in normal haemostatic mechanisms which decrease the risk of haemorrhage at delivery. These changes include an increase in clotting factors and a dampening of fibrinolysis favouring thrombosis. Risk factors for thromboembolism in pregnancy include:

1. High maternal age
2. Multiparity
3. Obesity
4. Immobility
5. Previous history of thromboembolism
6. Operative delivery
7. Blood disorders (rare)
8. Use of stilboestrol to suppress lactation.

Blood group O appears to confer some protection against thromboembolism. The recurrence rate of deep venous thrombosis (DVT) or pulmonary embolus (PE) in women who have had thromboembolic disease in previous pregnancies is 5–10%.

Assessment

Women with a history of thromboembolism should be identified in the booking clinic. Suspected thromboembolism occurring during pregnancy or the puerperium should be actively investigated to reach a definitive diagnosis. Clinical diagnosis of DVT is unreliable and venography or ultrasonography should be arranged. Clinical suspicion of PE should be confirmed by a ventilation-perfusion scan of the lungs. Chest X-ray, ECG and arterial blood gas measurement may also be helpful. Anticoagulation should be commenced when thromboembolism is suspected without waiting for confirmation.

Management

PE/DVT during pregnancy

1. Commence intravenous infusion of heparin 40 000 i.u./day; continue for 5–7 days.
2. Change to subcutaneous heparin 10 000 i.u. b.d. and continue until the end of the puerperium.

History of previous DVT/PE

Prophylactic anticoagulation should be considered because of risk of recurrence. There is no consensus about who to treat and which regimen to follow and the benefits of anticoagulation should be balanced against the risks of fetal and maternal side-effects (see below). Regimens which have been used include:

1. Continuous subcutaneous heparin through pregnancy and the puerperium.
2. Subcutaneous heparin until 13 weeks; warfarin between 13 and 36 weeks; subcutaneous heparin from 36 weeks until the end of the puerperium.
3. Dextran 70 in labour followed by heparin (subcutaneous) or warfarin during the puerperium.

Anticoagulation with either heparin or warfarin is associated with risks for both mother and fetus. Heparin does not cross the placenta and it has a short half-life. Its actions are readily reversible by protamine sulphate. However, it is associated with maternal thrombocytopenia and prolonged administration causes bone demineralization. Warfarin crosses the placenta and can cause chondrodysplasia punctata, microcephaly and optic atrophy in the fetus. Later in pregnancy it can cause fetal intracranial haemorrhage. Therefore warfarin is avoided in the first trimester and from 36 weeks onwards. Warfarin has a long half-life and its effects cannot be rapidly reversed in the event of a complication such as antepartum haemorrhage. Breast-feeding is not contraindicated in women taking heparin or warfarin.

THYROID DISEASE

Interesting facts

Thyroid disease has been estimated to complicate 0.5% of all pregnancies. It is usually pre-existing but may appear for the first time in pregnancy.

HYPOTHYROIDISM

The main causes of hypothyroidism are idiopathic, Hashimoto's thyroiditis, and postablative hypothyroidism.

Assessment

The clinical diagnosis of hypothyroidism may be difficult during pregnancy but may be suggested by inappropriate weight gain, cold intolerance or skin changes. There may be a goitre and reflexes may be sluggish. Laboratory investigations show a low free thyroxine (T4) level and a raised thyroid stimulating hormone (TSH) level. Total serum T4 is low for pregnancy but may be within the normal range for the non-pregnant woman.

Management

Thyroxine should be given as a single daily dose. Thyroid function should be checked as the pregnancy progresses. Breast-feeding is not contraindicated.

HYPERTHYROIDISM

Hyperthyroidism in pregnancy is usually due to Graves' disease. Untreated hyperthyroidism is associated with an increased incidence of preterm labour and low birth weight and a raised perinatal mortality rate. Women who have had surgery for Graves' disease may still have thyroid stimulating autoantibodies which can cross the placenta and cause neonatal thyrotoxicosis.

Assessment

The symptoms of hyperthyroidism may mimic the normal changes of pregnancy and include heat intolerance, palpitations, emotional instability, and fatigue. A goitre may be present. TSH is undetectable while free T3 and T4 are elevated.

Management

The aim of management is to control maternal hyperthyroidism while allowing the development of normal thyroid function in the fetus. Both drug therapy and surgery have been used. The thiourea derivatives, carbimazole and propylthiouracil, are in common use and their main action is to inhibit synthesis of T3 and T4. These drugs cross the placenta and may effect the fetal thyroid causing transient hypothyroidism at delivery. There is no contraindication to breast-feeding.

24. Labour—first stage

J. Rymer

Expectations of the examiners

The candidate is expected to understand the mechanism of labour and the management of normal and abnormal labour. The principles of active management of labour are essential to modern obstetrics.

Definitions

Labour is defined as the process by which the fetus, placenta, and membranes are expelled from the birth canal. The first stage of labour commences when regular uterine contractions are associated with cervical change, and concludes with full dilatation of the cervix.

Interesting facts

Previously labour was said to be normal when spontaneous delivery occurred within 24 hours of the onset of spontaneous regular contractions. However, as the complications of labour are directly related to its duration, labour is now deemed normal if spontaneous delivery occurs within 12 hours.

Physiology

In pregnancy, the uterus is in a relaxed state and must expand to accommodate the growing fetus. However, when labour commences, it must contract regularly and forcibly so that the cervix progressively effaces and dilates allowing the fetus to descend through the birth canal.

In labour, the myometrial smooth muscle contracts at regular intervals, resulting in intrauterine pressures of 50–75 mmHg. The wave of excitation, and hence the resulting contraction, normally passes downwards from the fundus of the uterus. As the muscle contracts, it also retracts (the muscle does not relax to its original length, but stays at a shorter length). Successful parturition involves regular and effective uterine contractions and a responsive cervix. Cervical ripening is characterized by softening, effacement and dilatation, but the hormonal control of this

217

process is still not understood. Prior to term, the release of prostaglandins causes an increase in the water content of the cervix and breakdown of cervical collagen. PGE_2 has a marked effect on cervical ripening. During labour, prostaglandins and oxytocin interact in the generation of uterine contractions.

Mechanism of normal labour

Descent. Significant descent of the head into the pelvis occurs in most primigravidae in the later weeks of pregnancy. In multigravidae descent may not occur until the onset of labour.

Engagement. This occurs when the maximum diameter of the head has passed through the pelvic brim. It may occur before labour commences, and the head usually engages in the occipitotransverse.

Flexion. This is a continuous process during labour. With full flexion the posterior fontanelle is easily palpable on vaginal examination through the dilated cervix, and the most favourable diameter presents.

Internal rotation. This is rotation of the head inside the pelvis, and it occurs because of the shape of the birth canal, the position of the head, and the inclination of the levator ani. Usually the rotation is anterior, so that the denominator (the occiput) swings from left occipitotransverse (LOT) to direct occipitoanterior (OA).

Extension. The head remains flexed until the vertex reaches the perineum. As the head 'crowns' it extends, following the axis of the birth canal.

External rotation (restitution). The head reverts to the position it previously held before internal rotation occurred (occipitotransverse).

Lateral flexion. The anterior shoulder appears, followed by the posterior shoulder. Delivery of the trunk is then achieved by lateral flexion.

Assessment

The diagnosis of labour is made when regular uterine contractions are associated with cervical change. As the cervix effaces the operculum (mucus plug in the cervix) is released (a 'show'). Each obstetric unit should be clear on its criteria for the diagnosis of labour, and the delivery suite should be reserved for women in active labour.

History

Specific questioning should involve:
1. Contractions
   a. Time of onset
   b. Frequency
   c. Duration

2.   Presence of a show
3.   Rupture of the membranes.

Examination

1.   Abdominal palpation is performed to assess:
      a. Gestation
      b. Lie of the fetus
      c. Presentation
      d. Descent of the head (Fig. 24.1).
2.   Vaginal examination:
      a. Speculum examination if there is any question as to whether liquor is draining. Nitrazene reaction has been used to indicate the presence of liquor but is unreliable.
      b. Digital examination should assess the softness, length, and dilatation of the cervix, and the station (relative to the ischial spines) of the presenting part.
3.   Fetal well-being:
      a. Fetal movements
      b. CTG (ideally for 20 minutes)
      c. Presence of meconium in the liquor.

Management

If the diagnosis of 'labour' is made then the membranes should be ruptured provided that a cord presentation has been excluded. This enables the colour of the liquor to be assessed, and aids the progress of labour. The best way to record the progress of labour is to use a partogram, i.e. a visual representation of progress in labour. This should include a record of:

1.   The date and time of admission.
2.   Cervical dilatation. This is marked in centimetres at zero time (on admission) and at subsequent examinations.
3.   Descent of the head. Determined by abdominal palpation of the number of 'fifths' of the head palpable above the brim and vaginal assessment of the relationship of the presenting part to the ischial spines (station).
4.   Contractions
      a. Frequency
      b. Duration
      c. Strength: assessment of strength of contractions by palpation is unreliable.
5.   Fetal heart rate.
6.   Colour of the liquor and time and manner of membrane rupture.
7.   The use of syntocinon.

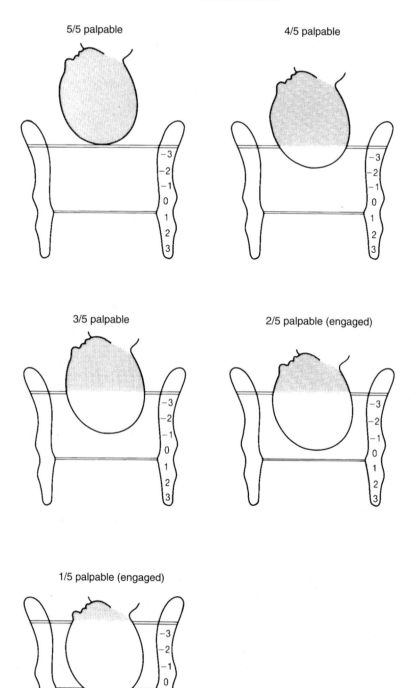

Fig. 24.1 The abdominal palpation of the fetal head can be described in 'fifths' of the head palpable above the brim.

8. Maternal status
   a. Blood pressure
   b. Pulse
   c. Temperature
   d. Urinalysis
   e. Medication.

Progress in labour

The regular assessment of progress is the key to good management. In primigravidae, delivery should be achieved within 12 hours. The minimum rate of cervical dilatation acceptable in primiparous women is 1 cm/hour. Delay in progress may be due to:

Inefficient uterine action (primary dysfunctional labour). In primiparous women this is common. The earlier the diagnosis is made the more chance there is of correcting it and achieving a normal delivery. Once diagnosed, a syntocinon infusion should be commenced and progress assessed regularly. (See Appendix VI for partograms.)

Secondary arrest. If the fetal head is partially extended it does not fit into the lower uterine pole well and this is more common in primiparous women especially with an occipitoposterior position. These women generally have a bad start to labour, and may present with inefficient uterine action. Premature rupture of membranes is common. The head remains high and deflexed and there may be severe backache. The sinciput reaches the pelvic floor first and therefore rotates anteriorly, i.e. the occiput is posterior. The larger occipitofrontal diameter of the head presents (10 cm), making its passage through the pelvis more difficult.

Cephalopelvic disproportion (see Ch. 25.) In multiparous women, labour is more rapid and inefficient uterine action is rare. Delay in a multiparous woman may be due to obstruction, with subsequent uterine rupture if not recognized.

Posture during labour

The woman should adopt the most comfortable position bearing in mind that aortocaval compression must be avoided. Early in the first stage women may want to mobilize, but most adopt a recumbent position once labour is established.

Oral intake

Women in labour have delayed gastric emptying and this will be exacerbated by narcotics and fatigue. It is advisable to allow clear fluids and no food. H_2 antagonists should be given 6-hourly.

Support during labour

Labour is a stressful event and a woman requires support from a person known to her and a midwife who ideally remains with her throughout her labour.

Active management of labour

The aim of active management is to ensure that all women in their first pregnancy deliver a healthy child after a labour less than 12 hours. A woman's first experience will determine her obstetric future both emotionally and physically.

The principles of active management are:

1. Antenatal education
2. Regular assessment of progress in labour
3. Presence of a support person throughout labour (ideally, the *same* person throughout)
4. Early correction of abnormal progress
5. Provision of suitable analgesia.

If active management is correctly applied, the caesarean section rate is reduced.

25. Labour—second stage

J. Rymer

Expectations of the examiners

The candidate will be expected to have a thorough knowledge of what is normal and abnormal in the second stage of labour. The importance of the correct timing of intervention should be appreciated.

Definition

The second stage of labour commences with full cervical dilatation and concludes with delivery of the fetus.

Interesting facts

In primigravidae the average length of the second stage is 40 minutes, and in multiparae, 20 minutes.

Physiology

The uterus continues to contract and force the fetus through the cervix. At full dilatation the cervix has retracted past the presenting part and is no longer palpable. Contractions are usually stronger but occur less frequently than in the first stage. If the normal mechanism of labour is occurring, the head rotates internally as it descends and when the pelvic floor becomes distended the 'bearing down' reflex occurs.

Assessment

Full dilatation is diagnosed by vaginal examination. The position and station of the fetal head should be noted.

Management

When the bearing down reflex occurs the woman will want to 'push' (in the absence of an effective epidural). After breathing in, the glottis is closed, and the patient pushes down with the aid of the diaphragm and abdominal wall muscles. Two or three bearing down efforts are made with each contraction. It is essential that the woman receives constant attention during the second stage to detect signs of fetal or maternal distress.

Once anal dilatation occurs, normal delivery should follow shortly afterwards. The woman is prepared for delivery, and the accoucheur assists the delivery by ensuring that the fetal head remains flexed, and that the head is delivered in a controlled manner. If needed, an episiotomy is performed (ideally with some form of pain relief) as the head distends the perineum. Once the head is delivered the oropharynx is suctioned. The head restitutes and is then grasped and pulled downwards (towards the maternal sacrum) so that the anterior shoulder is delivered. The trunk is then laterally flexed upwards (towards the maternal umbilicus) so that the posterior shoulder is delivered, rapidly followed by the trunk. Great care of the perineum must be taken at all times.

If a spontaneous vaginal delivery has not occurred within 1 hour of full dilatation then the vaginal examination should be repeated. In primigravid women, if there has been no progress, then a syntocinon infusion should be commenced and a repeat vaginal examination should be performed in 1 hour. If there is no progress and the head is too high for an instrumental delivery, then a caesarean section is performed. If progress has occurred, then an instrumental delivery may be performed, or the second stage may be allowed to continue depending on the fetal and maternal condition. In multiparous women, it is dangerous to use syntocinon for second stage augmentation alone, due to the risk of uterine rupture.

If the position of the head is occipitoanterior and does not descend with augmentation (in primigravidae), this suggests true cephalopelvic disproportion.

If the position of the head is occipitoposterior, the station of the head will determine whether a vaginal delivery is possible. This can either be performed with rotational forceps, e.g. Kjellands or vacuum extractor (see Ch. 28), or with lift-out forceps if the head is low enough.

Cephalopelvic disproportion

In the past, slow progress in the first stage of labour was wrongly termed cephalopelvic disproportion, whereas now the most likely diagnosis is considered to be inefficient uterine action and this is treated with an oxytocin infusion.

If progress still fails to occur, then a tentative diagnosis of cephalopelvic disproportion can be entertained, provided the head is not occipitoposterior. If these strict criteria are applied to make the diagnosis, 1 in 250 primigravidae will have cephalopelvic disproportion, and if allowed to labour subsequently, 50% will deliver vaginally.

True cephalopelvic disproportion is rare, and the diagnosis can only be made in retrospect. Once this diagnosis has been made it will strongly influence the mode of delivery in subsequent pregnancies.

In parous women cephalopelvic disproportion can occur due to either a larger fetus, or a reduction in pelvic capacity, or both. The uterine action in these cases will be vigorously reactive and the risk of uterine rupture is considerable, especially if oxytocin is used. The diagnosis rests on features such as delay in descent of the presenting part, exaggerated moulding and unremitting uterine activity.

SUMMARY

A prolonged second stage of labour requires sensible management if maternal and fetal trauma are to be avoided.

26. Labour—third stage

J. Rymer

Expectations of the examiners

A thorough knowledge of the normal and abnormal third stage is essential. The candidate should appreciate that proper management of the third stage is of vital importance in reducing the incidence of postpartum haemorrhage, retained placenta, and consequent maternal morbidity and mortality.

Definition

The third stage commences with the delivery of the baby and finishes with delivery of the placenta.

Interesting facts

Postpartum haemorrhage is the most common cause of serious blood loss in obstetrics. It is an important cause of maternal mortality, accounting for 53% of maternal deaths from haemorrhage in England and Wales (Report on Confidential Enquiries into Maternal Deaths 1991–93).

Physiology

The continuation of uterine contractions, and the reduction of surface area of the uterine cavity cause the placenta to separate from the uterine wall. As separation occurs there is some retroplacental bleeding which contributes to the separation process.

There are two processes which help to control excessive bleeding from the placental bed:

1. The interlacing bundles of muscle in the uterine wall contract and twist compressing the vessels as the uterus decreases in size.
2. Normal coagulation, i.e. release of thromboplastins, platelet aggregation, and fibrin formation.

Haemostatic processes may be less efficient in the following circumstances:

226

Table 26.1   Risk factors for postpartum haemorrhage.

Past history of a postpartum haemorrhage
Grand multiparity
Uterine overdistension (e.g. large baby, twins)
Antepartum haemorrhage
Coagulation disorders
Poor uterine contractions
Prolonged labour
Large placental bed (e.g. rhesus disease)
Operative delivery

1. Dysfunctional labour
2. Uterine overdistension, e.g. multiple pregnancy
3. Anaesthetic agents, e.g. halothane
4. Morbid adherence of the placenta.

Assessment

Risk factors for a postpartum haemorrhage should be identified in the patient's previous obstetric history (see Table 26.1) or current pregnancy.

Management

The policy for management of the third stage varies between obstetric units. As the anterior shoulder is delivered an ecbolic is administered i.m. or i.v. in the form of oxytocin ± ergometrine (see Table 26.2). The placenta is usually delivered by the Brandt–Andrews technique. The cord is held with the right hand and downward traction is applied while the uterus is lifted upwards with the left hand placed suprapubically. If the placenta does not advance then it is usually still attached to the uterus. If the placenta is not delivered after 30 minutes then a manual removal is required (see 'Complications' below). Once the placenta has been delivered the fundus is briefly massaged to ensure that it contracts. The genital tract must be inspected for any lacerations and repaired appropriately. The placenta should be examined to ensure completeness and normality.

An assessment of the blood loss should be recorded.

Table 26.2   Time from administration to action on the uterus for the various oxytocic drugs.

Drug	Administration	Time
Oxytocin	i.v.	30 s
Ergometrine	i.v.	40 s
Oxytocin	i.m.	2.5 min
Ergometrine + oxytocin	i.m.	2.5 min
Ergometrine	i.m.	7 min

Complications

Postpartum haemorrhage

A primary postpartum haemorrhage is defined as a blood loss ≥ 500 ml within 24 hours of delivery. The incidence of postpartum haemorrhage is 5% of deliveries.

Aetiology

1. Uterine atony
2. Local trauma to vagina or cervix
3. Retained placenta or products of conception
4. Other:
   a. Uterine inversion
   b. Uterine rupture
   c. Defective coagulation.

Management. The assessment and treatment should take place simultaneously.

Examine the fundus. If it is high and soft then uterine atony and/or retained products are the cause of the bleeding. The fundus should be massaged to expel clot and ensure maximum retraction. In severe haemorrhage, bimanual compression with the uterus compressed between a vaginal and an abdominal hand can be used. If the fundus is not palpable then uterine inversion should be suspected and an immediate vaginal examination performed. The placenta and membranes should be checked to ensure they are complete.

Resuscitation. An i.v. line of large bore (14 g or greater) should be inserted while the initial examination is taking place (two lines in severe cases). Blood should be sent for FBC, clotting studies and 4 units of whole blood cross-matched. Initially, crystalloid or plasma substitute should be infused as quickly as required.

Examination of the genital tract. If the fundus is retracted and bleeding is continuing then careful speculum examination should be carried out and vaginal or cervical lacerations repaired appropriately.

Further measures. Further management depends on the findings and response to the measures already mentioned.

1. Uterine atony. In most cases this will respond to massage and the bleeding will settle. A syntocinon infusion should be commenced (40 i.u. syntocinon in 500 ml of crystalloid over 2–4 hours) or ergometrine 0.5 mg i.m. can be given if the patient has no history of cardiac disease or hypertension at any stage in pregnancy. If these measures are not successful, the uterine cavity should be examined under general anaesthesia (or epidural/spinal if one is already in situ) to remove any retained products. If bleeding continues, then prostaglandin injected directly into the myometrium is usually effective but, if not, then surgery should be performed without delay.

Internal iliac artery ligation is often discussed but may not effectively control bleeding and hysterectomy should be undertaken sooner rather than later.

2. Retained products/placenta should be removed with great care under anaesthesia. It is important that maximum uterine retraction is maintained until removal and this is best accomplished by syntocinon infusion and fundal massage if necessary.

3. Uterine rupture. If an EUA reveals a hole in the uterus then a laparotomy must be performed. If possible the tear is repaired, but if haemostasis cannot be achieved then a postpartum hysterectomy or internal iliac ligation (or embolization) can be performed.

Retained placenta

If the placenta is not delivered within 30 minutes then preparations should be made for a manual removal. This can be performed under spinal, epidural, or general anaesthesia.

Uterine inversion

The fundus of the uterus descends through the cervix usually with the placenta still attached. This has become a rare complication with the use of oxytocics and the Brandt–Andrews technique. Management involves immediate reduction if possible. If this is ineffective, then an i.v. line must be inserted, blood cross-matched, and the hydrostatic method of reduction attempted. Sterile saline is run into the upper vagina while the forearm occludes the introitus. If this fails, then abdominal surgery is required.

Amniotic fluid embolism

The patient suddenly collapses and a severe coagulation defect develops. If recognized, the patient needs to be ventilated, given steroids, and the coagulation defect corrected. The diagnosis is usually made at post-mortem.

Causes of postpartum collapse

1. Haemorrhage
2. Pulmonary embolism
3. Amniotic fluid embolism
4. Eclampsia
5. Others.

SUMMARY

If the third stage is managed appropriately the incidence of postpartum haemorrhage will be reduced.

27. Fetal monitoring in labour

J. Rymer

Interesting facts

The aim of fetal monitoring in labour is to detect fetal hypoxia so that resulting perinatal morbidity and mortality can be prevented. The reaction of the fetus to hypoxia is variable and dependent on its individual reserve. Therefore each fetus should be assessed for its relative risk of developing hypoxia in labour and surveillance during labour managed accordingly.

Methods

There are various methods of monitoring a fetus during labour:

Note the colour of the liquor. Meconium staining may result from an episode of hypoxia which causes vagal stimulation of the gut, relaxing the anal sphincter. Thick fresh meconium is considered an ominous sign. The absence of liquor is associated with IUGR and the fetus should be treated as if the liquor is meconium stained until proven otherwise.

Auscultation of the fetal heart using a Pinard's stethoscope. This is an intermittent form of fetal monitoring and should be employed during and immediately after contractions to detect accelerations or decelerations in the fetal heart rate. It is useful in low-risk patients with no identifiable abnormalities.

Sonar pulse detector (sonicaid). This is also an intermittent form of fetal monitoring and should be used in a similar way to the Pinard stethoscope.

Continuous fetal heart rate monitoring. This method involves either an abdominal transducer, which detects the fetal heart movements ultrasonically, or an electrode attached to the fetal scalp which records a signal from the fetal heart (Fig. 27.1). The abdominal transducer is less accurate. Most recording instruments also record uterine activity — cardiotocograph (CTG). The CTG should always be interpreted in the light of the clinical details in each case, e.g. the colour of the liquor, the stage of labour, and the drugs administered to the mother.

a

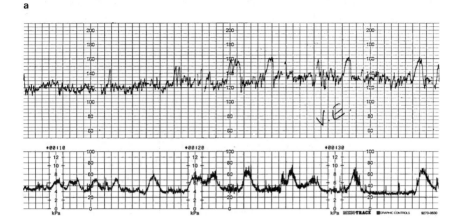

b

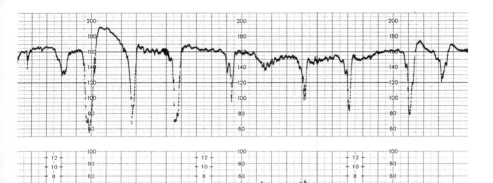

Fig. 27.1   Cardiotocographs (CTGs). a, Normal reactive trace; b, early decelerations.

Fetal heart rate patterns

Normal. The normal baseline heart rate is between 110 and 160 beats/minute. Accelerations of 10–15 beats/minute for at least 15 seconds indicate a healthy fetus. Baseline variability should be 5–25 beats/minute.

Baseline tachycardia. (FHR >160/minute.) Associated with certain drugs, prematurity, hypoxia, or maternal pyrexia.

Baseline bradycardia. (FHR <110/minute.) Between 90 and 110 is only significant if there are decelerations or decreased variability. It may be due to postmaturity, hypoxia, or heart block. Severe bradycardia (<90 beats/minute) is usually associated with a preterminal condition in the fetus.

Loss of baseline variability. A normal heart rate shows irregular accelerations and if this variation is lost it may indicate hypoxia or fetal sleep rate (95% last <40 minutes).

Increase in baseline variability. This can occur in high fetal activity states, acute or acute on chronic hypoxia.

Early decelerations (Fig. 27.2). These decelerations begin with the onset of a contraction and return to the baseline by the end of the contraction. They do not drop more than 20–40 beats and are associated with compression of the fetal head and are not a sign of fetal distress.

Late decelerations (Fig. 27.3). The low point of the deceleration occurs after the peak of the contraction and the fetal heart rate is slow to

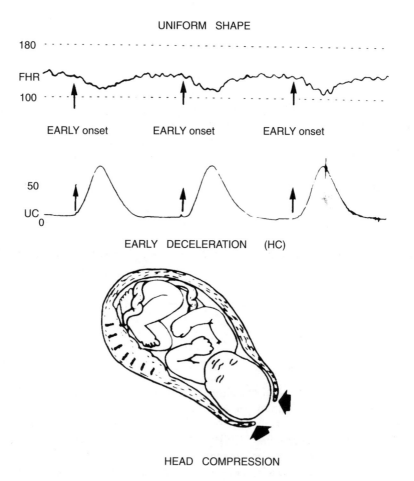

Fig. 27.2 Head compression and early deceleration (HC).

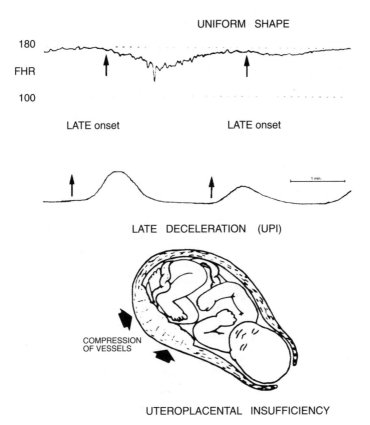

UNIFORM SHAPE

180

FHR

100

LATE onset   LATE onset

LATE DECELERATION (UPI)

COMPRESSION
OF VESSELS

UTEROPLACENTAL INSUFFICIENCY

Fig. 27.3   Uteroplacental insufficiency and late deceleration (UPI).

recover. The greater the lag-time between the end of the contraction and the return of the fetal heart rate to its normal baseline, the more serious is the hypoxia likely to be. Late decelerations are usually associated with fetal hypoxia and fetal blood sampling is indicated if labour is to proceed.

Variable decelerations (Fig. 27.4). These are steep sided and variable in shape and timing. They may be associated with cord compression. They can be identified as mild or moderate (<60 dropped beats for <60 seconds) or severe (>60 dropped beats for >60 seconds).

Management

In the low-risk mother it is acceptable to use intermittent monitoring. Interpreting continuous FHR recordings is difficult and the whole clinical picture must be taken into account. If the fetal heart tracing suggests fetal distress then various steps can be taken:

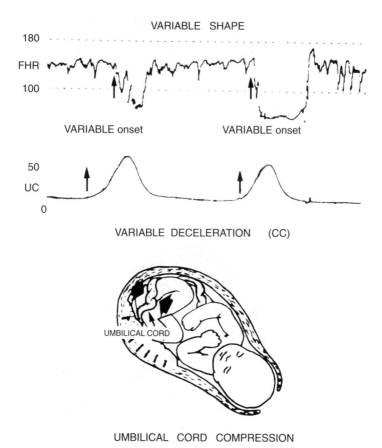

Fig. 27.4 Umbilical cord compression and variable deceleration (CC).

1. *Delivery*, e.g. if a woman is in early labour with thick meconium-stained liquor and there are persistent late decelerations, then abdominal delivery is advised.
2. *Fetal blood sampling*. This should be regarded as complementary to continuous FHR recording. If the latter facility is used alone then the caesarean section rate will be higher due to false positive diagnoses (Table 27.1). Fetal blood sampling should be repeated at least hourly as long as the CTG remains abnormal. Increase the frequency of sampling if the CTG deteriorates. The rate of fall of pH between samples should be noted. A large fall (>0.01 units/hour in first stage or >0.02 units/hour in second stage) is significant and may indicate delivery even if both pHs are within normal range. A fetus will attempt to maintain its pH for as long as possible but once buffering capacity is exceeded pH can fall very quickly.

Table 27.1   Interpretation of fetal blood sampling.

pH	Interpretation
>7.25	Normal Allow labour to continue
7.20–7.25	Borderline If delivery is anticipated within 1–2 hours proceed but repeat pH in 1 hour
<7.20	Abnormal Deliver immediately

3. *Resuscitation.* If the cause of acute fetal distress is due to a correctable maternal condition, then appropriate measures should be undertaken.
   a. The patient should adopt a lateral position with the foot of the bed higher than her heart.
   b. Augmentation should be discontinued and, in rare cases, uterine action should be inhibited using a tocolytic drug.
   c. Maternal hypotension should be corrected.
   d. The mother should be given oxygen.

SUMMARY

The currently available methods for intrapartum monitoring are still unreliable and interpretation of continuous fetal heart rate patterns is difficult and must be used in conjunction with fetal blood sampling.

28. Obstetric intervention

J. Rymer

INDUCTION OF LABOUR

Expectations of the examiners

The candidate should be familiar with the common indications and current methods of induction.

Interesting facts

Historically, induction of labour was mainly performed to ensure a small baby in cases of severe pelvic deformity.

Indications

Labour can be induced for numerous maternal and/or fetal reasons. When considering induction, two factors must be considered: (1) the risk to the mother or fetus if the pregnancy continues, versus (2) the risk of preterm delivery and complications of induction. The absolute contraindications are:

1. Placenta praevia
2. Abnormal lie
3. Known cephalopelvic disproportion.

Assessment

Important factors that must be considered prior to induction of labour are:

1. Gestation
2. Maternal well-being
3. Fetal well-being.

In order to determine the method of induction the maternal abdomen must be palpated noting the presentation of the fetus, and whether the head is engaged or unengaged. A vaginal examination should be performed. The consistency, position, length, and dilatation of the cervix should be documented and the station of the presenting part (see Bishop's score in

Table 28.1 Bishop's score (inducibility rating).

		1–2	3–4	5–6
Dilatation	0	1–2	3–4	5–6
Score	0	1	2	3
Length of the cervix (cm)	3	2	1	0
Score	0	1	2	3
Station	–3	–2	–10	+1 +2
Score	0	1	2	3
Consistency	Firm	Medium	Soft	
Score	0	1	2	
Position	Posterior	Mid	Anterior	
Score	0	1	2	

Total score = 0–5 unfavourable
6–13 favourable

Table 28.1). If the cervix is unfavourable the chances of a good response to labour induction are low.

Method

If the presenting part is not high and an artificial rupture of membranes (ARM) is technically possible, then the patient should be transferred to the labour ward, and an ARM performed under aseptic conditions. This can be performed with an amnihook or Kocher's forceps, and after the membranes have been ruptured, they should be swept back to release further prostaglandins. Some patients will spontaneously commence labour if left alone, but the majority require augmentation. A syntocinon infusion is used, either immediately or after a period of time, initially at a low dose, and increasing every 15 minutes, until regular contractions are established. The fetal heart rate must be monitored — in most centres this is done continuously, and the cervical dilatation should be assessed regularly.

If the cervix is unfavourable, then prostaglandins can be used. The current trend is to use intravaginal preparations, e.g. pessaries or gel. The state of the cervix is reassessed after an interval, and if possible the membranes are ruptured. If the cervix remains unfavourable, a further dose of prostaglandin can be used. The dosage and timing of prostaglandin administration are very variable.

Complications of induction

1. Fetal distress
2. Maternal distress
3. Precipitate delivery
4. Operative delivery
5. Iatrogenic prematurity

6. Uterine rupture
7. Amniotic fluid embolism
8. Water intoxication (if high doses of syntocinon and in conjunction with excessive fluid)
9. Diarrhoea, nausea, vomiting (systemic effects of prostaglandins).

Summary

Induced labours have a higher incidence of operative deliveries, and the recent trend has been away from induction. The decision for induction must include the consideration of risks and benefits to both mother and fetus.

FORCEPS DELIVERIES

Expectations of the examiners

The candidate should be familiar with non-rotational forceps, e.g. Wrigley's and Neville Barnes', and be able to discuss the indications and prerequisites for forceps delivery. The candidate should also have a basic understanding of Kjelland's forceps but would not be expected to use these rotational forceps.

Interesting facts

A pair of forceps consists of two instruments, each a mirror image of the other. There are four components: a blade, a shank, a lock, and a handle. Each blade has a cephalic and a pelvic curve (Figs 28.1, 28.2).

Indications for use

There must be a maternal and/or fetal reason to expedite delivery:
1. Fetal
   a. Distress
   b. Aftercoming head of breech
2. Maternal
   a. Delay in second stage
   b. Maternal disease, e.g. cardiac disease
   c. Dural tap.

Assessment

The following requirements must be satisfied before a forceps delivery can be performed:

1. Adequate analgesia
2. Bladder empty
3. No obvious cephalopelvic disproportion present

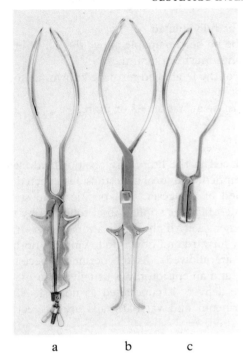

a   b   c

Fig. 28.1   Forceps in common use. a, Neville Barnes' forceps; b, Kjelland's forceps; c, Wrigley's forceps.

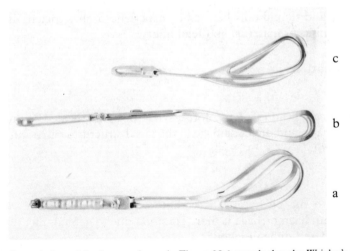

Fig. 28.2   Lateral view of the forceps shown in Figure 28.1 reveals that the Wrigley's and the Neville Barnes' forceps have a much larger pelvic curve than the Kjelland's forceps (b).

4. Cervix must be fully dilated
5. There must be no head palpable above the pelvic brim
6. The membranes must not be intact
7. The position of the fetal head must be known, i.e. occipitoanterior ± 15%
8. The head must be at station +2 or more.

Method

The patient is placed in the lithotomy position and cleaned and draped. The bladder is emptied, and local anaesthesia is injected at this point if it is the chosen method of analgesia. The position and station of the vertex arechecked. The left blade is applied first, followed by the right, and they should lock together easily if the application is correct. The direction of traction is initially forward and down, following the normal axis of delivery (only three pulls are allowed). As the perineum becomes distended, the head is extended, and an episiotomy is usually performed. The forceps are removed, and the delivery is conducted as normal. After delivery of the placenta, the perineum and vaginal walls are inspected, and any tears appropriately repaired.

Rotational forceps

Kjelland's forceps have a cephalic curve, but no pelvic curve, and a sliding lock to correct for asynclitism. They are used when rotation of the head is required and should only be used by experienced obstetricians as they can cause significant maternal and fetal injury.

Complications

Fetal

Incorrect application of the forceps has been implicated in intracranial haemorrhage, and direct damage to the facial structures can occur (e.g. eye, nose, skull).

Maternal

Trauma to the birth canal is common and uterine rupture can occur. Postpartum haemorrhage is more common due to genital tract trauma and prolonged and difficult labour.

VENTOUSE DELIVERIES

Expectations of the examiners

The candidate is expected to be able to recognize the instrument and understand the principles behind its use.

Definition

A vacuum extractor (Ventouse) is a suction cup connected to a suction device. A vacuum is created between the cup and the fetal scalp and traction is applied in the axis of the birth canal to expedite delivery.

Indications for use

The indications are the same as for forceps deliveries, but maternal effort is needed. Therefore, in situations where maternal effort must be avoided, e.g. cardiac disease, severe hypertension, the Ventouse is contraindicated.

An incompletely dilated cervix is not an indication in modern obstetrics.

Requirements for a Ventouse delivery

The same as for a forceps delivery.

Method

The patient is prepared as for a forceps delivery. The cup is placed over the posterior fontanelle, and a vacuum of 0.8 kg/cm^2 is created. Traction is applied in the axis of the birth canal, imitating the normal mechanism of labour. Delivery must occur within three pulls, as with forceps deliveries.

Complications

Mainly fetal scalp injuries:

1. Cephalhaematoma — bleeding beneath the periosteum
2. Subgaleal haematoma — bleeding beneath the galea caused by emissary vein rupture
3. Intracranial haemorrhage — this complication is rare and related to hypoxia and prematurity.

These can be avoided if the technique is used appropriately.
The Ventouse has specific advantages over the forceps:

1. It can be used with minimal or no anaesthesia
2. It occupies no space between the fetal head and the maternal tissues
3. There is less risk of maternal and fetal injury if used correctly.

CAESAREAN SECTION

Expectations of the examiners

The examiners will assume that the candidate has assisted at caesarean sections. The indications, risks, and complications of the operation should be known and the management of future deliveries.

Definition

A caesarean section is a surgical procedure whereby the fetus is delivered abdominally through a uterine incision.

Interesting facts

Although low, the maternal mortality following caesarean section is greater than the maternal mortality following vaginal delivery. A woman's obstetric future may be prejudiced by the presence of a uterine scar.

Indications

There are many indications for caesarean section and the commonest are listed below:

1. Fetal
   a. Fetal distress—this can either be antenatally or intrapartum
   b. Malpresentations and malpositions
   c. Multiple pregnancy
2. Maternal
   a. Failure to progress in labour
   b. Previous caesarean section—most obstetricians would deliver a woman who had two previous caesarean sections by an elective caesarean section
   c. Pre-eclampsia or eclampsia
   d. Cephalopelvic disproportion
3. Placental
   a. Praevia
   b. Abruption
   c. Cord prolapse.

With most of the indications listed above, other factors may need to be taken into account, e.g. gestation, stage of labour, parity.

Method

The operation can be performed under epidural, general, or spinal anaesthesia. The bladder is emptied and the woman is placed with a left lateral tilt to avoid supine hypotension. The abdomen is cleaned and draped. Most caesarean sections are performed through a horizontal suprapubic skin incision (Pfannenstiel). The various layers of the abdominal wall are divided to expose the lower segment of the uterus. A transverse incision is made in the lower segment and the presenting part is then delivered manually or with forceps (if cephalic), the baby's mouth is suctioned, and the rest of the body is extracted. The cord is clamped and cut, and the placenta is removed. The wound is then repaired in layers.

A 'classical' caesarean section involves a vertical skin incision (although it can be done through a transverse suprapubic skin incision) and a vertical incision in the upper segment of the uterus. This leaves a large scar on the uterus which is weaker in subsequent pregnancies. Most obstetricians would deliver a woman who had a classical caesarean with an elective caesarean in subsequent pregnancies.

Requirements

1. Ideally the patient should be starved and given an H_2 antagonist and an alkaline mixture prior to the operation (to neutralize the acid in the stomach)
2. The bladder must be empty
3. An intravenous line must be in place
4. An experienced anaesthetist must be present
5. Blood must be available.

Complications

Early

1. Anaesthetic problems, e.g. failed intubation, drug overdose, hypoxia, aspiration of gastric contents
2. Haemorrhage
3. Bladder and bowel damage
4. The original condition that caused the operation, e.g. pre-eclampsia, may worsen postoperatively.

Late

1. Infection, e.g. uterine, wound, chest
2. Thromboembolism
3. Haemorrhage
4. Urinary tract infection
5. Wound dehiscence
6. Psychological problems.

Very late

1. Infertility (following infection)
2. Uterine rupture in a subsequent pregnancy
3. Adhesion formation.

SUMMARY

The maternal morbidity and mortality for a caesarean section are higher when compared with a vaginal delivery.

29. Breech presentation and transverse lie

J. Rymer

BREECH PRESENTATION

Expectations of the examiners

Although the delivery of a breech presentation is a specialist area, the examiners will expect the candidate to understand the principles of antenatal and labour management. As a general practitioner, the candidate may well have to perform a breech delivery if it has not been diagnosed prior to delivery, or there is not enough time to call the flying squad as in preterm labour. There are several areas of controversy in the management of breech presentation, and the candidate could be expected to discuss these.

Definition

The word breech means 'the buttocks'. There are three types of breech:

1. Extended leg breech—the legs are flexed at the hip and extended at the knee (frank breech) (Fig. 29.1a).
2. Flexed leg breech—the legs are flexed at the hip and the knee (complete) (Fig. 29.1b).
3. Footling breech—one or both feet are below the buttocks (Fig. 29.1c).

Interesting facts

The incidence is 3–4% of all singleton pregnancies at term. The morbidity and mortality for a fetus in a breech presentation are considerably worse than for a vertex presentation. (Major contributors to this are prematurity, congenital anomalies, and birth trauma.)

Aetiology
1. Maternal
   a. Grand multiparity
   b. Uterine anomalies
   c. Pelvic tumours
   d. Bony pelvic abnormality.

244

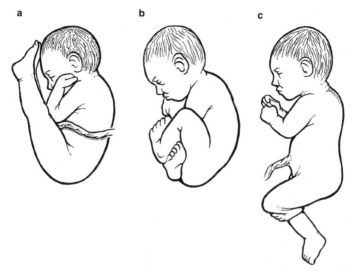

Fig. 29.1   Breech presentation; a, extended (frank); b, flexed (complete); c, footling.

2. Fetal
   a. Prematurity
   b. Multiple pregnancy
   c. Fetal abnormality
   d. Extended legs.
3. Placental
   a. Cornual implantation
   b. Placenta praevia
   c. Oligohydramnios
   d. Polyhydramnios.

The frequency of breech presentation decreases as pregnancy progresses.

A breech presentation does not become a concern until 36 weeks (except in preterm labour). External cephalic version may be performed after 36 weeks to convert the breech to a cephalic presentation.

The diagnosis of a breech presentation is made on palpation of the abdomen. The presenting part is wider and the head is felt in the fundus. The fetal heart is heard above the umbilicus.

If the position of the placenta is known, then a vaginal examination should be performed to exclude pelvic masses and gross abnormalities of the pelvic bones.

Investigations

An ultrasound scan should be performed for the following reasons:

1. To confirm presentation
2. To exclude a fetal abnormality

3. To determine placental position
4. To determine whether it is a flexed or extended leg breech
5. To assess the liquor volume
6. To estimate fetal weight.

X-ray pelvimetry is performed to exclude pelvic abnormality. The anteroposterior diameter of the pelvic inlet should be greater than 11.5 cm.

Management

Once ultrasound scan and pelvimetry have been performed, a decision on the mode of delivery should be made. Prior to 36 weeks unit policies vary. The ideal weight for a vaginal breech delivery is 2500–3500 g. Footling and flexed leg breeches are usually delivered by caesarean section, but in a multiparous woman a flexed leg breech may be allowed a trial of labour. Providing there are no maternal contraindications, an extended leg breech, without a fetal abnormality, between 2500 and 3500 g is favourable for a trial of vaginal delivery.

Most practitioners would not induce a breech presentation, as spontaneous onset of labour has the best prognosis. Once labour is established the membranes should be ruptured, and a fetal scalp electrode applied to the buttock. An epidural anaesthetic is ideal because of the need for an operative delivery. The fetus should be monitored continuously and progress in labour assessed regularly. The use of syntocinon augmentation in a breech presentation is controversial, and slow progress in labour (<1 cm/hour) is usually managed by a caesarean section.

Once full dilatation has occurred and the breech has descended to the perineum, then an episiotomy should be performed. As the breech continues to descend the sacrum is gently guided anteriorly, and the legs are stepped over the perineum (Pinard's manoeuvre). As the trunk descends the shoulders are delivered. If there is difficulty in delivering the shoulders then Lovset's manoeuvre must be performed. (Lovset's manoeuvre involves rotating the posterior shoulder anteriorly by rotating the trunk and then applying a downward traction. This enables the shoulders to descend below the pelvic brim and the arm usually appears spontaneously. If not, a finger can be hooked over the anterior shoulder and the arm brought down. The manoeuvre is repeated for the other arm.) The baby is allowed to hang until the nape of the neck is visible. The assistant then lifts the baby up and forceps are applied to the head to ensure a controlled delivery.

SUMMARY

Breech presentation is associated with increased perinatal morbidity and mortality, and must be considered a high-risk pregnancy.

TRANSVERSE AND OBLIQUE LIE

Expectations of the examiners

The candidate should be able to detect abnormal lie on palpation. The principles of management of a transverse and oblique lie should be known by the candidate. The management of cord prolapse is a common examination question.

Definition

The lie of the fetus is not in the longitudinal axis of the uterus.

Aetiology

1. Maternal
   a. High multiparity
   b. Uterine anomalies
   c. Pelvic tumours
   d. Pelvic contraction
2. Fetal
   a. Prematurity
   b. Multiple pregnancy
   c. Fetal abnormality
3. Placenta
   a. Placenta praevia
   b. Fundal placenta.

Assessment

On inspection the uterus appears wider than normal. The fundal height may be smaller than one would expect for the gestational age, and there is no presenting part in the pelvis. The back is lying across the maternal abdomen and the head is palpated in one or other flank. The fetal heart may be heard more laterally than normal.

As with a breech presentation, a vaginal examination should be performed (if the placental site is known) to exclude pelvic pathology.

Investigations

An ultrasound scan should be performed for the same reasons as in breech presentation.

Management

Transverse lie is uncommon. External cephalic version should not be attempted. If the transverse lie persists beyond 37 weeks then the woman should be admitted to hospital, because of the risk of cord prolapse. If a cause for the transverse lie is found, e.g. pelvic tumour or placenta praevia, then an elective caesarean section should be performed. If no cause is found then there are two accepted forms of management:

1. Await the onset of labour to see if the lie converts to longitudinal in labour. If it does, then the woman has a trial of labour. If it does not, then a caesarean section should be performed. If the lie converts to longitudinal prior to the onset of labour she can be allowed home or if the cervix is favourable, an artificial rupture of membranes (ARM) could be performed followed by syntocinon. In primiparous women this is very unlikely after 37 weeks, even when labour begins.
2. An elective caesarean section can be performed.

Cord prolapse

If a woman with a transverse lie has spontaneous rupture of membranes she must have an immediate vaginal examination to exclude cord prolapse. If the cord is felt then the woman must be put into the knee–chest position, or placed on all fours. The aim of adopting these positions is to use gravity to keep the presenting part from compressing the cord against the cervix. The examining hand must remain in the vagina to elevate the presenting part until the baby is delivered. (If there is to be a long delay between the time of cord prolapse and caesarean section, then 500 ml of fluid can be infused into the bladder via a Foley catheter which is then clamped.)

Urgent arrangements must be made to deliver the baby by caesarean section.

Delivery

A transverse lie that persists must be delivered by caesarean section. These can be difficult operations, especially if the fetal back is presenting.

A general anaesthetic is preferred to ensure maximum uterine relaxation. If there is no lower segment then a vertical incision should be performed in the uterus. After incising the uterus, a breech extraction is performed. A foot is grasped, the lie converted to longitudinal, and the feet and the remainder of the body are delivered.

A thorough inspection of the uterine cavity and the pelvis should be performed to attempt to determine a cause for the transverse lie.

SUMMARY

Transverse and oblique lie is uncommon and needs specialist referral. Women should be admitted from 37 weeks onwards. Cord prolapse is more common and is an obstetric emergency.

30. Twin pregnancy

J. Rymer

Expectations of the examiners

The candidate will be expected to be aware of the common antenatal complications of a multiple pregnancy. The overall management of multiple pregnancy should always be undertaken by a specialist unit.

Definition

A pregnancy with two fetuses.

Interesting facts

The incidence is 1 in 80 but this is increasing due to assisted conception techniques.

Pathophysiology

Twinning can either be monozygotic or dizygotic. Monozygotic twins result from the division of one conceptus, producing identical twins. Dizygotic twins result from the fertilization of two separate ova, and the twins have different genetic make-up. Dizygotic twins are always dichorionic and diamniotic, but monozygotic twins can vary from monochorionic and monoamniotic to dichorionic and diamniotic, depending on when division of the blastocyst occurred.

Aetiology

The frequency of monozygotic twins is constant at a rate of 1/250 births. However, the incidence of dizygotic twins is influenced remarkably by:

1. *Race.* In Nigeria twinning occurs 1 in every 19 births, compared to 1 in 155 births in Japan.
2. *Heredity.* A family history of twins, especially on the mother's side, is associated with an increase in the incidence of twin pregnancy.
3. *Increasing maternal age and parity.* Both of these factors are associated with a higher rate of twin pregnancies.

4. *Assisted conception.* The overall incidence of multiple pregnancies using these techniques is 2–3%. This is due to the induction of multiple ovulations and the replacement of more than one egg or embryo.

Assessment

At the booking visit, the history may include risk factors for multiple pregnancy as outlined above. 'Hyperemesis gravidarum' in the first trimester is more common, and on examination the uterine size may be larger than dates.

Investigations

An ultrasound scan should detect multiple pregnancies, although they can be missed.

The haemoglobin and the packed cell volume may be lower due to the exaggerated increase in plasma volume.

The α-fetoprotein levels in maternal serum will be higher, making interpretation difficult.

Management

Multiple pregnancy should not be regarded as a 'normal pregnancy', and patients should be seen more regularly in the antenatal clinic.

First trimester. An early scan (<14 weeks) should be performed for dating purposes. Severe hyperemesis warrants admission with intravenous hydration. Four-weekly visits are acceptable if there are no other complications.

Second trimester. A detailed anomaly scan should be performed at 18–20 weeks, as there is an increased incidence of fetal abnormalities.

Third trimester. After 28 weeks' gestation the patient should be seen at least every two weeks with regular ultrasound scans for growth assessment.

Routine admission at 28 weeks to 32 weeks has not been shown to decrease the incidence of preterm labour. Admission should be offered to the patient at any stage if she is unable to rest adequately at home.

In late pregnancy the commonest presentations are vertex, vertex (45%); vertex, breech (40%); but malpresentations are more common in multiple pregnancies.

Complications

Maternal

1. *Hyperemesis.* Severe cases require admission and intravenous hydration, but most settle by 12 weeks when the β-hCG levels begin to fall.

2. *Hypertension*. Not only does hypertension occur more often in multiple pregnancy but it tends to develop earlier, and be more severe.

3. *Gestational diabetes*. The diabetogenic state of normal pregnancy is exaggerated, increasing the incidence and severity of gestational diabetes.

4. *Anaemia*. The increase in plasma volume is much greater, exaggerating the 'physiological' anaemia of pregnancy. Iron and folate deficiencies are common because of the extra demands of a twin pregnancy.

5. *General discomfort*. Having a larger uterine mass puts added strain on the musculoskeletal system.

6. *Placenta praevia*. The incidence is increased in multiple pregnancies, presumably due to the increased placental area.

Fetal

1. *Prematurity* is the main factor in the increased wastage associated with multiple pregnancies. More than 50% of babies of multiple pregnancies are less than 2.5 kg compared with 6% of singletons. There are many contributing factors to the significantly increased incidence of preterm delivery in twin pregnancies:
    a. Overdistension of the uterus
    b. Increased incidence of pregnancy-induced hypertension
    c. Increased incidence of fetal abnormalities
    d. Increased incidence of abruption
    e. Increased incidence of malpresentation.

2. *Fetal abnormality*. There is an increased incidence of fetal malformation in monozygotic twin pregnancies.

3. *IUGR*. Growth retardation is common in twin pregnancies, especially when the placenta is monochorionic. One or both twins may be affected.

4. *Twin-to-twin transfusion*. The two placental circulations may form anastomoses in monochorionic twins. One fetus may become anaemic, and the other polycythaemic. The syndrome is usually diagnosed after birth, and either baby may require intensive care.

5. *Malpresentations*. Probably more common because of prematurity, increased incidence of fetal malformations, and mechanical restrictions of the uterine cavity.

Delivery

The decision on the mode of delivery depends on the presentation of the leading twin, and the presence of maternal or fetal complications. In the majority of cases, labour occurs spontaneously around 38 weeks.

The membranes should be ruptured as soon as labour is established. An intravenous line should be inserted, and blood should be grouped and saved. A fetal scalp electrode should be applied to the leading twin, and the second twin monitored externally.

An epidural is the optimal form of analgesia, as an operative delivery may be required.

Progress in labour must be assessed regularly as inefficient uterine action is common.

At delivery, two obstetricians, two paediatricians, an anaesthetist and midwifery staff should be present. Following delivery of the first twin, the cord is clamped and cut. The abdomen is palpated to ensure that the lie of the remaining fetus is longitudinal. (If the lie cannot be converted to longitudinal externally, then a caesarean section should be considered.) Fundal pressure is maintained, and the membranes ruptured during a contraction. Labour should resume, but if there are no contractions after 10 minutes, then a syntocinon infusion should be commenced. The second twin is then delivered. Breech extraction of the second twin may be necessary. The placenta is delivered, and a syntocinon infusion postpartum is advisable to prevent haemorrhage.

Complications

1. *Incoordinate uterine action.* This is a common occurrence in twins. There is debate as to whether labour should be augmented.
2. *Fetal distress.* The second twin is usually smaller and may not cope as well with the stress of labour.
3. *Prolapse of the umbilical cord.* The management depends on the circumstances: degree of cervical dilatation, the presence or absence of ruptured membranes, and the analgesia (see Ch. 29).
4. *Premature separation of the placenta.* If vaginal delivery can be achieved rapidly without harm to the fetus or the mother, then this should be performed. Otherwise, the fetus should be delivered by caesarean section.
5. *Locking.* This is rare but can occur when the first twin presents as a breech, and the second by the vertex. The chin of the first fetus locks in the neck and chin of the second cephalic fetus.

Postpartum

1. *Haemorrhage.* Due to the increased size of the placental bed, and the overdistension of the uterus, there is an increased risk of postpartum haemorrhage.
2. *Thromboembolic disease.* Twin pregnancies have an increased risk.
3. *Anaemia.* Due to the increased demand for iron in pregnancy and the greater blood loss.

SUMMARY

Twin pregnancies have significantly increased fetal and maternal morbidity and mortality. They are high-risk pregnancies and should be monitored carefully. The delivery should be conducted in a specialist unit. Only twin pregnancies have been discussed but the problems of a twin gestation are exaggerated by the presence of more fetuses. Most obstetricians would deliver pregnancies with three or more fetuses by caesarean section.

31. Obstetric analgesia and anaesthesia

G. Davis

Expectations of the examiners

Candidates will be expected to be able to advise women on the advantages and disadvantages of the different methods of analgesia and anaesthesia. The effects on mother and fetus, the complications and the management of the complications must be completely understood.

Definitions

Analgesia: loss of sensation to pain.
Anaesthesia: loss of all sensation including pain.

Interesting facts

There is a wide range of methods available for pain relief and the choice of a particular method will depend on a number of factors: mother's preference, severity of pain, stage in labour, methods available at the place of birth, and the presence of complications in the mother and/or fetus. Most women and their partners are anxious during labour and careful explanation and reassurance to reduce anxiety is an important aspect of the management of pain in labour. Patients vary widely in their tolerance of pain and their response to analgesia.

Pathophysiology

Source of the pain

Pain in labour is of two types: (1) intermittent and (2) continuous.

Intermittent pain is due to uterine contractions and is probably due to myometrial ischaemia at the peak of the contractions. The pain is most severe just prior to full dilatation (transition phase) when contractions are most intense and the cervix is dilating most rapidly. Sensation from the uterus and cervix is transmitted mainly in the sensory fibres of the T11 and T12 nerve roots, with smaller amounts in T10 and L1.

Continuous pain occurs in the lower back and suprapubically and the cause of this pain is not known. Lower back pain is more prominent with occipitoposterior positions.

In the second stage of labour, pain is associated with distension of the lower vagina and perineum. The perineum is innervated principally by the pudendal nerve (posterior two-thirds of vulva) with fibres passing to the S2, 3 and 4 nerve roots.

Pharmacokinetics in mother and fetus

Mother. Although liver production of various proteins alters markedly in pregnancy, it is unclear whether this affects the maternal handling of anaesthetic drugs in any way. Body fat increases by 4 kg on average during pregnancy, leading to a greater capacity to sequester lipid-soluble drugs.

Fetus. About one-seventh of the blood returning to the fetus from the placenta enters the left atrium directly. Any drugs in this blood are therefore available to affect the fetal brain. This is only likely to be significant with intravenous bolus injections, and conversely, six-sevenths of the umbilical blood flow passes through the fetal liver where drugs are metabolized.

Placental transfer

Like the blood–brain barrier, the placental barrier is composed of lipoproteins so the transfer of drugs depends on lipid solubility. Most agents which affect the central nervous system will therefore cross the placenta. Highly ionized drugs, such as muscle relaxants, do not cross the placenta.

Although there has been concern that exposure of pregnant women to trace quantities of anaesthetic gases may lead to abortion or fetal malformation, the evidence for this is inconclusive. During the first half of pregnancy intra-abdominal surgery increases the risk of miscarriage, but this is probably due to uterine manipulation rather than the anaesthetic agents.

PAIN RELIEF IN LABOUR

The different components of pain relief in labour are outlined in Table 31.1.

Although in this chapter interventional management is emphasized, perhaps the most important aspect of pain relief in labour is the individual woman's attitude. The ideal approach is for women to be healthy, relaxed, supported by labour partners, fully acquainted with the choice of methods available, free to make a choice, and with open minds should circumstances alter. It is the role of antenatal education to provide women with the opportunity to achieve such a state at the onset of labour.

Physical methods

The major advantage of these methods is that they are non-invasive and therefore not harmful to the fetus. They are useful early in labour and may

Table 31.1 Sources of pain relief in labour.

Education
  Antenatal classes
    Information
    Demonstrations

Environment
  Pleasant surroundings
  Supportive helpful staff
  Support of partner

Physical methods
  Massage
  Acupuncture
  Transcutaneous electrical nerve stimulation (TENS)

Pharmacological
  Analgesia
    Inhalational, e.g. nitrous oxide
    Narcotic, e.g. pethidine
    Regional analgesia: epidural, spinal, pudendal, perineal infiltration

---

act by overloading sensory inputs. Their major disadvantage is that they are often ineffective later in labour.

Inhalational agents

Entonox (50% nitrous oxide, 50% oxygen) is the only inhalational agent now available. The advantages of inhalational agents are that they are self-administered and safe for mother and fetus. The major disadvantage is that they are commonly used incorrectly leading to failure of this method.

In active labour, although contractions last approximately 60 seconds, the first 20–30 seconds are not usually as painful as the latter part of the contractions. It takes a similar period of time, 20–30 seconds, of deep panting using Entonox to achieve a blood level of nitrous oxide sufficient for analgesia. It is therefore important for the woman to begin rapid respiration with the onset of each contraction rather than waiting until the contraction is painful. Similarly, in the second stage of labour when pain is present throughout contractions, contractions must be anticipated by 30 seconds and inhalation commenced prior to the onset of the contraction if this method is to be successful.

Narcotic agents

Pethidine is the preferred narcotic for use in labour as it is less soporific than the other narcotics. Although it is a strong analgesic and is easily administered, there is a high incidence of side-effects and 40% of women in labour report no relief of pain. The side-effects are:

1. Dizziness
2. Drowsiness

3. Dissociated state of consciousness
4. Nausea
5. Vomiting
6. Hypotension.

Pethidine is usually given as a bolus i.m. injection of 100 mg which may need to be repeated. It is rare for a woman in labour to require more than two doses and, if the need arises, progress in labour should be reviewed. It is unlikely to cause significant delay in the active phase of labour. The effect . on the fetus is to depress heart rate variability and breathing movements and it causes respiratory depression and hypotonicity in the newborn. Respiratory depression is most likely to occur if a narcotic is given i.m. 2.5–3.5 hours prior to delivery. Respiratory depression is unlikely more than 6 hours after i.m. administration. Respiratory depression within 6 hours of narcotic administration is treated with a narcotic antagonist, most commonly naloxone 20 µg .i.m., repeated if necessary.

Because nausea and vomiting are common side-effects, narcotics are often given with an antiemetic. The antiemetic chosen varies considerably but is either an antihistamine, e.g. promethazine hydrochloride, an antidopaminergic (phenothiazine), e.g. prochlorperazine, or metoclopramide. The first two have sedative and anxiolytic properties and are sometimes preferred because of these effects.

The routine use of other sedatives, e.g. diazepam or barbiturates, is not acceptable in modern obstetric practice because of their prolonged effect on the neonate.

Epidural analgesia

The epidural (or extradural) space is the potential space lying outside the dura mater and containing blood vessels, lymphatics, and fat. The injection of local anaesthetics into this space produces analgesia in the spinal nerve roots to which the anaesthetic agents diffuse. Therefore, to provide effective analgesia in the first stage of labour the T10–L1 nerve roots must be blocked, while in the second stage of labour the sacral roots must be blocked. The use of epidural analgesia for caesarean section requires a more extensive block to at least T8 and sometimes even T6. There are two routes for epidural analgesia: caudal via the sacrococcygeal membrane or lumbar between adjacent vertebral spines. In obstetrics the latter route is now used almost exclusively.

Indications

1. *Pain relief.* This is the commonest reason.
2. *Hypertensive disorders.* Blood pressure is more easily controlled when an effective epidural block is present.

3. *Maternal heart disease.* The abolition of pain reduces stress and the bearing down reflex thereby relieving strain on the heart. Care is necessary, however, if the patient has a fixed cardiac output, e.g. mitral or aortic stenosis, and cannot compensate for hypotension.
4. *Cerebrovascular disease.* This is rare in pregnancy but epidural analgesia would be indicated in the presence of an intracranial aneurysm or angioma.
5. *Breech and twin delivery.* The presence of an effective epidural block allows the use of forceps to control delivery of the aftercoming head in a breech delivery or intrauterine manipulation of the second twin.

Contraindications

1. Recent antepartum haemorrhage: epidural analgesia may be associated with profound hypotension in the presence of significant blood loss.
2. Coagulation disorder: a clotting defect due to anticoagulants or coagulopathy (e.g. in severe pre-eclampsia) increases the risk of haemorrhage into the epidural space.
3. Sepsis at the injection site.
4. Sensitivity to local anaesthetic agents.
5. Lack of adequately trained staff.
6. Bony disorder of lower spine.
7. Active neurological disease.

In the presence of a uterine scar (previous caesarean section or hysterotomy), some obstetricians will not offer epidural analgesia. This is because of the concern that the epidural may 'mask' the pain of uterine rupture. This is a subject of debate and in most units epidural analgesia is used in the presence of a uterine scar.

Management

A fine plastic catheter is passed through an introducer which is inserted in the midline midway between two lumbar spinous processes — usually L2–3 or L3–4 (Fig. 31.1). Positioning of the patient is critical and the epidural catheter is inserted when the woman is lying in the left lateral position or, less commonly, sitting with her back flexed. The skin area is cleansed and the large bore Tuohy needle (introducer) is inserted after infiltrating the skin and subcutaneous tissues with local anaesthetic.

The commonest local anaesthetic agent used is bupivacaine. Bupivacaine is given (5–20 ml of 0.25%, 0.375% or 0.5%) in an initial test dose of 3 ml and then 5 minutes later the remainder is given. The purpose of giving a test dose is to ensure that the catheter has not inadvertently traversed the dura (a spinal block) or is in an epidural vein. Lignocaine is

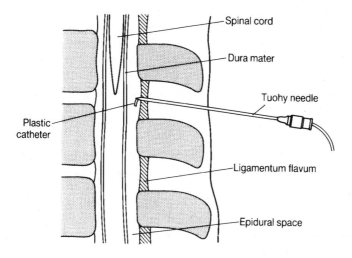

Fig. 31.1 The correct insertion of an epidural catheter. A Tuohy needle is pushed through the skin and ligamentum flavum into the epidural space. The plastic catheter is then passed through the needle, pushed a little further into space, and the needle is removed.

used less commonly and provides a shorter acting, dense block which is useful prior to instrumental delivery.

Observations

Prior to inserting the epidural catheter an i.v. line must be inserted and hypovolaemia corrected. The use of a 'preload' of 500–1000 ml crystalloid fluid is controversial. The fetal heart must be monitored continuously and maternal blood pressure and pulse recorded every 5 minutes for at least 15 minutes. An analgesic effect is not observed for 15–20 minutes and usually lasts 60–90 minutes. As soon as sensation begins to return the epidural catheter should be 'topped up'. Alternative methods are to give a continuous infusion of anaesthetic agent or intermittent boluses controlled by the woman (patient controlled analgesia, PCA). A low concentration (0.125%) of bupivicaine is infused, usually with an opioid such as fentanyl or pethidine.

Complications

1. Hypotension (drop in systolic blood pressure of >20 mmHg) is treated by ensuring that aortocaval compression is not occurring and administering 1 litre of Hartmann's solution or normal saline over 20 minutes. If these measures are ineffective or maternal or fetal distress occurs, ephedrine should be given, 5–10 mg i.v. This has an inotropic

and chronotropic action on the heart and does not cause placental vasoconstriction.

2. Total spinal block occurs with injection of the local anaesthetic agent into the intrathecal space. There is rapid, progessively ascending block of motor, sensory and autonomic nerves. This is manifested by marked hypotension, bradycardia and increasing respiratory distress which may culminate in apnoea. Treatment is to provide oxygen and vasopressors initially and, if complete respiratory paralysis occurs, artificial ventilation.

3. Failure to achieve adequate analgesia can usually be treated by injecting further anaesthetic, but if this fails the epidural catheter may have to be resited.

4. Dural puncture occurs in 1–2% of cases and results in a severe headache in 70% of these cases. The headache usually starts within 48 hours of delivery and lasts for 6 days if left untreated. If it is recognized at the time of insertion the catheter is resited and good analgesia achieved. An elective forceps delivery should be performed if delivery is not speedily effected. After delivery dural puncture is treated conservatively with bed rest, analgesia, and adequate fluids. If a severe headache persists after 24–36 hours a 'blood patch' is performed. To achieve a blood clot over the hole in the dura, 20 ml of the patient's blood is injected into the epidural space. The patient lies flat for 30 minutes and the headache is usually absent after this period.

5. Increased rate of forceps delivery. There is still considerable debate on this issue. The aggressive use of syntocinon in the second stage of labour will reduce the forceps rate. Despite syntocinon, there appears to be an increased rate of both straight and rotational forceps deliveries with epidurals but this does not increase the perinatal morbidity or mortality.

6. Local anaesthesic toxicity may develop with either accidental intravascular injection or excessive total dosage. Premonitory signs include a metallic taste, circumoral tingling, nervousness, and nausea. If untreated, these may progress to muscle twitching leading to convulsions, cardiovascular depression and cardiac arrest.

7. Other rare complications are meningitis and neurological sequelae.

The major advantage of epidural analgesia is that it is the only method of completely abolishing pain in labour (90% of patients have complete or substantial relief). The fetus is rarely affected and the patient is awake and alert. The major disadvantage is that it requires the presence of skilled personnel. Closer observation is also necessary and there is an increased incidence of operative delivery.

Caesarean section. As discussed above, caesarean section under epidural anaesthesia requires a more extensive block. The advantages are that the patient and her partner can see and be involved with the infant immediately; blood loss is reduced and the incidence of postoperative complications is reduced. The disadvantages are that the anaesthesia may not be sufficient necessitating general anaesthesia and, from the operator's point of view, the baby is more difficult to deliver as the patient's abdominal muscles may not be completely relaxed. Epidural infusion or PCA with opioids may be continued for 24–36 hours for postoperative analgesia.

Spinal analgesia

Spinal block is used primarily as a single injection intrathecally in the lumbar region for instrumental delivery, caesarean section or manual removal of the placenta. A small volume of a heavy form of local anaesthetic agent usually mixed with an opioid (e.g. 2.5 ml of bupivicaine with 200 mg morphine) is injected with the patient in the sitting position to minimize the spread of the agent cephalically. The block is effective in 3–5 minutes and the patient is observed as with epidural anaesthesia. The advantage of this method is that it is rapid and gives a dense block. The disadvantages are that if it is ineffective then there is no catheter to repeat the dose, cephalic spread with consequent respiratory depression may occur and hypotension is common. Despite these drawbacks, spinal anaesthesia is becoming more widely used because of its advantages.

Pudendal block

This is a suitable method of analgesia for non-rotational forceps or vacuum extraction. The pudendal nerve is blocked by infiltrating 5–10 ml of 0.5–1% lignocaine around the nerve on each side as it passes around the ischial spine. This is usually done vaginally or, rarely, through the perineum. The commonest problem is that there may be inadequate analgesia on one or both sides and perineal infiltration is often required.

GENERAL ANAESTHESIA

The major problems associated with general anaesthesia in the obstetric patient are regurgitation and aspiration of the stomach contents during induction of anaesthesia. Although this has been recognized for many years, it is still a major cause of avoidable maternal death. The reasons for the increased risk are:

1. General anaesthesia is often performed as an emergency procedure with the patient not starved.
2. There is delayed gastric emptying and relaxation of the lower oesophageal sphincter in pregnancy.
3. In labour, gastric emptying is even further delayed especially when opioids are given.

4. Oedema of the vocal cords is more common in pregnancy (due to pre-eclampsia).
5. The increase in body fat and breast size in pregnancy and the presence of an abdominal mass combine to make intubation technically more difficult.

Indications

1. Early pregnancy—abortion, termination of pregnancy, ectopic pregnancy, insertion of cervical suture.
2. Caesarean section.
3. Instrumental delivery—this is rarely necessary under general anaesthesia and should be used with great caution because of the risk of fetal trauma.
4. Obstetric emergencies—ruptured or inverted uterus, uncontrollable postpartum haemorrhage.
5. Manual removal of the placenta.

Preoperative medication

The drugs usually given preoperatively are contraindicated in pregnancy because of the effects on the fetus. Acidity of the stomach contents is reduced by giving H_2-receptor blocking drugs orally every 6 hours in labour and prior to elective surgery in pregnancy. Ranitidine is more commonly used as it has fewer side-effects than cimetidine. An alkali mixture, e.g. 15–30 ml magnesium trisilicate or sodium citrate, is given orally immediately prior to induction of anaesthesia.

Induction of anaesthesia

The patient is placed in the left lateral position during transport to, and in, the anaesthetic room. Oxygen is given by mask or mouthpiece for 3–5 minutes prior to induction. This reduces the effects on mother and fetus of the apnoeic period between the onset of paralysis and the initiation of ventilation.

Following the injection of the induction agent, cricoid pressure is immediately applied and maintained until the endotracheal tube is in place and its cuff inflated. The most commonly used induction agent is thiopentone (250–300 mg). This is followed immediately by suxamethonium to induce rapid paralysis to allow endotracheal intubation. Paralysis is continued throughout the operation and anaesthesia maintained with nitrous oxide in oxygen which is administered in a relatively high concentration until delivery has occurred. This mixture is supplemented with a volatile agent (e.g. halothane) in low concentrations.

Following delivery, syntocinon (5–10 mg) is given to ensure uterine contraction and the concentration of the inhalational agents is usually increased.

Complications

Because light anaesthesia is maintained prior to delivery, approximately 3% of patients will experience some degree of awareness of which about one-tenth will be painful. This dilemma is difficult to resolve because of the concern over neonatal drug-induced CNS depression. The use of volatile 0.5% halothane or an equivalent dose of isoflurane or enthrane virtually abolishes awareness.

Aspiration of gastric contents (Mendelson's syndrome) is the most important contributor to maternal morbidity and mortality associated with general anaesthesia. The syndrome is unlikely to occur if the pH of the gastric contents is >3.0, stressing the importance of prophylactic measures discussed above. Management involves bronchoscopy if solid material is aspirated, oxygen and bronchodilators, intravenous fluids, steroids and antibiotics, and artificial ventilation if necessary.

Other complications of general anaesthesia are:

1. Intraoperative
   a. Circulatory collapse
   b. Respiratory failure
   c. Cardiac failure
2. Postoperative
   a. Patient drowsy
   b. Respiratory infection
   c. Deep venous thrombosis/pulmonary embolus
   d. Gastrointestinal stasis.

32. Puerperium and breast-feeding

G. Davis

Expectations of the examiners

Problems arising in the puerperium are usually managed in the community and therefore by general practitioners. The examiners will expect candidates to have a good understanding of the normal course of the puerperium and practical remedies for any problems. The management of postpartum haemorrhage (PPH) is a frequent examination question as it is a life-threatening condition which is relatively common.

Definitions

Puerperium: the weeks following delivery in which the pregnancy-induced changes return to normal. By convention this is 6 weeks, although it may take longer for all the organs to return to normal.

Postpartum haemorrhage (PPH)
Primary: blood loss from the genital tract of 500 ml or more in the first 24 hours after delivery.
Secondary: blood loss from the genital tract of 500 ml or more at any time in the puerperium after the first 24 hours.

Puerperal pyrexia: temperature of 38°C or greater, or 37.4°C on three successive days, within 14 days of delivery or miscarriage.

Physiology

The pelvic organs never entirely return to normal after childbirth. The uterus weighs 1000–1200 g immediately postpartum, 500 g 1 week later, and has returned to the non-pregnant weight (50–70 g) by 6 weeks. It is not normally palpable abdominally after 10–14 days. The cervix never returns to normal and is slit-like and often irregular. Mature breast milk is produced by 7 days postpartum as a result of oestrogen withdrawal.

The increased production of plasma proteins which occurs in pregnancy rapidly returns to normal after delivery and this is complete by 3 weeks postpartum. The cardiovascular and renal systems have returned to their non-pregnant state by 6 weeks, except the renal collecting system which takes about 3 months. The cardiovascular system reverts quickly after delivery and is 50% back to normal by the third day after delivery.

Ovulation after delivery is extremely variable and affected by lactation. In non-lactating women, 10–15% will have ovulated by 6 weeks but in lactating women, ovulation is rare before 10 weeks. Menstruation often occurs prior to initial ovulation.

PRIMARY POSTPARTUM HAEMORRHAGE

See 'Labour—third stage' (Ch. 26).

SECONDARY POSTPARTUM HAEMORRHAGE

Secondary PPH is not usually as life threatening as primary PPH but can be very frightening to the patient.

Aetiology

1. Infection
2. Retained products of conception.

Assessment

1. History
   a. Amount of blood loss—as most cases occur at home this is often difficult to assess
   b. Method of delivery
   c. Completeness of placenta at delivery
   d. Fever
   e. Offensive lochia
2. Examination
   a. Temperature, other vital signs
   b. Height and tenderness of fundus
   c. State of the cervical os
3. Investigations
   a. USS will sometimes demonstrate retained products of conception but is usually not helpful in those cases where it is not clinically obvious
   b. FBC, cross-match
   c. Cervical swabs
   d. Blood cultures and other investigations as required if the patient is septicaemic.

Treatment

In most cases the diagnosis is clear. If the cervical os is open then evacuation of the uterus will be necessary. If the woman is febrile and/or toxic then 12–24 hours of intravenous antibiotics are required prior to the evacuation. A tender well-retracted uterus with a closed cervical os in an otherwise well woman should be treated with oral antibiotics, amoxycillin and metronidazole (200 mg t.d.s. in breast-feeding women).

PUERPERAL INFECTION

Interesting facts

This was the largest cause of maternal mortality until the 1930s when aseptic techniques, and then antibiotics were introduced. Puerperal fever was caused by the spread of group A streptococcus from patient to patient. Anaemia increases the susceptibility of women to infection postnatally.

Pathophysiology

Although infection may occur at any site, the puerperal woman is particularly susceptible to wound infection and infection of the reproductive, urinary and respiratory tracts, and the breasts.

1. The reproductive tract has usually been traumatized and there may be retained products or blood clot. In practice, the severity of infection is varied and may be complicated by pelvic vein thrombosis
   a. Mild infection confined to the vagina, cervix, and uterus
   b. Moderate infection with spread to the pelvic organs to give salpingitis and pelvic peritonitis
   c. Severe cases where generalized peritonitis and septicaemia develop.
2. The urinary collecting system is still dilated and the woman may have been catheterized during delivery.
3. General anaesthesia predisposes the woman to postnatal chest infection.
4. The breasts become engorged after delivery and bacterial contamination and infection may occur.
5. The presence of an abdominal wound after caesarean section is a focus for infection.

Bacteriology

1. Reproductive tract
   a. Endogenous organisms
      i. Coliforms
      ii. *Streptococcus faecalis*
      iii. Anaerobic streptococci
      iv. *Clostridium welchii*

    b. Exogenous organisms
       i. Haemolytic streptococcus (group A)
      ii. *Staphylococcus aureus*
2. Urinary tract
    a. *Escherichia coli* (90%)
    b. Others
       i. *Proteus*
      ii. *Klebsiella*
3. Breasts
    a. *Staphylococcus aureus* (> 90%).

Assessment

Women with puerperal pyrexia need a full history, physical examination, diagnosis of the source of infection, and appropriate treatment.

History

1. Method of delivery
2. History of trauma to birth canal
3. Time of onset of fever (infections in the birth canal usually give a rise in temperature 12–24 hours after delivery)
4. Site of pain
5. Any other symptoms suggesting incidental infection, e.g. sore throat.

Examination

A full physical examination should be made with particular attention to:

1. Signs of septicaemia
    a. Temperature
    b. Rapid, weak pulse
    c. Hypotension
    d. Pallor
    e. Altered consciousness
2. Chest—signs of infection
3. Abdomen
    a. The fundus may be tender and high if endometritis is present
    b. More widespread tenderness or peritonism is associated with severe puerperal sepsis
    c. The abdominal wound is the commonest site of infection after caesarean section
4. Vagina
    a. The perineum should be inspected
    b. If the cervical os is dilated then retained products are likely.

5. Lower limbs.

Deep venous thrombosis (DVT) is more common in the postnatal period and may cause pyrexia. The pelvic veins may be involved, particularly if sepsis is present.

Investigations

1. Midstream specimen of urine
2. High vaginal/endocervical swabs for culture
3. Blood cultures if temperature > 38°C
4. Other investigations if septicaemic
5. Venogram (or USS if available) if suspicion of DVT
6. Sputum if chest infection is suspected
7. Wound swab if abdominal delivery.

Treatment

1. *Reproductive tract.* Evacuation of retained products should be performed after 12–24 hours of i.v. antibiotics. Septicaemia will need appropriate circulatory support and often these patients are best managed in an intensive care unit. Treatment should begin before the infecting agent or its sensitivities are known, but after appropriate swabs have been taken.
    a. Mild
        i. Amoxycillin (oral)
        ii. Metronidazole (oral)
    b. Moderate
        i. Ampicillin (i.v.)
        ii. Metronidazole (pr)
    c. Severe
        i. Cephalosporin (i.v.)
        ii. Gentamicin (i.v.)
        iii. Metronidazole (pr).
2. *Urinary tract*
    a. Amoxycillin, or
    b. Nitrofurantoin—this is more effective than amoxycillin but there is a small risk of haemolysis in patients with G6PD (glucose-6-phosphate dehydrogenase) deficiency
    c. Pyelonephritis requires i.v. cephalosporin or ampicillin.
3. *Breast infection.* See 'Breast-feeding' below.
4. *Chest infection*
    a. Amoxycillin, or
    b. Erythromycin
    c. Other antibiotics as appropriate.

OTHER PROBLEMS

Thrombosis

There is an increased risk of thrombosis in the puerperium because of the hypercoagulable state of the blood (oestrogen effect) and other predisposing factors: pelvic trauma during delivery, bed rest, varicose veins. If there is any suspicion of DVT or pulmonary embolus, full heparin anticoagulation is indicated and urgent definitive investigation. Warfarin passes into breast milk but in such small quantities that breast-feeding is not contraindicated

Haemorrhoids

The venodilatation that occurs in pregnancy is exacerbated by the woman's expulsive efforts in labour and haemorrhoids are a common problem in the first few days postpartum. The treatment is conservative with the use of salt baths and proprietary soothing agents. Advice on a high fibre and fluid diet should be given. Prolapsed haemorrhoids should be replaced after each bowel movement. Surgery, except in extreme cases, should only be performed when the problem still persists 3 months after delivery.

Psychiatric complications

The 'blues' begin on day 2–3 after delivery in 50% of women. Clinical depression occurs in 5% and frank puerperal psychosis in 0.3%. The cause of these disturbances is unknown but the high incidence suggests a metabolic cause. Risk factors are:

1. Previous postpartum psychiatric disorder
2. Previous psychiatric history
3. Previous stillbirth or early neonatal death
4. Ambivalence about motherhood or relationship with her partner
5. Lack of social contacts
6. Major problem in the pregnancy or puerperium.

Features of the blues are lability of mood, anxiety, tiredness, and insomnia. They are best treated by education, support, and night sedation if sleeping is a problem. Any sign of more severe psychiatric disturbance should precipitate early referral to psychiatric services. Depression may become evident at any time up to 3–4 months postnatally and is recognized by tiredness, insomnia, psychomotor slowing, loss of confidence, and a withdrawal from relationships with partner and/or baby. Treatment involves restructuring the woman's daily life so that she has adequate rest, and counselling and specialist referral may be required.

Psychosis is rare, usually depressive in nature and can be life threatening to mother, baby or both. Urgent psychiatric referral and care is required and the best results are achieved if mother and baby remain together.

BREAST-FEEDING

Physiology

The principal hormone involved in milk biosynthesis is prolactin but complete development of the terminal alveolar cells of the breast into active milk secreting units also requires insulin, cortisol, oestrogen, and progesterone. During pregnancy, prolactin, which is secreted by the anterior pituitary, increases from 8 weeks to reach its maximum at term. Human placental lactogen (HPL) is secreted by the placenta in huge amounts and may have some lactogenic effect but its major role in pregnancy is in the regulation of lipolysis. Full lactation in pregnancy is prevented by high levels of progesterone which interfere with the binding of prolactin to its receptors in the glandular tissue of the breast.

During pregnancy, and for the first 3–4 days after delivery, only colostrum is produced, consisting of desquamated, epithelial cells and a transudate from maternal serum. The trigger for full milk secretion is the rapid clearance of oestrogen and progesterone which occurs after delivery. Prolactin levels also fall but more slowly. Suckling initiates milk 'let-down' by stimulating tactile sensors in the areolae which cause oxytocin release from the posterior pituitary. The blood-borne oxytocin causes the myoepithelial cells in the breast ductal system to contract and eject stored milk. Suckling also stimulates prolactin secretion which is necessary for the on-going synthesis of milk. Optimal milk production depends on the availability of thyroxine, insulin, cortisol, dietary intake of nutrients and fluid, frequent feeding and a supportive environment. As a general principle, 1% of any drug administered to the mother will cross to the infant.

Composition

Colostrum is a yellow fluid with a high content of antibodies, particularly secretory IgA. It contains more protein (desquamated cells) but less carbohydrate and fat than normal breast milk. Most of the protein is lactalbumin and casein with the lactalbumin providing the essential amino acids (Table 32.1).

Table 32.1 Composition of milk. (From T E Oppe 1974 Present day practice of infant feeding. DHSS Report on Health and Social Subjects. London, HMSO.)

	Human	Cow
Protein	1.0 g/dl	3.3 g/dl
Fat	3.8 g/dl	3.7 g/dl
Carbohydrate	7 g/dl	4.8 g/dl
Sodium	15 mg/dl	58 mg/dl
Calcium	33 mg/dl	125 mg/dl
Phosphorus	15 mg/dl	96 mg/dl
Energy	67 kcal/dl	66 kcal/dl

In extreme circumstances, the high levels of sodium and phosphorus in cows' milk may lead, respectively, to hypernatraemia in infants with diarrhoea, and low calcium and convulsions. Preterm babies need larger amounts of sodium, calcium, and phosphorus.

Management

Antenatal

Patients should be encouraged to breast-feed, and general health and diet should be maintained. Nipple shields may be of some value to women with inverted nipples. Daily antenatal care of the nipples is probably not of great benefit.

Postpartum

The mother and infant should have learned how to breast-feed by 3–4 days postpartum when normal milk production begins. It can be a stressful time for both partners so gentle reassurance, supervision and education by an experienced person is optimal. Mother and infant should be comfortable and the mother should have washed her hands. The nipple (including part of the areola) is fed into the baby's mouth and the nose is kept clear by the mother pressing a finger on the breast just above the baby's nose. The 'letdown reflex' occurs in the first 3 minutes and the infant obtains 90% of its feed in the first 3–5 minutes. When the infant is finished, the nipple is gently withdrawn and the baby is 'winded'. Feeding is most effective if the infant is fed when hungry rather than to a schedule.

Problems

Engorgement

This is due to the sudden secretion of milk on the third or fourth day and is best avoided by frequent feeding under supervision. Treatment is to use heat in the form of a shower or bath, analgesia, a firm, supportive brassiere, and reassurance. Sometimes expression of a small amount of milk relieves tension in the breast sufficiently for the infant to fix on the nipple adequately.

Infection

Mastitis. This usually occurs as a result of a cracked nipple or a blocked duct. There is a tender, inflamed wedge of breast tissue and a pyrexia. *Staphylococcus aureus* is the cause of 95% of mastitis, and it should be treated with flucloxacillin or erythromycin. Breast-feeding should continue unless this is too painful, in which case milk should be expressed from the affected breast.

Abscess. Abscesses usually develop if mastitis is not treated promptly or correctly. Fluctuance may be difficult to elicit but an abscess should be suspected if mastitis does not resolve with antibiotics. The treatment of the abscess is to stop breast-feeding from the infected side, continue expressing the milk and incision and drainage.

Nipples

Problems with nipples are one of the major reasons for women giving up breast-feeding and therefore should be treated assiduously.

Pain. Pain is experienced by 80% of women 2–4 days after delivery. This is usually associated with engorgement and is treated by more frequent, brief feeds, keeping the nipples clean and exposing the nipples to air (breast shields) and to sunlight.

Cracked nipples. Superficial cracks are treated as above, but with deep cracks the baby should be temporarily removed and the breast gently expressed by hand until it heals. Antiseptic sprays or creams are not useful.

Contraception

If breast-feeding is used exclusively and menstruation does not appear, ovulation usually does not occur before the 11th week postpartum. Menstruation resumes in 40–75% of women while still breast-feeding and ovulation occurs shortly after. The contraceptive effectiveness of lactation depends on the frequency of suckling, the use of supplemental feeding and the level of maternal nutrition (if low, the contraceptive effectiveness is greater). As oestrogens inhibit prolactin release their use in the postpartum period is contraindicated, although many women will continue to breast-feed normally if commenced on the combined oral contraceptive once breast-feeding is well established.

The other options for contraception are: progestogens (the progestogen-only pill (POP) or Depo-Provera), barrier methods, or IUDs. Most women opt for the POP which should be started in the first postpartum week. Its commonest complications are irregular bleeding and a higher failure rate compared to the combined pill or Depo-Provera.

Suppression of lactation

In most cases, this is achieved by not stimulating the breasts (no suckling), a firm supportive brassiere and analgesia if required. By 5–6 days postpartum the discomfort improves. Complete suppression of lactation can be achieved with bromocriptine 2.5 mg b.d. for 10–14 days followed by gradual withdrawal over the ensuing 7 days. Lactation suppression is indicated in perinatal death, adoption of the infant, severe breast problems, or active maternal tuberculosis. Routine use is not recommended because of the side-effects of nausea and vomiting and reports of hypertension, stroke and myocardial infarction associated with the postpartum use of bromocriptine.

OTHER PUERPERAL CONSIDERATIONS

Contraception

Contraception in breast-feeding women is discussed above. In women who are not breast-feeding, a small proportion will ovulate prior to the 6-week postnatal check, so contraception should be instituted in the first 3 weeks after delivery. In the non-lactating woman the choices are similar to those for the non-puerperal woman.

Vaccinations

All women lacking rubella antibodies should be vaccinated after delivery providing contraception can be assured for the ensuing 3 months. All rhesus-negative women delivering rhesus-positive babies should be given Anti-D prophylaxis (not strictly a vaccination) within 72 hours of delivery.

Postnatal examination

This is traditionally performed at 6 weeks postpartum as most of the pregnancy-induced changes in maternal physiology have returned to normal and it is an appropriate time for assessing the mother–infant interaction.

As mentioned above, contraception in the non-lactating woman should have been initiated prior to this visit. At the visit a brief history should be taken focusing on the maternal reproductive tract, breasts and the infant's feeding, behaviour and health. Maternal blood pressure should be checked, particularly if this has been a problem in pregnancy, and the breasts and lower genital tract examined. A smear should be performed if necessary.

33. Obstetric and gynaecological emergencies

J. Rymer

Expectations of the examiners

Emergencies are a common theme in examination questions and the candidate must be familiar with their immediate management, particularly shoulder dystocia and postpartum haemorrhage.

CORD PROLAPSE

Definition

After membrane rupture the umbilical cord prolapses into the vagina and may even protrude past the introitus. Cord presentation is when the cord is presenting and the membranes are still intact.

Interesting facts

If cord prolapse occurs in hospital the prognosis for the fetus is much better than if the event occurs in the community.

Aetiology

The presenting part is usually high allowing the cord to descend below it. Most cord prolapses occur with a malpresentation but they can occur with a cephalic presentation. They can occur with artificial (ARM) or spontaneous rupture of membranes but the prognosis is much better if it occurs with ARM, as the diagnosis is instantly made, and management can be instituted without delay.

Management

Once the cord is felt in the vagina the woman should be turned into the all fours position with her head down and buttocks elevated (or any other position that allows gravity to pull the head away from the cervix) so that the cord is not compressed between the cervix and the presenting part. The examining hand remains in the vagina to continue elevating the head away from the cervix, taking care to handle the cord as little as possible thus avoiding spasm of the cord vessels. Immediate help must be summoned to arrange a caesarean section. The hand remains in the vagina until the uterus is opened.

If a patient needs to be transported and there will be considerable delay, a Foley catheter can be inserted into the bladder and 500 ml of normal saline can be infused into the bladder to keep the presenting part out of the pelvis, thus alleviating compression of the cord.

Prognosis

If cord prolapse occurs in hospital and is rapidly diagnosed and dealt with appropriately then the outcome is usually good.

SHOULDER DYSTOCIA

Definition

As the fetus is delivering the shoulders are in the anteroposterior position and the anterior shoulder becomes impacted on the symphysis pubis.

Interesting facts

Time is of the essence as the fetus is unable to breathe while the thorax is compressed so management must be immediate.

Management

Shoulder dystocia tends to occur with large babies. If it is anticipated then senior staff should be present at delivery. The diagnosis is made when the head is delivering but there is delay in the delivery of the chin and it appears to recede. Without delay the woman should be put into the lithotomy position, or her legs elevated in such a fashion as to cause flexion of the sacrum. A large episiotomy should be performed and suprapubic pressure exerted by an assistant. The majority of shoulder dystocias will be corrected with these procedures. If the shoulders are still impacted then an attempt is made to deliver the posterior shoulder by rotating the shoulders so that they go from an anteroposterior position to a diagonal position in the pelvis, as the diagonal diameters are wider. If this cannot be achieved then the clavicles can be broken by snapping them between the acoucheur's second and third fingers. If the shoulders are still firmly impacted one can resort to symphysiotomy by infiltrating above the symphysis with local anaesthesia (not needed if an epidural is already sited and working adequately) and inserting a Foley catheter into the urethra. The catheter is then pulled to one side (to avoid urethral damage) and an incision is made over the symphysis downwards until the ligament is divided. The pelvis will immediately widen and delivery will follow.

Prognosis

This is entirely dependent upon the time delay between shoulder dystocia occurring and delivery of the baby. Trauma to the baby is common, e.g. Erb's palsy.

ANTEPARTUM HAEMORRHAGE (See Ch. 23)

Definition

Bleeding from the genital tract after the 24th week of pregnancy and before the delivery of the baby.

Interesting facts

Placenta praevia and placental abruption must always be considered as the diagnosis.

Management

This will depend on the amount of bleeding and the gestation. Assuming significant bleeding, the management is as with any haemorrhage — resuscitate the mother ensuring an airway, breathing and circulation. Once the mother is stable one needs to

1. Assess the amount of blood that has been lost and is being lost
2. Assess the status of the fetus.

If active bleeding is continuing then delivery must be considered. The mode of delivery will depend on diagnosis, gestation and fetal status. For example, if there is active bleeding with a major placenta praevia at 32 weeks then an emergency caesarean section must be performed; however, if there is active bleeding with a placental abruption at 32 weeks and the baby is dead, then an ARM and syntocinon would be appropriate.

Prognosis

DIC can develop with placental abruption or with any severe haemorrhage. After delivery in all cases of antepartum haemorrhage, the woman is at risk of postpartum haemorrhage and syntocinon must be given with the delivery of the anterior shoulder and then a 40 i.u. syntocinon infusion for 2–4 hours after delivery.

Fluid management in these women can be very difficult, so insertion of a CVP line in the early stage is helpful.

UTERINE RUPTURE

Definition

The uterus ruptures and this can either be a primary rupture where there has been no previous uterine surgery or trauma, or a scar dehiscence which can vary from the peritoneum to endometrium being ruptured, or the peritoneum remaining intact but the underlying uterine tissue has ruptured.

Interesting facts

Placental abruption and uterine rupture can present with similar symptoms and signs. When maternal collapse in labour occurs, one must consider uterine rupture.

Aetiology

Most cases are associated with a previous caesarean section scar, especially a classical scar. A primary rupture is usually associated with obstructed labour or injudicious use of syntocinon in a multiparous woman. Uterine rupture can also occur from traumatic instrumental deliveries and intrauterine manipulations. Cervical stenosis can obstruct labour, and if not recognized can cause the uterus to rupture.

Management

The symptoms of uterine rupture are usually pain (abdominal or shoulder-tip) and the signs include: fetal distress, signs of shock, alteration in uterine shape or fetal presentation, vaginal bleeding, haematuria and cessation of contractions. If the peritoneum overlying the previous scar is intact the signs may be subtle.

Resuscitation must be immediate and then a laparotomy. After delivery of the baby the uterus is then repaired or a hysterectomy is performed and this will depend on the site and extent of the rupture, the woman's condition, her age and parity.

Summary

Uterine rupture is an obstetric emergency which requires immediate resuscitation of the mother and urgent laparotomy.

UTERINE INVERSION (see Ch. 26)

Definition

The fundus of the uterus is inverted as the placenta is being pulled in a downward direction by cord traction.

Interesting facts

If correct management of the third stage is employed, uterine inversion should not occur.

Aetiology

Usually due to premature attempts to deliver the placenta without a suprapubic hand providing counter-traction to the uterus. It can be associated with morbid adherence of the placenta or a very short umbilical cord.

Management

Immediate replacement of the fundus to its original anatomical position and no attempt to remove the placenta should be made. The longer the delay the more chance that manual replacement will not be possible. When attempting immediate replacement, a fist is preferable to fingers to avoid uterine perforation. If replacement does not occur then the hydrostatic method is used. This involves filling the vagina with warm fluid maintaining a seal with a hand and a pack at the introitus. The pressure of the fluid, should push the uterus back to its original position. Once the uterus is in place, then the placenta can be removed manually. A syntocinon infusion should be instituted for at least 4 hours post inversion.

Summary

Uterine inversion must be corrected immediately and the placenta should not be removed until the fundus has returned to its anatomical position.

AMNIOTIC FLUID EMBOLISM

Definition

Amniotic fluid escapes into the systemic circulation and the thromboplastin causes an anaphylactic type reaction and a severe coagulation defect develops.

Interesting facts

The diagnosis is usually made at post-mortem.

Aetiology

It is usually associated with high parity, women >35 years, precipitate labour, intense uterine stimulation, overdistension of the uterus, uterine rupture, and DIC.

Management

The patient may present with acute dyspnoea and signs of cardiovascular collapse. The event is usually undiagnosed and fatal, but if recognized the patient must be given oxygen by a facial mask initially and then intubated and ventilated and given high-dose steroids. An attempt should be made to correct the coagulation defect. A massive postpartum haemorrhage may occur.

POSTPARTUM HAEMORRHAGE

See Chapter 26.

PULMONARY EMBOLISM

Definition

A thrombosis (usually from the legs or pelvis) embolizes to the lungs causing complete or partial obstruction of the pulmonary arterial blood flow to the distal lung.

Interesting facts

Pregnant women have an increased risk of thromboembolic disease and this is exaggerated in the presence of twins, polyhydramnios, or an operative delivery.

Clinical presentation

The presentation will depend on the size and location of the embolus, and if severe will present with acute collapse which may be accompanied by chest pain and shortness of breath.

Management

Women at high risk of pulmonary emboli should be given TED stockings and, depending on the history, prophylactic anticoagulation.

Basic resuscitation principles are followed, namely establish an airway, ventilate, and give fluids. Once the patient is stable then she should be fully heparinized. A positive diagnosis must be made on a VQ scan.

Prognosis

This will depend on the immediate management and the size and location of the embolus.

RUPTURED ECTOPIC PREGNANCY

Definition

The ectopic gestation has ruptured through the wall of the fallopian tube, or, if a cornual implantation, through the cornua of the uterus.

Clinical presentation

The woman may present in hypovolaemic shock due to the intraperitoneal haemorrhage. If she is cardiovascularly stable she may complain of symptoms of pregnancy, severe constant abdominal pain which was sudden in onset, and feeling faint on sitting or standing.

On examination she may be tachycardiac, hypotensive (or demonstrate postural hypotension) with a rigid abdomen.

Management

If shocked the patient needs resuscitation and then an immediate laparotomy. Blood should be taken for FBC and 4 units cross-matched. Decompensation may occur on entering the peritoneal cavity as the blood in the peritoneal cavity is often compressing the bleeding vessel(s). The site of bleeding must be found immediately and controlled. This can vary from oversewing the tube to total salpingectomy. Depending on the amount of blood loss and the condition of the patient, blood may need to be transfused.

Prognosis

Ectopic pregnancy is a cause of maternal mortality. In the latest triennial report (1991–93) there were nine reported ectopic deaths representing 4.2% of all direct and indirect deaths. Of these deaths, eight were directly due to the rupture of the ectopic pregnancy. However, as ectopic pregnancies occur in women of reproductive age group they tend to do well.

CERVICAL SHOCK

Definition

A vasovagal reaction caused by distension of the cervix producing bradycardia and hypotension.

Clinical presentation

Cervical shock can occur during insertion of an IUD, endometrial sampling, or hysteroscopy. If a woman is miscarrying either clots or products of conception can distend the cervix.

Management

The products of conception (or whatever is distending the cervix) must be removed immediately and the patient will instantly recover. This should be done before setting up an intravenous line and the usual resuscitation techniques. An urgent evacuation of the products should be arranged. If it occurs during IUD insertion, atropine either i.v. or i.m. should be administered.

TORSION OF AN OVARIAN MASS

Definition

The ovarian mass torts on its pedicle thus compromising its blood supply.

Interesting facts

Ovaries are as important and as vulnerable as testes and a torted ovarian mass should be managed with the same urgency as a testicular torsion.

Assessment

The patient may give a history of previous intermittent pelvic pain, urinary frequency, and other symptoms of a pelvic mass. When torsion occurs the presentation is that of severe colicky pain. On abdominal examination the patient is tender and may have rebound and guarding. Vaginal examination is exquisitely tender. An ultrasound examination may confirm the diagnosis.

Management

Depending on the size of the mass laparoscopic management may be possible and the mass untwisted and then removed laparoscopically. If not a laparotomy may be performed.

OVARIAN HYPERSTIMULATION

Definition

The ovaries are overstimulated leading to a syndrome resulting from many large ovarian follicles.

Clinical presentation

The situation usually occurs as a result of parenteral gonodotrophins. The patient may complain of lower abdominal pain, swelling of the abdomen, or shortness of breath, depending on the severity of the disease, and whether or not ascites and pulmonary oedema have developed.

Management

The aim is supportive therapy until the condition resolves but some severe cases require ventilation and intensive intravascular fluid management.

34. Home deliveries

I. Page

Expectations of the examiners

The candidate will be expected to be aware of the arrangements needed for home deliveries, and to appreciate under which circumstances women initially suitable for home delivery should be transferred to hospital care. In addition, the candidate should be able to perform a normal delivery, to recognize abnormalities that may occur in labour, and to resuscitate a mother or baby.

Epidemiology

The place of delivery was first recorded nationally in 1927, when 85% of births took place at home. Successive government committees advocated increasing the proportion of hospital deliveries so that by 1965 only 26%, and since 1987 less than 1%, of women have delivered at home.

The advantages that were claimed for hospital delivery are now being reassessed, and it is acknowledged that evidence to support the claim that the safest policy is for all women to give birth in hospital is inconclusive.

Assessment

Every woman has the right to have her baby at home, and health authorities are required (without exception) to ensure that a midwifery service for home births is provided. General practitioners are not required to provide care for women who wish to have a home delivery, but attend if summoned in an emergency.

An antagonistic approach to the woman's request for a home delivery by her general practitioner or hospital staff is unhelpful, as it will make her less likely to accept transfer to hospital delivery if problems do arise.

The assessment of suitability for a home delivery covers two aspects:

1. The anticipated 'normality' of the delivery for the mother and baby
2. The adequacy of facilities in the home.

Home facilities

These are usually assessed by the midwife who will be undertaking the delivery. The birth room should be capable of being heated to, and maintained at, about 22°C. It should be clean and well lit, with a work-top of some form for the midwife's equipment. If the woman intends to give birth on her bed, the mattress should be firm enough to allow the midwife access to the woman's perineum.

Ideally, a telephone should be present in the house to enable the midwife to summon help immediately if it is required. A neighbour's telephone is acceptable, providing there is easy and reliable access to it. Nowadays the midwife may have a mobile phone.

Hot water should be available, as should some means of warming the blankets and clothes the baby will wear (a hot water bottle is adequate).

Obstetric assessment

Guidelines regarding the place of delivery were laid down by the Maternity Services (Cranbrook) Committee in 1959 and are still broadly applicable. Their aim is to try to avoid transfer of the mother and baby during labour, as this may worsen the outcome. However, early transfer due to delay in labour is unlikely to effect outcome.

Where there is an apparent medical or obstetric contraindication to home delivery, the midwife and general practitioner should encourage the woman to have a consultant's opinion. Ultimately, if the woman decides to have the baby at home, the midwife *must* attend. She can call on *any* general practitioner in an emergency who should attend.

Height. Women under 152 cm (5 ft 0 in) have a higher perinatal mortality rate (PNMR), and a higher incidence of caesarean section in labour.

Age. Nulliparae under 18 years or over 30 years are known to have an increased PNMR, as do multiparous women over 35 years.

Parity. Nulliparae are known to have an increased incidence of prolonged labour which makes intrapartum transfer more likely. They are also more likely to develop pre-eclampsia, and to require induction of labour for prolonged pregnancy.

'Grand multiparae' have an increased risk of multiple pregnancy, placenta praevia, fetal malpresentation, and unstable lie. There is an increased risk of disproportion, which may present as uterine rupture or shoulder dystocia. Paradoxically, the uterus tends to relax more in the third stage, leading to an increased risk of postpartum haemorrhage.

Weight. Obese women are more difficult to assess as 'normal' in pregnancy and labour, and often have large babies. It is more difficult to treat them if problems arise.

Social class. This is becoming harder to assess, but social classes IV and V are at increased risk of maternal, fetal and neonatal problems.

Maternal disease. Any coexisting disease, such as hypertension or diabetes mellitus, is a contraindication to home delivery.

Previous uterine surgery. A scar in the uterus (previous caesarean section, hysterotomy, or myomectomy) is at risk of dehiscence in labour which requires urgent major surgery.

Obstetric history. Any woman who has suffered a previous perinatal loss is usually advised against home delivery. Similarly, previous low birth weight babies (when due to growth retardation) or difficult deliveries are contraindications to home delivery, as are problems in the third stage (postpartum haemorrhage, retained placenta) which have an increased risk of recurrence.

Current pregnancy. If the pregnancy becomes abnormal then care should be transferred to the hospital antenatally. Abnormalities can occur at any stage of pregnancy, and examples include isoimmunization, pre-eclampsia, antepartum haemorrhage, malpresentation (after 37 weeks), and fetal growth retardation.

Summary

A healthy woman, over 152 cm tall, under 35 years of age, having had a previously normal pregnancy and delivery, having her second to fourth baby, in social class I, II or III and with no current medical or obstetric problems, can be defined as 'low-risk' and home delivery viewed as acceptable.

Where a woman with a normal pregnancy goes into spontaneous labour at term she can expect a normal, safe outcome to her labour.

Advantages

Many of the claimed advantages for home delivery are difficult, if not impossible, to quantify as they refer to the way the mother feels about the birth. It is certainly true to say that being treated as an individual is more likely at home, as most hospitals have policies of management which have been designed to cope with the abnormal and do not need to be applied to low-risk cases. Some studies have shown there is a greater risk of medical intervention simply by being booked for hospital delivery, which would be avoided by home delivery.

Disadvantages

The incidence of serious, unexpected emergencies that can harm the mother or her baby is about 7%, even in low-risk cases. They include shoulder dystocia, neonatal apnoea, postpartum haemorrhage, and retained placenta. Most of them can, however, be managed safely by the attending midwife or general practitioner.

The major problems arise in those few cases where more specialized medical assistance and skill are required. In these cases there may be some considerable delay when awaiting the arrival of the local flying squad (if it exists), during which time the condition of the mother or baby may markedly deteriorate.

SUMMARY

Home delivery is now a rare event. It can be accepted for 'low-risk' mothers providing the attending midwife makes adequate arrangements for assistance in an emergency. A supportive approach from the woman's general practitioner (and obstetrician) will also be of value. In addition, the woman and her partner should have a full understanding of the risks and benefits of a home delivery.

35. Stillbirths

M. McDonald

Expectations of the examiners

The examiners will expect the candidate to understand the causes of stillbirth, know how to appropriately manage the event and arrange follow-up.

Definition

'Stillborn child' means a child which has issued forth from its mother after the 24th week of pregnancy and which did not at any time after being completely expelled from its mother breathe or show any other signs of life, and the expression 'stillbirth' shall be used accordingly (section 41; Stillbirth (Definition) Act 1992, HMSO).

Interesting facts

The definition of a stillbirth was altered by the 1992 Act to reduce the legal age of viability from 28 to 24 weeks' gestation. This has resulted in a 33% rise in the officially recorded stillbirth rate.

The perinatal mortality rate for the UK is 8.9/1000.

A Confidential Enquiry into Stillbirths and Deaths in Infancy (CESDI) was established in 1992. Conducted along similar lines to the Confidential Enquiry into Maternal Mortality, all fetal and baby deaths in the CESDI range are reported for England, Wales and Northern Ireland. From April 1996 responsibility for the enquiry rests with a consortium drawn from the Royal College of Obstetricians and Gynaecologists, the British Paediatric Association, the Royal College of Pathologists, and the Royal College of Midwives.

Risk factors

1. *Maternal*
   a. Age — adolescent and advanced maternal age
   b. Obstetric history — previous stillbirth
   c. Existing medical conditions, e.g. diabetes, renal disease
   d. Smoking

    e. Alcohol

    f. Narcotics abuse

    g. Diet — inadequate nutrition

    h. Infection, e.g. syphilis, parvovirus, listeria

    j. Rhesus incompatibility

2. *Fetal*

    a. Sex

    b. Multiple pregnancy

    c. Birth weight

    d. Fetal anomaly

    e. Chromosome abnormality

3. *Socioeconomic*

    a. Ethnicity

    b. Education

    c. Income

    d. Marital status

    e. Occupation.

Assessment

The death of the baby can occur during the pregnancy or in labour. An intrauterine death in pregnancy may be detected at a routine antenatal check up. The clinician may find that the fetal size is not consistent with gestational size. There may be absence of the fetal heart sounds. The woman may present with a history of diminished or absent fetal movements. Unfortunately, some women delay reporting the latter through a mistaken belief that the baby's movements slow down significantly at the end of pregnancy due to lack of space.

Investigations

1. *Maternal*

    a. An ultrasound scan to determine the following:

        i. Confirmation of clinical diagnosis of intrauterine death

        ii. Confirm the presenting part; in the case of a multiple pregnancy, to confirm the well-being of the other fetuses.

    A second medical opinion on ultrasound may be obtained to support the original diagnosis.

    b. Blood samples are required for:

        i. Full infection screen–TORCH

        ii. Prothrombin time

        iii. Kleihauer test

        iv. Screen for antiphospholipid syndrome if appropriate, e.g. second trimester loss.

        v. Coagulation screen

    c. Swab from the lower vagina to detect the presence of Group B
       β-haemolytic streptococci.

2. *Baby*
    a. Surface swabs for detection of Group B β-haemolytic streptococci
    b. Birth weight
    c. A full post-mortem examination (prior to a pathological post-
       mortem examination)
    d. Full skeletal X-ray even if parents are unwilling to have a post-
       mortem
    Additional tests may be requested by the pathologist or obstetrician,
    e.g. axilla skin sample for karyotyping, or specific blood specimens.

3. *Placenta*
    a. Weight
    b. Swabs for full infection screen.

Treatment

Intrauterine death

Intrauterine death is the death of a fetus after 24 weeks of pregnancy and
prior to the onset of labour. This allows some degree of preparation for the
parents.

Confirmation of the diagnosis needs to be presented in a manner which
encourages the woman (and her partner if possible) to ask questions. If the
maternal condition permits, she may choose the time of induction of
labour, allowing her to return home and make suitable arrangements for
other children and to collect her belongings for hospital confinement. In
the meantime the delivery suite will be informed of the planned induction.

The local policy for the induction of labour is followed, with particular
reference to guidelines on artificial rupture of the membranes. Many units
delay this until the woman is established in labour because of the risk of
infection.

Adequate information about her progress should enable the woman to
participate in her care appropriately and to make informed choices where
necessary. Interpreters should be utilized for non-English-speaking
women. Where possible, continuity of carers should be maintained, as this
will enhance the quality of care and reduce the feeling of loss of control
which many women experience at this time. Care of the partner or
companions should include the location of refreshments, the telephone,
and overnight accommodation.

Progress of labour is assessed by vaginal examination. If the onset of
labour has been spontaneous it may still be necessary to augment further if
delay occurs. Throughout labour adequate analgesia needs to be provided.
Sedatives may be prescribed to assist with the emotional pain.

If possible the midwife or doctor should try to prepare the woman for
the appearance of the baby, particularly if the fetus is likely to be

290 PREPARATION AND REVISION FOR THE DRCOG

macerated. Work undertaken by bereavement counsellors and support groups has revealed that women do appreciate seeing their baby, even with gross abnormalities. Many recount stories of how their imagination was much worse than the reality, of how they visited libraries to learn more. Gentle encouragement and sensitive handling of the situation can ensure that the experience assists them in remembering their dead child. Focusing on the details of the baby can help the parents enormously, such as the colour of the hair, the tiny hands with their fingernails, and so on.

The birth may be very traumatic for the woman as the reality of the situation can no longer be denied. The delivery is conducted as any labour. The placenta is saved for transfer to the mortuary with the baby.

Intrapartum death

Intrapartum death is a fetal death which occurs in labour, either during the first stage or at delivery. Fetal distress will indicate the potential danger to the fetus and appropriate action to relieve the situation may already have been taken, this can result in a stillborn baby delivered by caesarean section. The loss of a baby during labour affects not only the parents but can traumatize the midwives and doctors involved in providing the immediate care. Possible errors of management should be reviewed at a later date but the primary responsibility is to ensure that the mother is not in danger and to assist her through the remainder of the labour. A paediatrician may be present for the delivery to perform resuscitation if at all possible.

The parents should be informed immediately of the outcome of the birth. They are likely to be shocked and may not comprehend the events straight away. The situation needs to be explained to them as far as possible at this time.

Management following delivery

The baby should be given to the parents to hold and examine for themselves. Photographs should be taken of the baby and other mementoes such as a lock of hair or a footprint given to the couple. They may wish other family members to see the baby and be involved and this should be arranged. They should have the opportunity to spend as much time as they wish with the baby prior to transfer to the mortuary.

The practical arrangements following the birth include the completion of a stillbirth certificate. At an appropriate time when the woman has rested the doctor should discuss the post-mortem examination and obtain consent. They may have questions about the procedure and wish to see the baby afterwards. In most hospitals this would not be a problem, but the doctor should be aware of local policy, particularly if the body will be sent to another hospital for specialist post-mortem. Many pathologists now use

Strong glue or dental floss to repair the body, enabling the parents to view the baby afterwards.

Completion of clinical details is essential for the pathologist. When the baby is transferred to the mortuary, all clothing and sheets should be removed as they will speed up rate of autolysis.

The decision about disposal of the body generally rests with the parents and the doctor should be aware of the options available locally. This will be a hospital burial or cremation, or may be arranged privately by the couple. In order to make the choice the mother and her partner need to appreciate that if arranged by the hospital a shared, unmarked grave may be used although the baby will be in an individual casket, and there is unlikely to be a funeral service. A private funeral can be arranged according to the parents' wishes but they may need assistance in knowing who to approach locally. If cremation is chosen the doctor must complete the necessary form.

Discharge

The mother should decide her own time of discharge in consultation with medical and midwifery staff. Bromocriptine may be prescribed to suppress lactation. The GP and community midwife should be informed of the outcome of the pregnancy and the care to date. A follow-up appointment with the consultant obstetrician should be given for 6 weeks' time. In some units joint perinatal loss clinics have been established which provide an opportunity for the woman to return and meet with the obstetrician and a neonatologist. Appointment times need to recognize that there may be a number of questions to answer and explanations to give and the appointment provides an opportunity to go over the post-mortem findings in person.

SUMMARY

The management of stillbirth involves close liaison with other disciplines, including midwifery and social workers. Groups such as the Stillbirth and Neonatal Death Society (SANDS) provide a network of support for the parents who can access this via telephone links or group meetings at an appropriate time for themselves. For the staff left behind, the key issue is what lessons have been learnt from the experience: 'Could we have done something differently which would have had a better outcome?' The answer lies in regular auditing of perinatal loss, and perinatal mortality and morbidity meetings have a significant role to play in responding to this question. Reporting accurate information to CESDI will enable national audit findings to be published. Finally, staff should also remember that delivery of a stillbirth can be a distressing event for doctors and midwives, and preparation in handling sensitive situations of this nature should begin as early as possible.

36. Maternity benefits

I. Page

Expectations of the examiners

The candidate will be expected to be aware of the various benefits which are available to pregnant women and mothers.

Accuracy

Details of the benefits change with the Chancellor's budget each year. The details below follow the 1996 Budget.

DURING PREGNANCY

Dental treatment

Details are set out in leaflet D11—NHS dental treatment. Free dental treatment is available during pregnancy and for 12 months after delivery. It is also available for anyone receiving family credit or income support (see below). Form F1D, available from the dental surgery, should be completed even if the woman is receiving either family credit or income support to ensure she can receive free treatment for the full period if she should stop being eligible for the benefit.

Prescription charges

Details are set out in leaflet P11—NHS prescriptions. A prescription charge exemption certificate is available during pregnancy and for 12 months afterwards. Form FW8, which is available from GP surgeries or midwives, should be completed even if the woman is receiving family credit or income support (as with dental treatment).

Hospital fares

Although not strictly a maternity benefit, women receiving family credit or income support can claim public transport fares, petrol costs or occasionally taxi fares for their antenatal (and postnatal) visits. Details are set out in leaflet H11—NHS hospital travel costs. The claim is paid at the hospital on production of the benefit order book. If the woman has a low income she can apply to the agency benefits unit of the DHSS (using form AGI — Help with NHS costs) which may issue a certificate of entitlement.

Social fund maternity payment

Details are set out in leaflets FB8—Babies and benefits, and FB27 — Bringing up children? It is intended to help with expenses for the new baby, and can only be made to women receiving family credit or income support. The amount is £100.00 for each baby expected, adopted or born, but is reduced if the claimant or her partner hold over £500 in savings. Form SF100, available from antenatal clinics or Social Security offices, should be completed between 11 weeks before and 13 weeks after delivery.

Statutory maternity pay (SMP)

Details are set out in leaflets FB8—Babies and benefits, and NI17A—A guide to maternity benefits. Maternity pay is paid by the woman's employer.

To qualify, the woman must work for her employer for the 26 weeks up to the 15th week before her estimated date of delivery (EDD) and work 1 day of that week, and also earn enough (£61 per week) during the last 8 weeks to pay class 1 national insurance (NI) contributions.

If she is dismissed before the 15th week before her EDD because of problems in the pregnancy or premature delivery she may still be eligible for SMP.

SMP is paid for up to 18 weeks, starting anytime after 11 weeks before her EDD. It is not paid while the woman is working, but she can now work right up to her delivery without losing any of her benefit.

To claim SMP the woman must:

1. Inform her employer in writing at least 3 weeks before stopping work, that she intends to stop work because of pregnancy and intends to claim SMP.
2. Send her maternity certificate (form Mat B1 available from her midwife or doctor after 26 weeks of pregnancy) to her employer before the end of the third week in which she claims SMP.

SMP is paid at two rates. To qualify for the higher rate (6 weeks at 90% of earnings, then 12 weeks at the standard rate) a woman must have worked more than 2 years full time or 5 years part time. The standard rate is paid for the whole 18 weeks to women who have worked between 6 months and 2 years, and is £54.55 per week. Income tax and NI contributions may have to be paid on SMP.

State maternity allowance (SMA)

Details are set out in leaflets FB8—Babies and benefits, and NI17A — A guide to maternity benefits. This allowance is paid by the DHSS.

It is payable to women who have recently changed or given up their jobs, or who have recently been self-employed.

To qualify a woman must have paid class 1 or 2 NI contributions for at least 26 of the 66 weeks ending in the week before her EDD. As with SMP it is not paid if the woman is working.

To claim SMA, the woman must complete Form MA1, available from her antenatal clinic or Social Security office, and send it with her form Mat B1 to the Social Security office.

SMA is paid at a standard rate of £47.35 per week, but the higher rate of £54.55 is paid if the woman is in eligible employment in her qualifying week.

STILLBIRTHS

If the baby is stillborn (by definition after the 24th week of pregnancy) entitlement to the following benefits is not affected:

1. Free NHS dental treatment
2. Free NHS prescriptions
3. Social fund maternity payment
4. Statutory maternity pay
5. State maternity allowance.

AFTER DELIVERY

Child benefit

Details are set out in leaflets CH1—Child benefit, and CH7—Child benefit for children aged 16 and over. It is payable for every child under 16 (19 if in full-time education) living with the claimant.

Payment is usually by a book of orders which can be cashed at the Post Office every 4 weeks.

The claim form is available from Social Security offices and should be accompanied by the child's birth certificate.

Child benefit is £10.80 per week for the eldest qualifying child, and £8.80 for each other child.

One parent benefit

Details are set out in leaflets CH11—One parent benefit, and FB27 — Bringing up children? It is an extra benefit which is only payable for one child (usually the first).

Payment is usually by a book of orders which can be cashed at the Post Office every 4 weeks.

The claim form is in leaflet CH11, and the benefit is £6.30 per week.

Widow's mother's allowance

Details are set out in leaflet NP45—A guide to widow's benefits. It can be paid from the time of the husband's death for children for whom the woman receives child benefit, or from the time of delivery if she is widowed while pregnant.

If it is paid, then one parent benefit cannot be claimed.

The claim form (form BW1) is available from Social Security offices, and the allowance is £56.10 per week with an extra £9.80 per week for the first and £10.95 for each subsequent child.

OTHER BENEFITS

As family credit and income support have been mentioned in relation to most of the benefits payable during pregnancy, they are briefly described here. They are general, not maternity, benefits.

Family credit

Details are set out in leaflet FB27—Bringing up children?, and the claim form FC1—family credit is available from Post and Social Security offices.

It is a tax-free benefit for anyone bringing up one child (or more) and working at least 16 hours per week. The amount varies with income, and is usually payable if the net income is less than £90 per week with an extra allowance for each child. It is reduced by savings or capital over £3000. Once the rate has been assessed it remains constant for 26 weeks, regardless of changes in circumstances.

If family credit is paid the family is automatically entitled to:

1. Free NHS dental treatment
2. Vouchers for spectacles
3. Free NHS prescriptions
4. Refund of hospital fares
5. Social fund maternity payment.

Income support

Details are set out in leaflets FB27—Bringing up children?, and IS1—Income support, both available from Post and Social Security Offices.

It is a taxable benefit for people who do not have enough money on which to live, and who work less than 16 hours per week. The amount varies with individual circumstances, and is reduced if the claimants have capital or savings over £3000.

If income support is paid, the family is automatically entitled to the same benefits as those on family credit (see above).

37. Statistics

I. Page

Expectations of the examiners

The candidate will be expected to have an understanding of the epidemiology of perinatal and maternal morbidity and mortality as well as ethnic variations, and to understand the importance of accurate obstetric records in clinical audit.

BIRTH RATE

Definition

Total live and stillbirths per year per 1000 women aged 15–44 years.

Interesting facts

The general fertility rate (live births per 1000 women aged 15–44 years) is currently (1996) about 62 in the UK. All births are registered by a midwife (or doctor) with the local health authority within 36 hours, and the parents must notify the local registrar of births and deaths within 42 days of the birth.

ABORTION

This comprises spontaneous abortions (usually referred to as miscarriages) and induced (legal) abortions.

Definition

Termination of a pregnancy before 24 weeks' gestation with the expulsion of a dead fetus.

Interesting facts

The miscarriage rate is estimated to be about 15% of conceptions. The induced abortion rate is about 14 per year per 1000 women aged 14–44 years in England and Wales. Induced abortion may only be performed on premises approved by the Secretary of State under the 1967 Abortion Act. Less than 50% of induced abortions are carried out by the NHS. Over 80% of induced abortions are now performed within the first trimester of pregnancy.

STILLBIRTH RATE

Definition

Number of infants born with no signs of life after 24 weeks' gestation per 1000 total births (prior to October 1992 it was 28 weeks).

Interesting facts

The stillbirth rate in 1991 in the UK was 5.7, and is showing a downward trend.

NEONATAL DEATH RATE

Definition

Number of deaths, within 28 days of birth, of all live-born infants (regardless of gestation) per 1000 live births.

PERINATAL MORTALITY RATE

Definition

Number of stillbirths and first-week neonatal deaths per 1000 total births.

Interesting facts

The perinatal mortality rate (PNMR) has been recorded since 1930 in the UK and in 1994 was 8.9. It is showing a downward trend, with an acceleration in the rate of improvement.

Epidemiology

Age

PNMR is lowest in the age group 20–24 years. The higher rate in the under 20s reflects the greater number of primigravidae and unmarried mothers and poor acceptance of antenatal care. The increase in PNMR with maternal age reflects the greater incidence of maternal disease (such as diabetes and hypertension) and increased parity.

Parity

A 'J-shaped' curve (similar to that seen with age) is observed when comparing PNMR with parity, with the lowest PNMR occurring in women in their second pregnancy.

Race

Asians (Indians and Pakistanis) have an increased PNMR, reflecting a higher incidence of congenital abnormalities and a mean birth weight 300 g lower than that of Caucasians.

Black people (Africans and Caribbeans) have an increased PNMR due to sickle cell disease, a higher incidence of pre-eclampsia and eclampsia, a higher rate of twin births, and a mean birth weight 120 g lower than that of Caucasians.

Social class

PNMR increases between social classes I and V, with a further increase in unsupported women.

Multiple pregnancy

This predisposes to preterm delivery, pre-eclampsia and low birth weight and so has an increased PNMR. The problems become greater with each extra fetus.

Aetiology

There are three major determinants of perinatal mortality:

1. Congenital abnormalities
2. Low birth weight
3. Asphyxia.

However it is more useful to look at the causes as below.

Congenital abnormality

This group accounts for 20% of perinatal deaths in the UK, and most of the abnormalities are of the central nervous system. These can be detected in the second trimester by measurement of maternal serum α-fetoprotein, ultrasound examination of the fetus and amniocentesis where necessary. Other genetic and chromosomal abnormalities can be detected by chorionic villus sampling or amniocentesis. Termination of affected pregnancies (where the mother wishes) can be performed.

Isoimmunization

Perinatal deaths from haemolytic disease are now rare. The introduction of routine screening of maternal blood for blood group antibodies (in particular anti-D, anti-c, anti-Kell, and anti-Duffy) with follow-up by amniocentesis and assessment of the liquor bilirubin level, or by cordocentesis and fetal blood sampling, allows appropriate treatment to be given.

Pre-eclampsia

This excludes essential and renal hypertension which are usually considered a maternal disease, although both increase the risk of developing superimposed pre-eclampsia. Investigations are aimed at detecting fetal asphyxia and growth retardation, as well as ensuring maternal well-being.

Antepartum haemorrhage

Placenta praevia has little effect on PNMR as few babies require early delivery because of it, and those who are delivered early are usually in good condition.

Abruption is more common and accounts for about 20% of perinatal deaths due to asphyxia and prematurity. The risk of abruption increases with smoking and rising parity. It is associated with hypertension and raised maternal serum α-fetoprotein.

Mechanical

These perinatal deaths may be due to uterine rupture and cord accidents (which usually cause asphyxia) or birth trauma (as in breech delivery, forceps delivery, or shoulder dystocia).

Maternal disease

Diabetes mellitus is the maternal condition that causes most perinatal deaths. Others of importance are chronic renal disease, SLE or the presence of the lupus anticoagulant alone, and renal transplantation.

Miscellaneous

These are specific causes which cannot be ascribed to prematurity or asphyxia. Examples include the twin–twin transfusion syndrome, milk inhalation, and infections.

Unexplained

These are probably due to asphyxia, for which there may or may not be any evidence. Examples include unexplained intrauterine deaths, deaths from unexplained preterm delivery (including respiratory distress syndrome and intraventricular haemorrhage) and are categorized as being:

1. Term or preterm
2. Normal or small for gestational age.

Unclassifiable

A small group.

Prevention

One of the aims of antenatal care is to detect abnormalities early enough during the pregnancy to allow intervention to improve the outcome. This is relatively simple for congenital abnormalities where a careful history coupled with specific investigations, or general screening procedures for the whole population, can identify the abnormal fetus and so allow termination of the pregnancy where desired. It is not possible to cure most abnormalities at present, a situation that is unlikely to change for many years.

Isoimmunization with anti-D should be preventable with rhesus prophylaxis in all pregnant women at risk of sensitization. Care with blood transfusion will reduce the numbers who develop other antibodies.

There is no preventive measure against pre-eclampsia at present, although studies into the use of low-dose aspirin in patients at high risk have been promising. Early diagnosis and awareness of the risk to the fetus are essential. Treatment of the hypertension is of no benefit to the fetus, apart from allowing continuation of the pregnancy until the fetus is mature. Cigarette smoking makes the disease less common, but more severe when it does occur, and also increases the incidence of abruption ending in fetal death.

Fatal trauma to the fetus during delivery should be an avoidable event with correct intrapartum care, as should fatal cord accidents. There is no way of preventing antepartum cord accidents.

Ideally, maternal disorders should have been thoroughly assessed and controlled prior to the pregnancy. This is particularly the case with diabetes mellitus, where poor control increases the risk of congenital abnormality as well as increasing the risk of obstetric complications and sudden intrauterine death.

Provision of appropriate neonatal care facilities was emphasized by both the Sheldon Report (1971) and the Short Reports (1980 and 1985). For the high-risk pregnancy, arrangements should be made for delivery in a major obstetric unit with both special and intensive neonatal care units. If appropriate facilities are not available locally, then in-utero transfer is safer for the baby.

Improvement of social and environmental conditions is probably the most important factor in reducing the PNMR, as these are closely linked to both congenital abnormalities and low birth weight babies.

Summary

Perinatal mortality has fallen for a number of reasons and will fall further with improving socioeconomic conditions. Lack of appropriate care is apparent in up to one-third of perinatal deaths and therefore higher standards of obstetric care should result in a further reduction in PNMR. The special problems of the immigrant population must be remembered, and require further investigation. The Confidential Enquiry into Stillbirth and Deaths in Infancy (CESDI) may help in prevention of these deaths in the future.

MATERNAL MORTALITY RATE

Definition

Number of deaths of women while pregnant, or within 42 days of abortion or delivery, per 100 000 births.

Interesting facts

In the UK all maternal deaths are investigated by senior obstetricians, anaesthetists and pathologists and their findings are presented in the Confidential Enquiry into Maternal Deaths which is published triennially. This enquiry has operated since 1952 and details the causes of death and states whether care in each case could be said to be substandard.

The rate in the latest report (1991–93) is 6.0 per 100 000 maternities, and has halved every 10 years since the report began. Maternal deaths now constitute only 0.6% of deaths of females aged 15–44 years (in 1952–54 the figure was 4.0%).

Substandard care

This usually implies one of the following:

1. Failure to recognize predisposing factors
2. Failure to institute prophylactic measures
3. Deficiencies in routine antenatal care
4. Failure to recognize dangerous symptoms or signs
5. Delay in instituting proper management
6. Patient self-neglect.

Classification

The report divides the deaths into four groups:

1. Direct. Death due to an obstetric complication arising during pregnancy, labour or the postpartum period, e.g. amniotic fluid embolism.
2. Indirect. Death due to a pre-existing disease which was made worse by the pregnancy, e.g. maternal cardiac disease.
3. Fortuitous. Death due to factors unrelated to, and not influenced by, the pregnancy, e.g. road traffic accident.
4. Late. Deaths between 42 days and 1 year, due to direct or indirect maternal causes.

Demographic features

Age

Direct maternal mortality between 1991 and 1993 varies with maternal age. There was a marked increase in the rate in women aged over 35 years.

Parity

Direct mortality is lowest in women having their second baby, and rises with increasing parity.

Race

Maternal mortality in Britain is increased in women born outside the UK, particularly if they come from Bangladesh, India, or Africa. This is similar to PNMR.

UK area

There are wide variations in the maternal mortality rate in different areas of the UK but they do not correlate with the variations in PNMR.

Direct deaths

These account for 47% of the total, and their relative frequencies are shown in Table 37.1.

Pulmonary embolism

These deaths occurred equally during and after the pregnancy. Caesarean section increases the risk of fatal pulmonary embolism compared with vaginal delivery. The risk is also increased by obesity, immobilization,

Table 37.1 Causes of direct deaths in the UK: 1991–93

Cause	% of deaths
Pulmonary embolism	27.1
Hypertensive diseases	15.5
Ectopic pregnancy/abortion	14
Haemorrhage	11.6
Amniotic fluid embolism	7.8
Anaesthesia	6.2
Genital sepsis	7.0
Uterine trauma	3.1
Others	7.1

previous thromboembolism, and increasing parity. It is markedly higher in women aged over 35 years. There has been little change in the rate over the past 10 years. In many cases the diagnosis of venous thrombosis/embolism was not even considered, despite positive signs on examination. The RCOG now recommends risk assessment (for thromboprophylaxis) for all women having elective or emergency caesarean section, and has also made recommendations for prophylaxis against thromboembolism during the pregnancy.

Hypertensive diseases

Deaths from hypertensive disease were commonest in the first pregnancy. The causes of death were previously cerebral haemorrhage, oedema or infarction, but in 1991–93 ARDS was the commonest cause. Care was considered to be substandard in over three-quarters of the cases, with failure to control the blood pressure adequately and to deliver the patient expeditiously being the main points.

Haemorrhage

This had a fatal incidence of 6.4 per 1 000 000 maternities less than 1988–90 but still more than 1985–87. Three of the 15 cases were due to abruption, four to placenta praevia, and eight to postpartum haemorrhage. Care was deemed to be substandard in two-thirds of the cases. The risk increases with increasing age (particularly after 35 years) and parity, but is lowest in the second pregnancy.

Amniotic fluid embolism

This has a fatal incidence of 4.3 per 1 000 000 maternities. No cases developed symptoms before labour. The condition is commoner in women aged over 35 years but has no other consistent features. The mortality rate has not changed greatly during the past 15 years.

Ectopic pregnancy

The death rate from ectopic pregnancy has fallen despite the marked increase in the incidence of the condition. There was substandard care in all the cases, usually failure to perform a vaginal examination or consider the diagnosis. West Indian and Asian women are at increased risk.

Abortion

Five of the eight deaths were associated with legal induced abortion, the others following spontaneous miscarriage. The risk is increased in women aged over 35 years, but is not related to parity.

Anaesthesia

The number of anaesthetic deaths has decreased markedly, but their percentage contribution to maternal mortality has increased due to the increase in the number of obstetric anaesthetics given. Many cases reflected poor communication between obstetricians and anaesthetists, and failure to involve sufficiently senior anaesthetists in patients at increased risk of complications.

Genital sepsis

There were nine direct deaths, of which five occurred after surgery and four after vaginal delivery. Prophylactic antibiotics are now recommended for caesarean section.

Uterine rupture

The rate is decreasing, and there were no cases due to scar dehiscence in the last report. The need for early involvement of senior obstetricians in management of severe haemorrhage was emphasized.

Miscellaneous

There were nine cases in this group in 1991–93, of which two were associated with the use of ritodrine to suppress preterm labour. The RCOG has now issued guidelines for its use, to try and prevent future deaths.

Indirect deaths

These account for 36% of the total, and their relative frequencies are shown in Table 37.2.

Table 37.2 Causes of indirect deaths in the UK: 1991–93

Causes	% of deaths
Cardiac disease	37
CNS disease	25
Infection	8
CVS disease	3
Neoplasia	1
Others	26

Cardiac disease

Twenty-five per cent of these deaths were due to congenital defects, comprising either pulmonary hypertension or previous corrective surgery followed by episodes of bacterial endocarditis. Congenital defects are becoming a smaller part of cardiac-related deaths.

Seventy-five per cent were due to acquired disease. In the western world most of the acquired cardiac disease is the result of ischaemic change or aortic aneurysm, while in the developing countries rheumatic heart disease is more prevalent. The report noted that chest X-rays can, and should, be taken during pregnancy in patients with chest pain.

CNS diseases

Three-quarters of these deaths were due to intracranial haemorrhage, and the rest to status epilepticus in known epileptics. In this latter group it is possible that non-compliance with therapy was a factor.

Infections

Of the eight cases in 1991–93, five were due to fulminant streptococcal septicaemia with death of the woman within 24 hours of becoming ill.

CVS disease

Most of the deaths in this group were due to aneurysm rupture, and it has been suggested that there is a relationship between pregnancy and certain degenerative diseases of arteries.

Neoplasia

In most cases it is not certain that pregnancy has any direct effect on prognosis, apart from sometimes delaying treatment.

Fortuitous deaths

These account for the remaining 17% of maternal deaths covered by the Triennial Report. They are excluded from the international definition of maternal mortality.

Late deaths

These occur more than 42 days, but less than 1 year, after a pregnancy or delivery. They are reviewed in the Triennial Report and included in the new international definition (ICD 10).

Of the 46 late deaths in 1991–93, 10 were classified as direct, 23 indirect and 13 as fortuitous.

Caesarean section

Deaths associated with caesarean section are dealt with as a separate group in the Triennial Report as it is a major, and increasing, intervention in obstetric practice.

In 1991–93 there were 103 deaths following caesarean section. Of these, 63 were direct, 35 indirect and the remaining five fortuitous. Care was deemed to have been substandard in over half of the direct deaths. Death was commoner after an emergency procedure than after an elective one.

Prevention

The following recommendations have been abridged from the 1985–87 Triennial Report.

Hypertensive disease

Intervention with hypotensive agents should be considered earlier and premature delivery is often required. Signs of impending eclampsia should not be ignored.

Pulmonary embolism

There is a need for earlier detection of deep venous thrombosis. If thrombosis or embolism is strongly suspected then treatment with intravenous heparin should be started immediately. Thromboprophylaxis is appropriate for patients delivered by caesarean section.

Anaesthesia

More experienced anaesthetists and assistants should be available in maternity units, and particular care paid in the monitoring of dark-skinned patients.

Ectopic pregnancy

The diagnosis must be considered in all women aged 15–44 years with abdominal pain, especially if they have a history of subfertility, pelvic inflammatory disease, or tubal surgery (includes sterilization).

Haemorrhage

An experienced surgeon should perform caesarean sections for known placenta praevia. All maternity units should have a plan for the management of catastrophic haemorrhage, and access to expert advice in treating those women who refuse blood transfusion.

Sepsis

Acute genital tract sepsis should be considered as a cause of severe persistent shock, even in the absence of classical signs, and appropriate treatment instituted.

Epilepsy

Blood levels of anticonvulsants should be monitored throughout the pregnancy and puerperium to ensure the correct dose is being prescribed and taken.

Caesarean section

When problems arise a more senior surgeon or anaesthetist should be involved more quickly.

SUMMARY

Maternal mortality is falling due to the better health of the population and improvements in the obstetric care of the mother. As half of the direct deaths showed evidence of substandard care there is still room for improvement. It should be remembered that a vaginal delivery is usually safer for the mother than a caesarean section.

C. MISCELLANEOUS SUBJECTS

38. Neonatal medicine

A. Duthie

Expectations of the examiners

Candidates should be knowledgeable in the resuscitation and subsequent management of the newborn baby. They should be competent to examine the neonate, recognize abnormalities, and deal with feeding difficulties.

ANTICIPATORY CARE

Approximately 70% of infants requiring resuscitation are born following a complicated pregnancy or labour. A paediatrician should be present at delivery in the following situations:

1. Preterm infants <36 weeks' gestation and other small babies
2. Malpresentations
3. Fetal distress and meconium staining
4. Rhesus incompatibility
5. Instrumental or operative deliveries (excluding Wrigley's forceps lift-outs)
6. Narcotic analgesia given to the mother within 4 hours prior to delivery
7. Multiple births
8. Antenatal evidence of malformation
9. Other requests.

The candidate should be competent to resuscitate babies in the event of unforeseen emergencies.

RESUSCITATION

Immediately after birth, the baby should be dried gently but thoroughly and a rapid assessment made of respiratory effort, heart rate, colour, peripheral perfusion, muscle tone, and movement. The Apgar scoring system, devised by Dr Virginia Apgar in 1953 (Table 38.1), is still widely used. It does have limitations, but scores at 1 and 5 minutes give a measure of the need for, and response to, resuscitation. Babies with impaired breathing or apnoea

Table 38.1 The Apgar score (at 1 and 5 minutes).

	Score		
	0	1	2
Heart rate	Absent	<100/min	>100/min
Respiratory effort	Absent	Gasping, shallow, weak, irregular	Regular, crying lustily
Muscle tone	Limp	Some flexion	Active, well flexed
Reflex/irritability	None	Grimace	Cough/cry
Colour	Pale/blue	Body pink Extremities blue	Pink

should be resuscitated according to the recent guidelines of the working party of the Royal College of Paediatricians and Child Health and the Royal College of Obstetricians and Gynaecologists as outlined in Figure 38.1.

If the liquor is heavily meconium stained, there is a risk of meconium aspiration and subsequent severe respiratory difficulties. At delivery, these babies should be managed as outlined in Figure 38.1b.

CARE OF THE NORMAL BABY IN THE DELIVERY ROOM

The umbilical cord

The umbilical cord is usually clamped once the baby is delivered. No advantages/disadvantages to delayed clamping have been proven. The method used should be foolproof to avoid massive haemorrhage, e.g. forceps replaced by a commercial, sterile, disposable cord clamp.

Temperature control

The newborn baby is at risk of hypothermia because of:

1. High heat losses by conduction, convection and radiation.
2. Evaporation from a wet skin.
   (These losses are exacerbated by the baby's high surface area to volume ratio.)
3. Impaired ability to increase the metabolic rate immediately after birth.

Hypothermia may worsen hypoxia, acidosis and hypoglycaemia (especially in preterm infants) and induce expiratory grunting. To prevent this:

1. The delivery room should be warm (20–25°C) and exclude draughts.

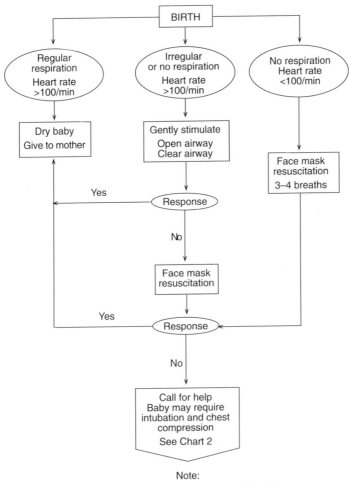

Fig. 38.1a Basic neonatal resuscitation (From Resuscitation of babies at birth: A report of a joint working party of the Royal College of Paediatricians and Child Health and the Royal College of Obstetricians and Gynaecologists 1997, pp 57 and 58. BMJ Publishing Group, London, with permission).

2. The baby should be dried and then wrapped with separate dry, warm towels following delivery.
3. Direct physical contact between mother and baby is a means of thermoregulation but, ideally, exposed parts of baby should be dry and covered.
4. Immediate bathing should be discouraged.

The baby should then be nursed in his/her *neutral thermal environment*, i.e. where body temperature is normally maintained, heat production is at

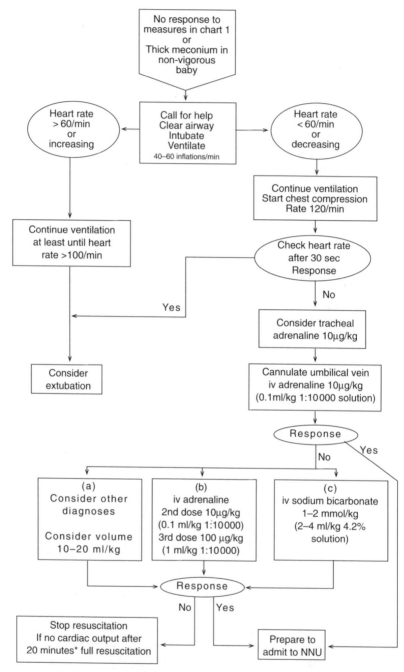

Fig. 38.1b Advanced neonatal resuscitation (Source as for 38.1a).

a minimum and there is no sweating. This is usually achieved by dressing the infant, wrapping him (or her) in covers in a cot which is situated in a warm room. Energy available for growth is then optimal.

Vitamin K$_1$

This vitamin is given as prophylaxis against haemorrhagic disease of the newborn, a potentially fatal disease which occurs more commonly in wholly breast-fed babies. A recent report from the UK, although inconclusive, suggested an association between intramuscularly administered vitamin K$_1$ and childhood cancer. This has been disputed by large studies from the USA and Scandinavia. Although vitamin K$_1$ is less effective when given orally, current recommendations are that all babies receive 0.5 mg vitamin K in two divided doses following birth and breast-fed babies should receive further doses of 0.5 mg at 7 and 28 days. It should be noted that the intramuscular preparation currently administered orally in the UK has not as yet been assessed or licensed for this use by the UK Licensing Authority.

Measurement

The baby's weight and occipitofrontal head circumference should be documented following birth, although the latter is often inaccurate at this early stage because of moulding during labour. Measurement of the ankle–crown length by tape measure is useless and may be misleading in follow-up. A stadiometer should be used for complete accuracy.

Labelling

In hospital, name tags are attached to ensure correct identification of all babies.

Bonding

The parent(s) and child should be left alone together as soon as feasible and, if the baby's condition allows, mother and baby should remain together unless the mother requests otherwise. Putting the baby to the breast shortly after delivery may help to promote breast-feeding.

CARE ON THE POSTNATAL WARD

Routine observations

These include recordings of:

1. Temperature
2. Heart rate
3. Respiratory rate

4.   Bladder and bowel activity
5.   Weight.

Temperature and heart rate

An abnormally high (>38°C) or low (<35.5°C) temperature or a tachycardia (heart rate >160/minute), which is sustained longer than 1 hour may be indicative of neonatal sepsis. The baby should be examined carefully.

Respiratory rate

In a normal term infant this should not exceed 60 breaths/minute. Other signs of respiratory distress include:

1.   Expiratory grunting
2.   Central cyanosis
3.   Subcostal/intercostal/sternal recession
4.   Tracheal tug
5.   Nasal flaring.

Respiratory distress in a term baby should be treated as neonatal sepsis (likely Group B β-haemolytic streptococcal infection) until proven otherwise. Further causes of respiratory distress to then consider are outlined in Table 38.2.

Transient tachypnoea of the newborn is a diagnosis based on suspicion when other more dangerous diagnoses, particularly infection, have been excluded. It is attributed to delay in the clearance of fetal lung fluid and is seen more commonly following caesarean section particularly in the absence of labour. Chest X-ray typically shows hyperinflated lung fields, prominent perihilar vascular markings and fluid in the horizontal fissure of the right lung.

Bladder activity

Delay in the passage of urine (>48 hours after birth) is rare in a healthy baby without obvious physical signs, e.g. enlarged, palpable kidneys or bladder. Urine is quite likely to have been passed unnoticed during delivery.

A poor, dribbling urinary stream in boys is indicative of congenital, posterior urethral valves.

Urate crystals may be normally precipitated as red streaks on the nappy and should not be mistaken for haematuria.

Bowel activity

Meconium is the viscid, green-black material passed in the first 2–3 days after birth. This changes to 'milk stools', the bright, mustard-yellow, soft and seedy motions of breast-fed babies and the firmer, paler yellow/brown

Table 38.2   Causes of respiratory distress in the term baby.

Infection—acquired before or during passage down the birth canal. Beware a history of prolonged rupture of membranes >24 hours and preterm labour

Organisms: Group B β-haemolytic streptococcus, *E. coli, Staphylococcus aureus, Listeria monocytogenes*, Klebsiella, Enterobacter, *Streptococcus pneumoniae* and others

Meconium aspiration

Congenital anomalies:

Upper airways obstruction, e.g. choanal atresia, Pierre Robin syndrome, laryngeal stenosis or web formation, pharyngeal tumours, external compression by vascular rings, neck tumours, e.g. goitre, etc.

Tracheo-oesophageal fistula ± oesophageal atresia.

Diaphragmatic hernia

Lung defects including

Congenital lobar emphysema

Congenital cystic adenomatoid malformation of the lung

Sequestered lobe

Pulmonary lymphangiectasia

Pulmonary agenesis/hypoplasia

Spontaneous pneumothorax

CNS depression, e.g. associated with intrapartum asphyxia

Intercostal or diaphragmatic paralysis, associated with:

Erb's palsy

Neuromuscular disease, e.g. myasthenia gravis, congenital myopathy

Cardiac failure

Metabolic disease with acidosis, e.g. organic acidaemias

Transient tachypnoea of newborn

motions of those bottle-fed. Meconium consists of swallowed amniotic fluid, desquamated intestinal epithelial cells and intestinal secretions including bile. Delay in its passage beyond 48 hours of birth is abnormal and may indicate intestinal obstruction or Hirschsprung's disease. A pale, putty-coloured 'milk stool' in a jaundiced baby should raise the suspicion of obstructive jaundice and extrahepatic biliary atresia should be excluded.

Weight

All normal term babies will lose weight in the first days of life as their energy expenditure and fluid loss is greater than their intake, but this should not exceed 10% of the birth weight. As feeding becomes established, weight should increase and birth weight be regained at 7–10 days of age. Thereafter, babies should gain weight at 20–30 g/day (1 oz/day except on Sundays!) until 6 months of age.

Cord care

Daily cleaning with alcohol-impregnated swabs and the application of hexachlorophane-containing powder to prevent colonization by potential pathogenic organisms is advocated by many units; others simply wash the cord with soap and water during baths. The clamp may be removed by the fourth or fifth day.

Skin care

Initial cleaning involves removal of vernix, dried blood and meconium especially from the flexures. The first full bath can be delayed for 1 or 2 days, the baby then being washed with a high fat baby soap. No special skin care is needed other than the application of a barrier cream, e.g. zinc and castor oil to protect the perineum and baby oil to the dry and cracked skin of postmature babies.

Parentcraft

This period of postnatal care offers the opportunity to help inexperienced mothers and fathers feed, bathe, change, dress and care for their newborn and so increase their confidence in handling their baby.

Feeding

In 1995, the Department of Health stated that: 'of the 64% of women nationally who breast-feed at birth, 12% will have stopped by the time they leave hospital. 20% will have stopped at the end of two weeks. By the end of 6 weeks the proportion of women in England and Wales who breast-feed is only 40%.' Sixty-five per cent of babies born in England and Wales were initially breast-fed but a third of these were bottle-feeding by 6 weeks of age. Breast-feeding offers the following advantages:

1. There is convincing epidemiological evidence that even in developed countries, where formula feeds can be prepared under sterile conditions, breast-feeding significantly reduces the risk of gastrointestinal, respiratory and urinary tract infections and, in preterm infants, also of necrotizing enterocolitis. Human milk (especially colostrum) contains factors active against infection which include:
    a. Maternal plasma immunoglobulins, IgG, IgM, IgE
    b. Secretory IgA specific to antigens in the maternal gastrointestinal and respiratory tracts, including potential pathogens to which the baby is likely to be exposed
    c. The bacteriocidal enzyme, lysozyme
    d. Lactoferrin, which competes for iron in the gut with certain bacteria, e.g. *E. coli*, and inhibits their growth
    e. Antiviral agents, e.g. interferon
    f. Phagocytes, lymphocytes, neutrophils, cytokines and complement.
2. Breast milk contains several hormones in greater concentration than in maternal serum, e.g. calcitonin, epidermal growth factor and

prostaglandins E and F. The effect of these hormones on gut mucosal development and activity is unknown.

3. Breast-feeding alone for 6 months lessens the risk of cows' milk protein intolerance. Whether breast-feeding protects against the development of eczema or asthma is still debated, although there are grounds to suggest it is important in those genetically at risk.

4. A lower incidence of sudden infant death syndrome has been demonstrated in breast-fed babies in New Zealand. In the UK, published studies have not shown a clear relationship between the two. Despite this, the Chief Medical Officer recommends encouragement of breast-feeding as a preventative measure.

5. The water, fat and protein content of breast milk changes throughout a feed giving a completely balanced diet. The fat and protein are more easily and completely absorbed than those in formula milks.

6. It is cheap and convenient.

7. There is no risk of hypernatraemia as occurs with formula feeds if reconstituted incorrectly.

8. Evidence is accumulating that the long-term benefits of breast-feeding may include a significant advantage in the child's cognitive function and a reduction in the risk of juvenile onset diabetes mellitus and maternal breast cancer.

Contraindications to breast-feeding

Maternal factors
Severe systemic disease, e.g. cardiac failure, chronic respiratory disease, neoplasia if on chemotherapy or exhausted.

Infection, e.g. tuberculosis, septicaemia, bilateral breast abscesses, HIV positivity in this country (there is a small risk of transmission of the virus via milk to the baby; in developing countries, failure to breast-feed carries a higher risk of infection in an immunocompromised baby).

Inverted nipples which do not respond to local treatment.

Treatment with drugs which may be secreted in sufficient quantity to seriously affect the baby (Table 38.3).

Baby factors
Inborn errors of metabolism where milk is harmful. e.g. phenylketonuria (breast-feeding is not contraindicated but is restricted), galactosaemia, alactasia.

In summary there are very few contraindications to breast-feeding and the advantages far outweigh the disadvantages even in our society. Mothers should be encouraged to breast-feed and be supported in their action. Provision of sensible and consistent advice is of paramount importance in this support.

Table 38.3 Drugs which may be secreted in breast milk in sufficient quantity to potentially seriously affect baby (this list is not exhaustive and further reference should be made to the British National Formulary).

	Drug	Comments
Anticoagulants	Phenindione	
Antibiotics	Chloramphenicol	Levels could be monitored in baby
	Ethosuxamide	
	Isoniazide	
	Metronidazole	Interrrupt feeding for 24 hours after an initial single large dose. Then use a daily dosage regimen
	Tetracyclines	
	Trimethoprim	
Immunosuppressives	Cyclosporin	
Radioactive isotopes		Interrupt feeding until radioactivity cleared
Antiarrhythmics	Amiodarone	
	Atenolol	
Anti-inflammatories	Indomethacin	
	Gold salts	
Antidepressants	Doxepin	
	Lithium	Levels could be monitored in baby
Antimalarials	Dapsone preparations	
Antimigraine	Ergotamine	
Others	High-dose oestrogen	
	High-dose vitamin A + D	

Feeding practice

Healthy term babies exercise autonomous control over feeding and will self-regulate their milk intake if fed 'on demand'. As a guideline, the recommended intake for bottle-fed babies on each day following birth is:

Day 1	60 ml/kg birth weight
Day 2	90 ml/kg birth weight
Day 3	120 ml/kg birth weight
Day 4 and onwards	150 ml/kg body weight (if greater than birth weight)

Examples of formula feed used in the UK are:

Manufacturer	*Whey-based*	*Casein-based*
Wyeth	SMA Gold cap	SMA White cap
Farleys	Ostermilk	Ostermilk 2
Cow & Gate	Premium	Plus
Milupa	Aptamil	Milumil

These milks, particularly those that are whey-based, have a reduced protein content compared to that in breast milk. The proportion of the more digestible lactalbumin to casein is higher in whey-based milks. They also have a lower salt content and are advised for bottle-fed babies up to 6 weeks of age. All are fortified with additional iron and vitamins D and K.

Feeding problems

Maternal (breast-fed babies)

Retracted nipples. Compression of the areola or use of Waller shells may help

Cracked and sore nipples. Consider the use of a nipple shield or if it is too painful, rest that nipple from baby but continue to express milk from that side, allowing breast-feeding to continue on the other side. Application of a bland ointment, e.g. Kamillosan, may be useful.

Acute mastitis. Regular breast-feeding should continue and baby should start with the affected side to empty that breast.

Breast abscess. Breast-feeding is contraindicated.

Breast engorgement (usually transient). Advise the expression of 20–30 ml of milk pre-feed to reduce the tension in the breasts sufficiently to allow baby to fix on.

Incorrect feeding technique. For effective breast-feeding there must be good apposition of the baby's tongue and lower jaw to the breast tissue behind the nipple, where the lactiferous sinuses are located. Poor milk intake will result in a hungry baby who is unsettled and cries incessantly. Frequent, small, green, 'mucous' motions may be passed and there may be pyrexia ('dehydration fever') and hypoglycaemia. Appropriate help and advice should be given. Complementary bottle feeding is not recommended as it has been shown to be a major contributor to failure of breast-feeding.

Baby

Not interested in feeding, i.e. refusing feeds, feeding for short periods infrequently or using a weak suck.

Examine carefully to ensure baby is generally well and to exclude:

1. Infection
2. Respiratory distress
3. Congestive cardiac failure
4. Primary neuromuscular problems
5. Dysmorphic syndromes, e.g. Down syndrome
6. Metabolic disorders
7. Congenital adrenal hyperplasia.

A strong suck reflex develops from approximately 35 weeks' gestation, hence premature babies may not suck so effectively.

A poor suck may follow a history of:

1. Birth asphyxia with poor Apgar scores and need for resuscitation
2. Difficult delivery
3. Sedation from intrapartum or antenatal drug therapy or from drugs excreted in breast milk.

Difficulty sucking, implying a mechanical problem, may occur with:

1. Cleft palate, including submucous palatal clefts
2. Micrognathia
3. Nasal obstruction, e.g. choanal atresia, excessive nasal secretions (usually transient in the first few days of life)
4. Maternal breast engorgement
5. Respiratory distress, where baby has difficulty sucking and breathing at the same time.

'Wind'. Breast-fed babies may gulp and swallow excessive air if the initial flow of milk is fast. This will similarly occur in bottle-fed babies where the hole in the teat is too large. If it is too small, baby will have to suck extremely hard to obtain the milk. Bottle-fed babies inevitably swallow more air as they take in the last few drops of milk or if the milk level falls below the level of the hole in the teat. Excessive swallowed air can cause abdominal discomfort with crying and regurgitation and may be avoided by gently rubbing or patting the baby's back whilst held upright or prone ('winding') during and after feeds.

Vomiting. This is common in the first days of life as the baby develops coordination between sucking, swallowing, and breathing.

Persistent vomiting suggests gastro-oesophageal reflux but ensure that the feeding technique is correct and that baby is clinically well as it is also a symptom of:

1. Infection
2. Cerebral disorder — intracranial haemorrhage, hydrocephalus
3. Metabolic disorders, e.g. galactosaemia
4. Congenital adrenal hyperplasia
5. Thyrotoxicosis
6. Cardiac failure
7. Withdrawal from maternal narcotic addiction
8. Intestinal obstruction, e.g. duodenal, jejunal or ileal atresia or stenosis; meconium ileus; volvulus with malrotation of the large gut; necrotizing enterocolitis; Hirschsprung's disease; intestinal duplications or cysts.

Beware vomitus which is:

1. Frothy—indicative of oesophageal atresia with tracheo-oesophageal reflux
2. Bile stained—suggests bowel obstruction distal to the ampulla of Vater
3. Blood stained—usually due to ingested maternal blood swallowed during delivery or from a cracked nipple but may, on occasions, be indicative of upper gastrointestinal bleeding secondary to oesophagitis, gastritis, haemorrhagic disease of the newborn and,

rarely, peptic ulceration, enterogenous duplications and cysts and haemangiomata.

Examination of the newborn

This enables screening for hidden abnormalities including congenital heart disease or dislocated hips but also allows time for parents to voice any concerns about their baby and to give reassurance about minor abnormalities and normal variants.

A great deal of information can be gained by looking at the infant lying in the cot, for example:

1. Colour — should not be cyanosed or pale
2. Posture — the term infant will lie with hips, knees and elbows strongly flexed, will wriggle spontaneously, stretch and yawn and should be observed to move all limbs
3. Dysmorphic or other obvious abnormal features
4. Evidence of respiratory distress (see 'Routine observations' above).

As the baby is handled and undressed, further information will be gleaned about muscle tone, movement, posture, and response to stimuli.

Skin

Minor variants include:

Dry, cracked and peeling skin of postmature infants.

Peripheral cyanosis of hands and feet which is common in the first 48 hours of life and may become more obvious on exposure.

Traumatic cyanosis—'blue' discoloration of the face, head and neck produced by masses of petechiae and caused by facial congestion during delivery when the umbilical cord may have tightened around the neck.

Harlequin change—flushing of one half of the baby with a clear demarcation from the normal side down the midline.

Mongolian blue spots—patchy blue-black coloration of the skin over the buttocks and lower back, which should not be mistaken for bruising as it is a normal finding in all babies, particularly non-Caucasians.

Milia—tiny sebaceous retention cysts producing pinhead sized, white spots scattered mainly over the nose.

Erythema toxicum (urticaria neonatorum)—a very common, variable, blotchy, erythematous rash which may be associated with yellow pinhead pustules (sterile). It occurs in the first week of life, is harmless and of uncertain cause.

Vascular naevi

Capillary haemangiomata—small defects of dermal capillaries which produce pale-pink patches on the nape of the neck, forehead, upper eyelids (salmon patches or stork marks). These gradually fade. Port-wine stains are larger and darker and grow with the child. If they occur in the distribution of the trigeminal nerve and do not cross the midline, there is the possibility of an associated intracranial vascular anomaly with epilepsy and/or hemiplegia (Sturge–Weber syndrome).

Cavernous haemangiomata (strawberry naevi). These are rarely present at birth but develop in the first 2 weeks as a bright red spot at any site which then increases rapidly in size over 3–9 months. They do eventually resolve and should not be treated unless in a site which is potentially dangerous, e.g. the eye.

Jaundice. Onset within 2–4 days after birth is extremely common and likely to be 'physiological' with an increased unconjugated (indirect) bilirubin level due to:

1. A high bilirubin load on the liver from relative polycythaemia in the baby and shortened survival of fetal red cells.
2. Decreased hepatic uptake of bilirubin.
3. Immaturity of uridine diphosphate glucuronyl transferase which conjugates bilirubin with glucuronic acid.
4. Deficiency of hepatic carrier proteins.

The bilirubin level peaks by day 3–4, then falls steadily and is normal by 11–14 days of age.

Beware the following abnormal situations:

Onset of jaundice within the first 24 hours of life. The most likely causes include:

1. Excessive red cell haemolysis due to rhesus, ABO or other blood group incompatibility
2. Infection
3. Increased red cell breakdown from
   a. Extensive bruising
   b. Cephalhaematoma
   c. Polycythaemia.

These will result in an unconjugated hyperbilirubinaemia and baby is at risk of kernicterus which may cause later athetoid cerebral palsy, developmental delay, high tone deafness, or even death. Graphs are available which indicate the level of unconjugated bilirubin at which treatment with phototherapy or exchange transfusion should be commenced, taking into account the baby's age, gestation, and health. Levels for intervention are substantially lower if the baby is premature and/or sick.

Investigations at this stage, to elucidate the cause, should include:

1. Full blood count with differential, reticulocyte count and blood film
2. Mother and baby's blood group
3. Coombs' test

4. Urine for culture
5. If baby is unwell then a full infection screen, obtaining blood, cerebrospinal fluid and urine (preferably by suprapubic aspiration) for culture, should be performed.

If the response to treatment is poor then rare causes of early onset jaundice should be considered and investigated appropriately. They include:

1. Congenital infection with cytomegalovirus, rubella, herpes, toxoplasmosis or hepatitis A, B, C
2. Metabolic causes, e.g. galactosaemia
3. Red cell structural abnormalities, e.g. hereditary spherocytosis
4. Red cell enzyme abnormalities, e.g. pyruvate kinase or glucose-6-phosphate dehydrogenase (G6PD) deficiency
5. Congenitally absent or defective bilirubin uridine diphosphate glucuronyl transferase activity in Crigler–Najjar syndrome.

Note the dangers of phototherapy which include:

1. Retinal damage
2. Dehydration through increased insensible water loss and passage of loose motions
3. Thermal instability
4. Rashes
5. Bronzing if the direct (conjugated) bilirubin level is raised.

Ensure therefore that babies under phototherapy wear eye shields for protection and have a good fluid intake.

Prolonged jaundice > 14 days. Although the most common cause of prolonged jaundice is breast-milk jaundice in breast-fed babies, it is important to consider other causes and extrahepatic biliary atresia should be excluded as a priority. In this condition, surgery to correct obstruction to the flow of bile is more likely to be successful in preventing chronic liver disease with cirrhosis and the need for liver transplantation if performed early (before 8 weeks of age). Babies must have their total and direct (conjugated) bilirubin levels measured. Breast-milk jaundice is characterized by an unconjugated hyperbilirubinaemia. In contrast, in extrahepatic biliary atresia conjugated bilirubin levels will be raised and there may, in addition, be a history of dark urine and pale motions to indicate biliary obstruction.

Other causes of a prolonged, conjugated or mixed conjugated/unconjugated hyperbilirubinaemia include:

1. Infection (congenital or acute as above)
2. Metabolic disease, e.g. galactosaemia, tyrosinaemia, fructosaemia
3. Endocrinopathies, e.g. hypothyroidism, hypopituitarism
4. Genetic disorders, e.g. α-1-antitrypsin deficiency, cystic fibrosis

5. Intrahepatic biliary hypoplasia (may be syndromic i.e. Alagilles)
6. Increased enteropathic circulation of bile secondary to intestinal obstruction
7. Other obstructive causes including choledochal cyst
8. 'Neonatal hepatitis' — a diagnosis of exclusion after full investigation
9. Rarities, e.g. Zellweger's, Wolman's, Niemann–Pick type 3.

The first-line investigations for any baby with a prolonged jaundice are therefore:

1. Measurement of total and direct bilirubin levels
2. Check the colour of the baby's motions!

If there is any suspicion of obstruction then an abdominal ultrasound scan should be performed and referral made (preferably to a specialist centre) for consideration for colloid liver scanning and liver biopsy. Other more specific investigations can be performed as the clinical picture then dictates, but initial tests should probably include:

1. Biochemical liver function tests
2. Full blood count and film
3. Urine for culture, or if the baby is unwell, a full infection screen
4. Clinitest and clinistix of urine for reducing substances
5. Thyroid function tests.

Head and neck

Head shape. This may be markedly affected by moulding during delivery and this returns to normal within several days. Caput succedaneum is the oedematous thickening of the scalp over the presenting part. Distinguish from cephalhaematoma where a collection of blood between periosteum and skull bones produces a tense, smooth swelling limited by the suture lines (Fig. 38.2).

An asymmetrical head with flattening of one side of the occiput and the opposite forehead and face (plagiocephaly) may be produced by long-term moulding in utero. Brachycephaly with flattened occiput and a reduced AP diameter of the skull is seen in Down syndrome and a prominent occiput in Edward syndrome.

Fontanelles and sutures. The anterior fontanelle is of variable size and eventually closes by about 18 months of age. The posterior fontanelle is small (0.5–1 cm diameter) and is usually closed by 3 months of age. A third fontanelle, formed by widening of the sagittal suture between the anterior and posterior fontanelles, occurs normally but is more common in Down syndrome. A tense, full or bulging fontanelle suggests raised intracranial pressure, as does undue separation of the sutures (up to 1 cm is normal). The sutures may be over-riding (producing a 'step-up' feel) secondary to moulding. This should be distinguished from the rarer

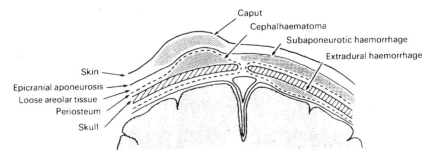

Fig. 38.2   Layers of the fetal skull illustrating possible sites of haemorrhage.

'ridging' of the suture line which occurs with premature fusion of that line (craniosynostosis).

Abrasions or lacerations of the scalp may be caused by fetal scalp electrodes or fetal blood sampling during labour.

Facies

May be typical for example of Down syndrome, infant of a diabetic mother etc.

Ears

Abnormalities of shape, size or position and the presence of auricular pits, skin tags or accessory auricles may be indicative of dysmorphic syndromes. The ears are low set if the top of the helix lies below a line drawn at right angles to the facial profile from the outer canthus of the eye.

Nose

Bilateral, complete nasal obstruction as occurs in choanal atresia causes marked respiratory distress as babies are obligate nose breathers. Transient increased nasal secretions blocking the small neonatal nose may cause mild distress. Nasal flaring may be a sign of respiratory distress (see 'Routine observations' above).

Eyes

Eyes may be abnormal in:
1. Size — small in microphthalmia; prominent in congenital glaucoma.
2. Slant, e.g. mongoloid in Down syndrome.
3. General appearance, e.g. sunsetting of the iris in raised intracranial pressure.

Conjunctival haemorrhages are common following birth, as are mildly 'sticky' eyes with a mucopurulent discharge. If this worsens, swabs should be taken to exclude pathogenic infection, particularly with gonococcus or chlamydia.

Pupils may be irregular if there is a defect in the iris (coloboma). This may be associated with a retinal defect. Congenital cataracts are usually excluded when the normal red, retinal reflex is obtained on direct ophthalmoscopy. This method is not foolproof however, as cataracts may develop after birth. For more detailed examination of the lens a +20 dioptre ophthalmoscope lens should be used. Cataracts may be:

1. Familial (usually autosomal dominant)
2. Part of a syndrome, e.g. Down
3. Of metabolic cause, e.g. galactosaemia
4. Associated with congenital infection, e.g. rubella, toxoplasmosis.

Immediate referral to the ophthalmologist is indicated.

Mouth and tongue

Obvious abnormalities include macroglossia (e.g. in hypothyroidism, Beckwith–Wiedemann syndrome) and micrognathia. Facial palsy, caused by direct pressure on the nerve by forceps or by compression on the maternal sacrum during delivery, may only be evident when the baby cries or grimaces.

A cleft lip (unilateral, bilateral or of more complex deformity) will be obvious but small soft palate clefts and submucous palatal clefts can easily be missed unless the palate is both directly viewed and palpated.

Other minor abnormalities include:

1. Sucking blisters on the lips
2. Epithelial (Epsteins) pearls — tiny white spots on the hard palate
3. High arched palate, e.g. in Marfan's syndrome
4. Ranula — mucus retention cyst on the floor of the mouth
5. Neonatal teeth — should be removed if loose to avoid inhalation.

Neck

The neck may be webbed in Turner's syndrome or swollen with a:

1. Cystic hygroma
2. Congenital goitre
3. Sternomastoid tumour — a firm swelling anywhere along the length of this muscle, usually with an associated torticollis with the head turned away from the side of the lesion. It represents a small haematoma or fibrous malformation.

Loss of continuity, swelling or crepitus of the clavicles may indicate a fracture.

Chest

The shape and movement may be abnormal, e.g. bell-shaped in pulmonary hypoplasia, tachypnoea with intercostal recession in respiratory distress. Palpation of the precordium will reveal thrills, ventricular heave, and will locate the apex beat (displaced in dextrocardia, diaphragmatic hernia, pneumothorax). Auscultation will reveal abnormal heart sounds and heart rate and will exclude any heart murmur. Breath sounds should be vesicular and air entry equal over both lung fields. Very occasionally, bowel sounds may be audible with a diaphragmatic hernia.

The breasts may be engorged and lactation may occur in both males and females. This is normal unless there is associated erythema indicative of mastitis.

Abdomen

Major defects, e.g. gastroschisis, omphalocele, will be evident at birth. A distended abdomen will be evident on inspection, as will visible peristalsis and erythema at the base of the umbilical cord ('umbilical flare').

The cut end of the cord should show two arteries and one vein (a single artery is only very occasionally associated with renal abnormalities).

An umbilical hernia may be large and unslightly but rarely causes complications. Surgery is rarely indicated before 2 years of age as the majority will close without intervention.

Urine discharging from the umbilicus indicates a persistent patent urachus and requires surgical treatment.

Abnormal masses may be palpated. A soft liver edge is often palpable 1–2 cm below the costal margin and the spleen is often 'tippable'. It is abnormally large if palpable greater than 1 cm below the costal margin. In a well-relaxed baby, the kidneys are usually palpable.

The inguinal region—indirect herniae may be visible (surgical referral needed). The femoral pulses should both be palpable and if not, it is important to determine the blood pressure in all four limbs to exclude coarctation of the aorta.

The anus. This should be directly visualized to determine position and patency so as to exclude an imperforate anus. Examination should not be deterred by the presence of meconium as a fistula will allow the passage of meconium whilst the anus remains imperforate.

Genitalia

In males true micropenis associated with hypopituitarism is rare. More commonly, it may appear deceptively short when buried in suprapubic fat. The position of the urethral meatus will be abnormal in hypospadias, which may or may not be associated with chordee (curvature of the shaft of the penis). These babies should not be circumcised as the foreskin will be required for later surgical correction. At full term, both testes should be palpable. Hydroceles usually resolve spontaneously.

In term females the labia minora should be covered by the labia majora. Virilization, e.g. in congenital adrenal hyperplasia, produces an enlarged, prominent clitoris. A white (occasionally blood-stained), mucoid vaginal discharge is normal, as are small skin tags and mucoid cysts around the vaginal opening.

Ambiguous genitalia. Chromosome analysis should be requested urgently and these results awaited before the sex of the baby is given to the parents.

Spine

Major spina bifida will be obvious at birth. Swellings, sinuses, 'birthmarks' or hairy patches over the vertebral column may indicate an underlying vertebral or spinal cord abnormality. Sacrococcygeal pits are common. Their bases should be intact to distinguish them from dermal sinuses which communicate through to the theca (risk of meningitis unless dealt with surgically). The spine should be straight.

Limbs

Ensure movement is symmetrical and posture and shape normal.

Birth injuries

A fractured humerus or clavicle will result in paucity of movement of that arm, the former often with obvious deformity.

Brachial plexus injury with contusion of:

1. The upper roots from downward traction of the arm or shoulder will produce paralysis of the muscles supplied by the cervical nerves, C5 and C6, i.e. Erb's palsy (Fig. 38.3) with lack of arm movement and characteristic 'waiter's tip' posture, or,
2. The lower roots by upward traction on the arm produce paralysis of muscles supplied by C8 and T1, i.e. the intrinsic muscles of the hand and flexors of the wrist and fingers with Klumpke's palsy.

Wrist drop may result from pressure or traction on the radial nerve as it spirals around the upper humerus.

Excessive moulding in utero (especially with oligohydramnios) may produce abnormal posture of the feet and ankles, e.g. talipes calcaneovalgus or equinovarus (postural or true type). A calcaneovalgus foot will usually correct spontaneously. In postural talipes equinovarus, the foot can always be straightened passively (gentle abduction and dorsiflexion of the foot should result in the little toe touching the outside of the leg). Referral to an orthopaedic surgeon is needed for true talipes equinovarus.

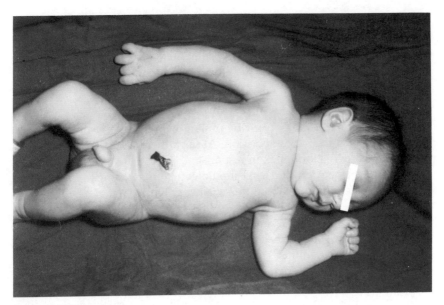

Fig. 38.3 Erb's palsy.

Hands and feet

Dysmorphic features include polydactyly, syndactyly, brachydactyly, clinodactyly, hypoplastic nails, single palmar creases, the characteristic clenched hand and position of the thumb with 'rocker bottom' feet in Edward syndrome, oedematous dorsum of the feet in Turner's syndrome etc.

Hips

Congenital dislocation of the hip is more common in girls than in boys, in those delivered in the breech position, and if there is a family history. There is an association with oligohydramnios, myelomeningocele and other neuromuscular abnormalities. It is important to detect this at birth as early intervention will usually be curative. The following tests are used:

Ortolani's test will detect a dislocated hip. The hips and knees are flexed. With the examiner's middle fingers over the outer aspect of the thighs, their tips on the greater trochanters and with the thumbs over the inner aspects of the thighs, the baby's legs are gently pulled away from the pelvis, abducted and externally rotated. Gentle pressure is applied anteriorly and medially on the greater trochanter and if the hip is dislocated, a definite 'clunk' is felt as the femoral head slips forwards into the acetabulum.

Barlow's test will detect a dislocatable hip. The pelvis on one side is stabilized. The other leg is held as above. The hip is brought in to an adducted position and then pushed posteriorly and laterally with the thumb (a dislocatable femoral head will 'clunk' out of the acetabulum).

If there is any doubt about hip stability then ultrasound examination is indicated and referral to an orthopaedic surgeon, who has a specialist interest in such problems, should be made.

Neurology

Muscle tone can be assessed by pulling baby gently by the wrists and hands to sit from the supine position. At term there will still be some head lag but the elbows should flex in response.

In ventral suspension, the head should come up in line with the body for a few seconds and limbs should flex against gravity.

Primitive reflexes. Assessment is usually limited to obtaining the Moro reflex: the baby's head is lifted from the supine position and supported in the examiner's hand. It is then allowed to drop suddenly backwards a short way. There should be rapid outward flinging of the arms, opening of the hands and extension of the legs, followed by a slower return to the normal position. If a neurological problem is suspected, then other primitive reflexes, e.g. the palmar, plantar, asymmetrical tonic neck response, stepping and walking reflexes should be elicited.

Biochemical screening tests

All babies born in the UK are currently screened for phenylketonuria (PKU) and hypothyroidism. A small blood sample is obtained by heel prick on days 5–9 of life and is allowed to dry as blood spots on blotting paper as provided in the standard 'Guthrie cards'. The baby should have been on a normal milk intake prior to testing.

Screening for cystic fibrosis is performed in some health regions by measurement of immunoreactive trypsin levels from one of the blood spots.

Any positive result obtained on a screening test must be checked by more sophisticated laboratory investigation.

Immunizations

Tuberculosis (TB)

It is recommended that in communities where TB is of high prevalence, BCG vaccination be given to all babies following birth.

Hepatitis B

The following immunization regimen is recommended for all infants of mothers who are hepatitis B surface antigen positive (if the mother is hepatitis B 'e' antigen negative, and hepatitis B 'e' antibody positive, then only (2) below is needed):

1. Hepatitis B specific immunoglobulin 200 i.u. (200 mg) intramuscularly within 12 hours of birth and
2. Hepatitis B vaccine 10 mg intramuscularly at birth (on the contralateral side), at 1 month and 6 months of age. Baby's antibody status should be checked at 1 year of age and a booster dose of hepatitis B vaccine given if antibodies are undetectable at this stage.

SPECIAL PROBLEMS

Potential neonatal problems may be anticipated before delivery in certain situations and the paediatrician should then be alerted. Consider the following:

Pre-existing maternal disease

Selected examples are described below.

Diabetes mellitus

During pregnancy the fetus is subjected to an excessive carbohydrate load with resultant pancreatic islet cell hyperplasia and hyperinsulinaemia. Insulin is an anabolic hormone which stimulates growth and, together with altered release of insulin-like growth factors, produces a baby who is large for gestational age. This macrosomic baby may have an enlarged heart (risk of hypertrophic cardiomyopathy) and liver and typical facies with bulging cheeks, plethora and hirsutism. Although this is most commonly seen if maternal diabetic control is poor during pregnancy, it can still occur when control has been good. The main hazards to be anticipated in the baby are:

1. A difficult vaginal delivery with an increased risk of shoulder dystocia and birth injury.
2. An increased risk of hyaline membrane disease because of delayed maturation of the pulmonary surfactant system.
3. Severe hypoglycaemia with jitteriness and fits when the rich source of maternal glucose stops at birth and there is still a circulating hyperinsulinaemia. High levels of glucose supplementation may be required.

There is an increased risk of congenital anomaly (particularly anencephaly, meningomyelocele, congenital heart disease, and sacral agenesis with or without agenesis/hypoplasia of the femora) in infants of diabetic mothers.

Thyroid disease

The transplacental passage of thyroid stimulating autoantibodies may cause overt neonatal thyrotoxicosis in 1 in 100 infants of mothers with Graves' disease. Most affected infants have a palpable goitre, and proptosis and lid retraction may be evident at birth. Symptoms of irritability, hyperactivity or jitteriness, tachycardia and occasionally cardiac arrhythmias with cardiac failure, excessive appetite with diarrhoea, weight loss or poor weight gain, excessive sweating or flushing, hepatosplenomegaly with thrombocytopenia, bruising or petechiae may develop soon after birth or some days or weeks later.

Antithyroid medication given to the mother during pregnancy may inhibit the fetus' own thyroid hormone synthesis and cause a goitre if baby responds with increased secretion of thyroid stimulating hormone (TSH). Breast-fed babies of mothers on antithyroid treatment should have their thyroid function monitored fortnightly for the first 2 months and monthly thereafter if all is well.

Narcotic analgesic addiction

Infants of narcotic analgesic drug addicts are at risk of being small for gestational age, of delivering prematurely and of developing withdrawal symptoms with jitteriness (occasionally with generalized, clonic convulsions), irritability, sweating, sneezing, a high-pitched cry, diarrhoea, vomiting and poor feeding, usually starting 24–48 hours following birth.

Problems in the baby recognized antenatally

Congenital abnormalities

Congenital abnormalities such as diaphragmatic hernia and gastroschisis may necessitate antenatal transfer of the mother to a unit where specialist neonatal advice, including surgical treatment, is immediately available.

Small for gestational age baby

The definition varies: a baby whose birth weight is either more than 2 standard deviations below the mean or below the 10th centile for that gestational age.

Dysmorphic features may suggest a chromosomal abnormality. Hepatosplenomegaly with thrombocytopenic purpura suggests congenital infection.

Potential neonatal problems include:

1. Increased risk of birth asphyxia, particularly if there have been adverse intrauterine conditions such as placental insufficiency.

2. Hypoglycaemia because of lack of adequate glycogen stores and relative hyperinsulinaemia. Early, regular feeding should be instituted and blood sugar levels monitored. Nasogastric tube feeding may be needed.
3. Hypothermia (see 'Temperature control' above). This is potentially a greater problem in these babies because of lack of subcutaneous fat.
4. Polycythaemia with an increased risk of
   a. Cerebral vein thrombosis
   b. Cardiac failure with
      i. Pulmonary hypertension
      ii. Pulmonary haemorrhage
      iii. Jaundice requiring phototherapy
      iv. Necrotizing enterocolitis
      v. Renal vein thrombosis.
5. Hypocalcaemia which may result in jitteriness and fits.

Preterm baby

Definition: a baby born before 37 completed weeks' gestation irrespective of birth weight.

Potential neonatal problems include:

Respiratory distress syndrome (hyaline membrane disease) due to deficiency of pulmonary surfactant, which acts to reduce surface tension within the alveolar sacs and prevents their complete collapse during expiration. Exudation of plasma and other blood constituents from the congested pulmonary capillaries produces an amorphous 'hyaline' membrane which lines the terminal bronchioles and alveoli, preventing gas exchange. Signs of respiratory distress (see 'Routine observations' above) develop within 3–4 hours of birth (sooner in very preterm infants). The natural history depends on the disease severity and gestational age but, in general, the condition improves from 36 to 48 hours of age as the proteinaceous material and cellular debris in the alveoli are removed by macrophages and surfactant is produced. Supportive therapy including oxygen, ventilatory support, artificial surfactant and inotropic support may be needed in the interim. Long-term ventilation and oxygen therapy increases susceptibility to chronic lung disease of prematurity (bronchopulmonary dysplasia).

Infection. There is increased susceptibility in preterm infants.

Intraventricular haemorrhage (IVH). This is the most common cerebral complication. Haemorrhage may be limited to the subependymal layer or germinal matrix of the cerebrum or extend into the ventricles with subsequent dilatation if the reabsorption or flow of CSF is impaired. Venous infarction, usually secondary to a severe IVH, will result in haemorrhagic necrosis of periventricular white matter with a high risk of subsequent neurological impairment.

Pathogenesis is complex involving the following factors:

1. Intravascular — impaired autoregulation of cerebral blood flow in preterm infants and episodes of increased cerebral venous pressure, both affect cerebral perfusion.
2. Extravascular — poor vascular support in the germinal matrix in premature infants.
3. Vascular — fragility of the germinal matrix vasculature.
4. Platelet and coagulation factors.

If preterm labour and delivery cannot be avoided, prevention of IVH involves avoiding prolonged labour, difficult or traumatic delivery, and birth asphyxia. It also involves careful neonatal care and handling postdelivery, to prevent hypothermia and respiratory distress, systemic hypo- or hypertension, with provision of appropriate ventilatory support (with early paralysis if necessary) to prevent episodes of hypoxia, hypo- or hypercapnia. The arterial partial pressure of carbon dioxide, Pa_{CO_2}, is normally a major regulator of intracranial vascular resistance and hence cerebral blood flow.

Jaundice. Comparatively low levels of unconjugated hyper-bilirubinaemia will produce kernicterus in the preterm baby with an increased risk of later athetoid cerebral palsy. Intervention with phototherapy and exchange transfusion is required at progressively lower levels of bilirubin with increasing immaturity.

Hypothermia. See 'Temperature control' above.

Fluid and electrolyte imbalance from immaturely functioning kidneys.

Feeding difficulties with functional intestinal obstruction and increased risk of necrotizing enterocolitis.

Apnoeas and bradycardias.

Persistent patent ductus arteriosus which may require surgical ligation.

Retinopathy of prematurity. This is a vasoproliferative retinopathy which may result in total retinal detachment and blindness. Excessive oxygen administration has been implicated in its pathogenesis.

39. Sexually transmitted infections in women

S. E. Barton

Expectations of the examiners

The candidate will be expected to understand the general principles of the diagnosis and management of sexually transmitted infections (STI). These include the following:

1. Appropriate history taking and clinical examination.
2. Where possible, the relevant tests that should be performed to obtain a microbiological diagnosis prior to commencing therapy.
3. The finding of one STI suggests that others may also have been acquired. As several conditions may be totally asymptomatic (e.g. cervical gonorrhoea or chlamydial infection, latent syphilis, vaginal condylomata acuminata), it is essential that both clinical examination and laboratory investigations screen for a wide range of infectious diseases.
4. The management of STI should include advice and education of the patient as well as contact tracing of partners. This will help to prevent reinfection after treatment, as well as reduce the reservoir of infection within the community. Often the presentation of a woman with a suspected STI will provide a valuable opportunity for her to receive advice about contraception.

It is essential that the candidate has a clear understanding of which clinical conditions can be managed by general practitioners, and which should be referred to departments of genitourinary medicine or gynaecology for specialist assessment and therapy.

Definition

A major problem with producing a satisfactory definition of a STI is that certain organisms produce an entirely local genital condition (e.g. trichomoniasis, genital warts), whereas others may cause severe systemic disease (e.g. secondary syphilis, AIDS). Moreover, not all STI are *always* transmitted by sexual contact (e.g. vertical transmission of congenital syphilis or HIV infection) and the question of whether to include conditions which are associated with sexual activity, but not necessarily transmitted, such as bacterial vaginosis, is a vexed one.

Interesting facts

Women with sexually transmitted infections can present with four manifestations:

1. Vaginal discharge
2. Pelvic inflammatory disease
3. Genital lesions (ulceration or condylomata)
4. Systemic infections.

Individual infectious agents can cause disease in more than one of these categories and most can also be asymptomatic.

This chapter will consider each of these broad clinical categories in turn, describing the common causes of each and their management.

VAGINAL DISCHARGE

Pathophysiology

The normal vaginal secretions of a premenopausal adult woman consist of desquamated vaginal epithelial cells, vaginal wall transudate, cervical mucus, a variable volume of fluid from the upper genital tract, and microorganisms (mainly Döderlein's lactobacilli). There is an individual and often cyclical variation in the amount of these secretions, as well as considerable variation in different women's perceptions of what constitutes a 'normal discharge'.

Aetiology

The causes of an alteration in vaginal discharge are summarized in Table 39.1. Several of these may coexist, for instance a woman who has recently commenced sexual activity may also have begun to take the pill, have vaginal candidiasis and tried douching with antiseptics to treat this. Such cases mean that accurate history taking, careful clinical examination and obtaining suitable specimens for laboratory tests are essential to make a correct diagnosis.

Non-infectious causes of alterations in vaginal discharge include the hormonal changes which occur at puberty and the menopause, as well as changes during the menstrual cycle. Retained foreign objects usually present with an offensive vaginal discharge, with the cause often being a piece of tampon. Chemical vaginitis usually occurs with the use of antiseptic douches, but also as a reaction to the use of perfumed or disinfectant bath additives. Non-infectious, gynaecological causes are less

Table 39.1   Aetiology of altered vaginal discharge.

Non-infectious
Physiological
   Puberty
   Menstrual cycle
   Sexual activity
   Pregnancy
   Menopause

Pathological
   Foreign body
   Chemical vaginitis
   Drug-related
   Gynaecological

Infectious
Vaginal
   Candida albicans
   Trichomonas vaginalis
   Bacterial vaginosis
   Others
      Human papillomavirus
      β haemolytic streptococcus

Cervical
   Neisseria gonorrhoeae
   Chlamydia trachomatis
   Herpes simplex virus

common and include genital tract neoplasms, and uterine prolapse and vaginal fistulae.

The commonest infectious cause of a symptomatic vaginal discharge is the yeast *Candida albicans*. More than 50 000 cases of vaginal candidiasis are treated in STI clinics annually in the UK and many more are self-treated or treated by GPs. In a small percentage of cases, other candidal species or *Candida glabrata* may be the yeast involved, but the clinical picture is similar. Another frequently identified cause is *Trichomonas vaginalis*, a flagellated protozoon, which accounts for 25% of cases of vaginal discharge in the USA.

In the considerable number of women who present with vaginal discharge, but have no evidence of either of these infections, a diagnosis of bacterial vaginosis is often made; however, a specific aetiological agent has not been identified for this condition (see below). Rarer causes of vaginal discharge include streptococcal infection or that associated with extensive vulvovaginal warts (although this is often due to secondary infection).

Infection of the columnar epithelium of the endocervix by *Neisseria gonorrhoeae* or *Chlamydia trachomatis* (serotypes D–K) can result in vaginal discharge alone, be complicated by pelvic pain and systemic symptoms, or be completely asymptomatic (see 'Pelvic inflammatory disease' below). Herpes simplex virus (HSV) infection may produce a vaginal discharge secondary to cervical lesions during a primary or recurrent episode; indeed, it is important to note that cervical and vaginal HSV lesions can occur in the absence of any externally visible, vulval lesions (see 'Genital lesions' below).

Assessment

Points in the history which may suggest particular infectious causes of an increased vaginal discharge include the following:

1. Pregnancy, diabetes mellitus, immunosuppression, recent antibiotic treatment, itchy vulval irritation or superficial dyspareunia suggest candidiasis.
2. New sexual partner, copious irritant discharge and malodour suggest trichomoniasis.
3. Presence of an IUD, malodorous vaginal discharge and dyspareunia suggest bacterial vaginosis. However, as no specific historical features are pathognomonic for any particular infection, clinical examination is essential.
4. Vulvovaginal erythema and oedema, vulval excoriation and the presence of curdy discharge with white/yellow plaques suggest candidiasis.
5. Excessive, often frothy yellow/green malodorous discharge suggests trichomoniasis.
6. Thin, adherent, homogenous, grey/white, offensive smelling discharge suggests bacterial vaginosis.

Despite these typical appearances, reliance on clinical diagnosis will often be misleading or miss the presence of multiple infections.

Investigations

A vaginal smear on a microscope slide can be Gram stained to demonstrate typical Gram-positive ovoid spores or tubular pseudohyphae of *Candida albicans*. Sabouraud's media can be inoculated to provide culture confirmation.

A drop of discharge on a slide, suspended in saline under a coverslip, can be examined as a wet mount preparation. This may reveal the presence of motile, flagellated trichomonads. Although this is a very reliable method of diagnosing trichomoniasis, this can be confirmed by using Whittington–Feinberg culture medium.

The diagnosis of bacterial vaginosis is based on the finding of typical 'clue cells' in a Gram-stained vaginal smear. These are characteristically granular epithelial cells, with coccobacillary organisms attached to their surface giving a 'salt and pepper appearance'. No microbiological test has been shown to be diagnostic of bacterial vaginosis and women without symptomatic bacterial vaginosis can have *Gardnerella*, *Mobiluncus* and anaerobes detected. In addition, the vaginal discharge will have a pH >5 and release a characteristic 'fishy' odour on mixing with 10% KOH. The pH of vaginal discharge is also raised in trichomoniasis, but is usually <4.5 in cases of candidal infection; this can be a quick and helpful guide to diagnosis. Ideally though, all women with vaginal discharge should have a full range of microbiological tests performed on vaginal and cervical samples (to exclude gonococcal and chlamydial infection).

Treatment

Vaginal candidiasis may be treated topically using an imidazole derivative, such as clotrimazole (500 mg × 1 or 200 mg × 3 nocte) or econazole (150 mg × 1 or × 3 nocte). These may be administered as vaginal creams or pessaries and will produce a cure in over 90% of cases. The availability of these treatments 'over the counter', without prescription, means that many women will have tried these remedies before they present to a doctor. In these cases, and in women with recurrent infection or a history of sensitivity to topical antifungals orally administered, '1-day' therapies such as 150 mg fluconazole stat, or 200 mg itraconazole b.d. for 1 day, are valuable options.

Metronidazole (400 mg b.d. for 5 days) is the treatment of choice for trichomoniasis. The same dose has proven efficacy against bacterial vaginosis; however, therapy utilizing 2% clindamycin gel intravaginally for 7 days has been shown to be of equivalent efficacy without the systemic side-effects of oral therapy. Unfortunately, relapses of bacterial vaginosis after treatment by either modality occur in a significant minority of women. The use of prophylactic therapy and the evaluation of potential benefits of vaginal applications such as Aci-jel are anecdotally reported as being helpful.

As *T. vaginalis* has been found to infect the male urethra and cause some cases of non-specific urethritis (NSU), it is important that the male partners of infected women are treated to prevent reinfection. However, there is less evidence to support such contact tracing for cases of candidiasis and bacterial vaginosis. This is only usually performed in cases of recurrent infection. Indeed, a further problem lies in the high prevalence of apparently asymptomatic women with laboratory evidence of these two conditions. Whilst further research is awaited on the local immune responses to candidal carriage and the role of *Gardnerella vaginalis* and anaerobes in bacterial vaginosis, most authorities do not advocate treating asymptomatic women.

All women with vaginal discharge should also be given simple advice on wearing looser cotton underwear, avoiding irritant soaps or bath additives and general health information.

Summary

Vaginal discharge is a common presenting complaint which merits a proper clinical assessment and accurate diagnosis to ensure the correct management.

PELVIC INFLAMMATORY DISEASE

Definition

Pelvic inflammatory disease (PID) is an infection of the endometrium, fallopian tubes and/or contiguous structures which is usually attributed to the ascent of microorganisms via the cervix and vagina.

Interesting facts

It is estimated that nearly 100 000 women in the UK develop PID each year. After one episode of infection, 12.8% of women will suffer from tubal infertility; after three episodes, this figure rises to 75%. In addition, chronic pelvic pain, dyspareunia, pelvic adhesions and an increased subsequent risk of ectopic pregnancy add to the morbidity associated with this condition.

Pathophysiology

It is unknown why only 10% of women with gonococcal or chlamydial cervical infection will develop PID. The barriers to the ascent of microorganisms include cervical mucus, which forms a mechanical barrier in the narrow endocervical canal, and contains lysozyme and immunoglobulins (especially IgA). Cyclical menstrual shedding of the endometrium may also contribute to preventing the establishment of uterine infection. In addition, the uterotubal junction as well as the downward flow of tubal mucus appear to act as further mechanical barriers to ascending infection.

Except in the few cases where infection is spread intra-abdominally (e.g. from an infected appendix), all of these barriers have to be passed by an ascending pathogen. This is often precipitated by trauma to the cervix and uterus as occurs in spontaneous and induced abortions, childbirth, or surgical procedures, especially the insertion of an IUD.

There is some evidence that spermatozoa and the motile protozoon, *Trichomonas vaginalis* may play a role in carrying *N. gonorrhoeae*, *C. trachomatis* or other microorganisms, into the upper genital tract. Once infected by one organism, the local damage to the fallopian tubes may result in an increased susceptibility to infection by other microorganisms, such as anaerobes and coliforms.

Aetiology

The question of whether PID is caused by a single or multiple infectious agents is unanswered. The current consensus view is that most commonly *N. gonorrhoeae* or *C. trachomatis* (types D–K) initiate an attack, but are often later replaced by opportunistic bacterial invaders, such as the anaerobic species *Peptococcus* and *Bacteroides*. The detection of *Mycoplasma hominis*, *Ureaplasma urealyticum* and even herpes simplex virus from the fallopian tubes of women with PID has implicated these agents as pathogens, but further evidence is awaited. Finally, it is important that pelvic tuberculosis is not forgotten as an occasional cause of PID. It rarely presents as an acute infection nowadays, but it is essential to exclude it as a cause of infertility and pelvic pain, especially in women from higher-risk groups.

Assessment

The spectrum of symptoms and signs present in cases of PID is very wide, and although bilateral low abdominal pain and an increased vaginal discharge are common presentations, no clinical picture is reliable. Because of this, gynaecologists will only make an accurate clinical diagnosis of PID in two-thirds of cases. This may be partly improved by using strict diagnostic criteria:

1. Abdominal tenderness, with or without rebound tenderness
2. Cervical motion tenderness ('excitation')
3. Adnexal tenderness.

All three must be present with at least one of the following:

1. Gram-negative intracellular diplococci seen on microscopy of endocervical secretions
2. Fever >38°C
3. Leucocytosis >10 000/mm^3
4. Purulent material in peritoneum on laparoscopy or culdocentesis
5. Pelvic abscess on clinical examination or ultrasound.

The inaccuracy in clinical diagnosis of PID, as well as the potentially fatal error of missing important differential conditions such as ectopic pregnancy, has led some authors to recommend that all women with pelvic pain should have a diagnostic laparoscopy performed. However, few centres have facilities for this and most will only perform laparoscopy on the most severe cases or those who do not respond to 48–72 hours of antibiotic therapy. Early laparoscopy allows the microbiological sampling of the peritoneum and tubal fimbriae, which may give a more accurate guide to the causative organisms than samples from the vagina or cervix.

Investigations

In all cases of suspected PID, endocervical swabs should be taken for culture of *N. gonorrhoea* and the detection of *C. trachomatis* (by culture, EIA or PCR tests). The addition of a urethral swab will increase the sensitivity of detecting *N. gonorrhoea*. High vaginal swabs are only useful for the detection of associated candidiasis, trichomoniasis or other vaginal infections. A full blood count and differential white cell count should be performed.

As part of the investigations to exclude other differential diagnoses in women with acute pelvic pain, a midstream specimen of urine for microscopy and culture, a pregnancy test and an ultrasound examination are often indicated.

Treatment

Bed rest and adequate analgesia are essential. Initial antibiotic therapy should be active against the range of pathogens commonly implicated in PID. As no single agent is suitable for this purpose, a combination of the following is suitable:

1. For *N. gonorrhoea*: oral ampicillin 3.5 g and probenecid 1 g stat or if high risk of penicillinase producing (PPNG) strains, use either spectinomycin 2 g i.m. stat or ciprofloxacin 250 mg orally stat.
2. For *C. trachomatis*: doxycycline 100 mg b.d. or erythromycin 500 mg q.d.s. for 14 days or a stat dose of azithromycin 1 g.
3. For anaerobes: metronidazole 400 mg t.d.s. for 7 days.

The most important component of outpatient therapy is the need for regular reassessment every 2–3 days to assess the clinical response to treatment.

In hospitalized patients, a broad spectrum agent such as gentamicin 80 mg i.v. 8-hourly is often added to a parenteral version of the above regimen. Women with severe cases of PID (i.e. febrile with generalized abdominal tenderness) need admission to hospital as well as those in whom the diagnosis is uncertain, those unable to tolerate oral therapy, those who do not respond to oral therapy, and those with suspected complications such as tubovarian abscesses.

In addition to treatment of the patient herself, it is essential that her recent sexual partners are examined and treated for evidence of STI. One study found that 68% of the partners of women with chlamydial PID had evidence of urethritis, as did 12% of partners of women without *Chlamydia* detected.

Summary

The clinical diagnosis of PID is often inaccurate, especially if a diagnostic laparoscopy is not performed. It is essential that endocervical specimens for

N. gonorrhoea and *C. trachomatis* are taken prior to commencing appropriate antibiotic therapy. By earlier and more accurate diagnosis, frequent clinical reassessment and contact tracing of sexual partners, the severe morbidity of PID may be reduced.

GENITAL LESIONS

GENITAL ULCERATION

Interesting facts

Genital (HSV) herpes simplex virus infection is the STI which has shown the greatest rise in incidence in the past decade. Most new infections are transmitted from an asymptomatic source partner. Genital ulceration is an important factor in the transmission of human immunodeficiency virus (HIV) infection.

Pathophysiology/aetiology (see Table 39.2)

Although recurrent genital HSV infection is often a mild and self-limiting condition, primary episodes may be severe and require hospital admission. Most genital infections are due to HSV type 2, but up to 20% of cases are caused by type 1, which usually infects the perioral area and can be tramitted during orogenital sexual contact. A primary attack occurs in patients with no previous exposure to type 1 or 2, who lack any neutralizing antibody. These are usually the cases with extensive genital lesions and severe systemic complications. In those who have previously acquired neutralizing antibody, commonly via a perioral HSV type 1 infection, the 'first episode' of genital infection is usually milder.

Table 39.2 Differential diagnosis of genital ulceration.

Non-infectious
    Physical or chemical trauma
    Erythema multiforme
    Stevens–Johnson syndrome
    Behçet's disease
    Lichen planus
    Crohn's disease
    Vulval malignancy

Infectious
    Herpes simplex virus
    1° or 2° syphilis
    Lymphogranuloma venereum
    Granuloma inguinale
    Varicella zoster
    Scabies/pediculosis pubis

The frequency and severity of recurrent HSV infections is worse in patients infected by HSV type 2 and in those patients with immunosuppression. However, the cause of the wide variation in rates of recurrences amongst otherwise healthy individuals is being increasingly attributed to psychoneuroimmunological factors.

Assessment

Careful history taking of any previous episodes, a typical prodrome of itching, dysuria, painful groins and legs and blistering prior to ulceration strongly suggest recurrent HSV infection. The use of new soaps or antiseptics, recent drug ingestion, previous dermatological problems and recent foreign travel as well as a full sexual history, are all also important.

Clinical examination must include thorough inspection of the lower genital tract and perianal region, as well as a general physical examination with a diligent search for lymphadenopathy or coexistent oropharyngeal lesions or other skin rashes.

In the UK, painful genital ulceration is usually herpetic in origin whereas painless ulcers are syphilitic: solitary ulceration suggests a 1° chancre and multiple ulcers 2° syphilis. However, as these infections can and do coexist, it is essential that tests for both are performed on women with genital ulceration.

Investigations

All new cases of genital ulcers should have samples taken for viral culture of HSV. If facilities exist, a specimen of serum expressed from the ulcer should be obtained and examined by dark ground microscopy to search for the live organisms of *Treponema pallidum*. Whether this is done or not, it is mandatory to obtain a venous blood sample for syphilis serology, which should be repeated 6 weeks later in cases of a suspected 1° chancre. The times of appearance of positive serological tests for syphilis are shown in Table 39.3.

The Venereal Disease Research Laboratory (VDRL) test is a non-specific test which is often used in conjunction with the TPHA in screening antenatal patients for syphilis. It can be complicated by a biological false-positive reaction following acute viral infections, typhoid or yellow fever immunizations and autoimmune conditions such as disseminated lupus erythematosus and rheumatoid arthritis. Thus it is essential that any positive test is repeated and combined with clinical examination before any

Table 39.3 Syphilis serology; time from exposure to positivity.

Fluorescent treponemal antibody test (FTA)	3–4 weeks
Venereal diseases research laboratory (VDRL) test	3–5 weeks
Treponema pallidum haemagglutination assay (TPHA)	8–10 weeks

treatment is commenced. In patients with a history of overseas travel or sexual contacts from the third world, it may be indicated to take cultures for *Haemophilus ducreyi*, a Gram-negative facultative anaerobe which causes chancroid and blood for serological diagnosis of *Lymphogranuloma venereum*, which is caused by *Chlamydia trachomatis* serotypes L_1, L_2, and L_3.

It is essential that a full screen for other STI is obtained from all patients who present with genital ulceration, which is usually best performed in departments of genitourinary medicine.

Treatment

Primary and first episode cases of genital HSV infection should be treated with a systemic antiviral therapy. No difference in efficacy, but a variety of oral dose frequencies are available, e.g. acyclovir 200 mg 5 × day, valaciclovir 500 mg b.d., and famciclovir 250 mg t.d.s. This will diminish the symptoms and new ulcer formation as well as reduce the risk of complications such as urinary retention occurring. This latter complication should be managed by analgesia, urinating into a warm bath, local anaesthesia and, only if all else fails, suprapubic catheterization. Counselling and advice are important to provide in these patients.

In recurrent HSV infection, most patients will be able to tolerate two to three annual episodes of slight genital discomfort with simple measures, such as saline bathing, wearing loose underwear and avoiding sexual contact until the lesions have healed. However, in cases where the attacks are very frequent (>one per month), severely painful or in those patients suffering extreme psychosexual problems because of their HSV recurrences, continuous prophylactic acyclovir (200 mg orally q.d.s. or 400 mg b.d.) may be prescribed as suppressive therapy. Despite its low toxicity, it is essential that women receiving acyclovir use adequate contraception, as it is not licensed for use in pregnancy.

HSV in pregnancy

The major risk of transmission of genital HSV to a neonate occurs in a mother having primary genital herpes. It is generally regarded that swabbing women for viral isolation if they report a past history of genital herpes is an ineffectual measure in preventing neonatal herpes. Interventional approaches are currently under evaluation — screening women for serology (type specific) and then testing the sexual partners for HSV antibodies (i.e. identifying the highest risk couple for neonatal transmission) or in women with a recent history of acquiring genital herpes recommending women to be delivered by caesarean section or taking acyclovir in the third trimester.

Syphilis should be treated by aqueous procaine penicillin 600 000 units/ day, intramuscularly, for 15–20 days, or in patients allergic to penicillin, by a 30-day course of erythromycin or oxytetracycline (500 mg q.d.s. orally). Patients with primary and secondary syphilis should be warned of the Jarisch–Herxheimer reaction, a self-limiting febrile illness (thought to be related to the release of treponemal toxins and immune complex formation) which may be lessened by oral aspirin therapy. However, as more serious complications of therapy can occur in patients with later stages of cardiovascular or neurosyphilis, such cases should only be treated as inpatients under medical supervision.

Although contact tracing is desirable in new cases of genital HSV infection, for syphilis this is mandatory and patients should be referred to the health adviser at the local genitourinary medicine clinic to facilitate this, as well as the appropriate serological follow-up of the index patient.

Summary

Genital ulceration is an increasingly common problem in the UK. The range of disease extends from microscopic, solitary painless ulcers to multiple, severely painful systemic disease. Whatever the presentation, the correct diagnosis will only be obtained by careful clinical investigation and appropriate follow-up. Much of the morbidity of genital herpes relates to psychosexual problems which need to be addressed by the suitability of clear information and supportive counselling.

GENITAL WARTS

Pathophysiology/aetiology

Genital warts are caused by human papillomavirus (HPV). The lesions produced range from large exophytic warts (often types 6 and 11) to flat subclinical lesions (often types 16 and 18) which are only visible on colposcopic examination. All epithelia in the lower genital tract may be infected by HPV, often by multiple types. HPV types 16 and 18 infection of the cervical epithelium has been strongly implicated in the aetiology of cervical neoplasia. A less convincing association has also been proposed between vaginal and vulval HPV infection and premalignant conditions at these sites (VAIN (vaginal intraepithelial neoplasia) and VIN). In view of the association of HPV with CIN, it has been recommended that women with a history of genital warts should have more frequent cervical cytology performed (i.e. annually); however, evidence suggests that the prevalence of CIN in women with a history of warts is no different to that found in women with any other STI.

The main differential diagnoses of genital warts are from molluscum contagiosum, caused by a pox virus, and condylomata lata, the classical lesions of secondary syphilis. Occasionally benign skin tags, sebaceous cysts or pigmented naevi can also confuse the diagnosis.

Assessment

A history of slow growing, painless, vulvovaginal lumps is highly suggestive of genital warts. This is one of the few STI to be diagnosed solely from their clinical appearance. However, a third of women who present with genital warts will have another STI present on more detailed investigation.

The lesions of molluscum contagiosum are also characteristic, being pearly white, umbilicated papules which may also be found on other parts of the body; they are transmitted by close, but not always sexual, contact.

Condylomata lata are coalescent, large fleshy masses of the papular lesions of 2° syphilis found in moist body areas. Other signs of 2° syphilis are usually present.

Investigations

A thorough examination of the lower genital tract, using a colposcope if available, is necessary to document the distribution of HPV infection present. A cervical cytology smear and a full screen for other STI should be performed.

In cases of 2° syphilis, dark ground examination of a smear from the condylomata lata will reveal spirochaetes and serological tests will be positive.

Treatment

External genital warts can be treated by chemical (25% podophyllin or trichloroacetic acid, washed off after 4 hours) or physical destruction (cryocautery, diathermy, laser). Internal warts should only be treated by physical methods due to the increased risk of side-effects with chemical agents, such as local ulceration and systemic absorption of podophyllin causing peripheral neuropathy and hypokalaemia. Moreover, podophyllin must be avoided in pregnancy due to the high risk of teratogenicity.

All methods have shown initial cure rates of between 70 and 90%, but whatever method is used, the long-term recurrence rates approach 50%. One of the reasons for treatment failure and early recurrence has been identified as poor compliance with therapy. In particular, the need for patients to reattend clinics for applications of chemicals such as podophyllin and trichloroacetic acid can often impose great strains on the patient's ability to take time off work. Recently, podophyllotoxin (warticon condyline, warticon-fem) has been licensed for self-treatment of external genital warts. For patients who are able to clearly understand and follow instructions for twice daily applications of podophyllotoxin to their clearly visible external genital lesions, this form of treatment may provide a way of ensuring greater compliance with repeated applications of chemical therapy. Less successful innovations in therapy which have been evaluated include immunostimulants (e.g. isoprinosine or α-interferon) which have been tried both alone and as adjuvants to local therapy. Used as sole treatment, immunostimulants seem to have very low efficacy while as adjuvants to physical destructive therapy in patients with recalcitrant condylomata acuminata, especially if this is secondary to systemic immunosuppression, there seems to be a place for this therapy under specialist supervision.

The value of contact tracing the male partners of women with genital warts serves to screen them for HPV and other STI. The value of condom use by the male partner during, and for some time after, treatment has been suggested, but there is little evidence for this.

Molluscum contagiosum is treated by either applying neat phenol on a wooden stick into the centre of each lesion, or by using cryotherapy or electrocautery.

Summary

Genital warts often serve as a marker for other STI. As no systemic anti-HPV agent exists, the treatment is local. Long-term cure rates are often poor. Genital HPV infection, like other STI, acts as a risk factor for the development of cervical neoplasia; hence regular cervical cytological sampling of all women with warts, or any other STI, must be recommended.

INFESTATIONS

Unless there is a high level of clinical awareness and a good light in the examination room, the detection of the ectoparasites which cause pediculosis pubis or scabies will be missed. In the former, *Phthirus pubis* ('crabs') themselves, or their eggs ('nits') are visibly attached to the base of pubic hairs and in the latter, if the typical burrows of the scabies mite are lifted with a needle and the contents placed in 10% KOH on a slide, *Sarcoptes scabiei* may be visualized on microscopy.

Scabies and pediculosis pubis should be treated by 25% benzyl benzoate or 1% γ-benzene hexachloride applications from the neck downwards. Sexual partners and close family contacts should be seen and also treated.

ASYMPTOMATIC/SYSTEMIC INFECTIONS

Aetiology

The three most important systemic infections which may be sexually transmitted are syphilis, hepatitis B, and HIV infection. All of these have asymptomatic phases in their natural history, all may be transmitted vertically by a pregnant woman, and all may be fatal.

Currently, despite large and continuing research efforts, only one vaccination effective to protect against a sexually transmitted systemic infection exists — hepatitis B. Recently, sexual transmission of infectious agents such as hepatitis C and human T-lymphotrophic virus-1 (HTLV1) have been described. Increased serological testing for these latter agents, accompanied by an increased awareness of their natural history, are currently being evaluated in different settings.

Assessment

Although each of these infections does produce well-described clinical syndromes, the initial infection and subsequent carriage may be completely asymptomatic. Thus, the diagnosis of these infections will often be missed unless serological screening is performed in patients presenting with another STI. It is important that the patient understands the nature of any screening test performed and is counselled before the result is known.

Investigations

Hepatitis B may only be diagnosed by serology. Within 4–12 weeks of infection, hepatitis B surface (HBsAg) and e antigens (HBeAg) appear in the serum. HBsAg is usually cleared by 4 months from the onset of the infection and this usually precedes the appearance of HBsAb, the antibody which confers long-term immunity. During this serological window, Hep B core antibody may be the only positive indication of infection. HBeAg is usually cleared rapidly unless a chronic carrier state develops. Liver enzymes must be checked at regular intervals, but no pattern is pathognomonic of hepatitis B virus infection.

Seroconversion for anti-HIV typically occurs 4–12 weeks after acute infection, although longer delays have been described. The earlier detection by HIV p24 antigen or PCR testing can be useful following a specific case (e.g. following a rape, a needlestick injury, or during pregnancy). All positive tests should be repeated, along with a full screen for other STI, a full blood count and CD4 lymphocyte count.

Treatment

Acute viral hepatitis B is usually self-limiting and management is usually supportive. Advice on a low fat, high energy diet, the avoidance of alcohol and bed rest is given and the patient's liver enzymes regularly checked until normal. In chronic hepatitis, advances in antiviral therapy continue to show a role for interferon and possibly specific antivirals. The contacts of patients who are infectious for hepatitis B should be seen and tested;

immunization should be offered to the non-immune. Vaccination against hepatitis B infection should be offered to all non-immune patients in higher-risk groups (e.g. female sex workers, those who travel to higher endemicity areas) and is essential for all medical, nursing and laboratory staff who come into contact with patients or their blood.

The management of symptomatic women with HIV infection is based on antiretroviral therapy using combinations of nucleoside and non-nucleoside analogues. In addition, where HIV-induced immunosuppression exists, prophylaxis against opportunistic infections (such as *Pneumocystis carinii* pneumonia) is recommended.

SYSTEMIC STI AND PREGNANCY

For many years, women attending antenatal clinics have been screened for syphilis and often hepatitis B infection, on serum samples obtained at their booking visit. In many units HIV antibody testing is offered as well. However, it is generally accepted that this must be accompanied by a clear informative pretest consultation. Several studies have demonstrated that decisions to proceed with a pregnancy amongst women identified as being HIV seropositive is seldom influenced by their knowledge of HIV infection. However, the data indicating that the use of AZT as antiviral by a pregnant woman and early treatment of her neonate diminishes the risk of vertical transmission, may influence more women to wish to know their HIV serological status.

Ideally, the time to diagnose asymptomatic infections, which may be transmitted vertically, is prior to the pregnancy, as part of comprehensive preconceptual care. This service is increasingly being offered, particularly in relation to HIV infection, by the developments and improvements in facilities of sexual health clinics, and an increase in the sites available where women may be tested for HIV and other infections.

Syphilis

Vertical transmission via the placenta is almost inevitable if the mother is suffering from secondary syphilis and is likely if she has a primary chancre, but becomes more unlikely with increasing duration of latent disease. In 30% of women with untreated early syphilis, the pregnancy will end in a second trimester spontaneous abortion or stillbirth. If a live infant results, it may rarely be born showing signs of early congenital syphilis, or more usually be born well, developing signs within the first few weeks, months or even years of life. With successive pregnancies, the outcome tends to improve.

Adequate treatment of maternal syphilis prior to a pregnancy will prevent any transmission to the fetus or infant. It should be remembered that infection of the mother may also occur during pregnancy and therefore screening at 14–16 weeks' gestation will not prevent all cases of congenital infection. Furthermore, if reinfection is considered a possibility during a pregnancy, then retreatment is essential.

Hepatitis B

Infection of a pregnant woman carries a maternal mortality risk of 1.8% and a 2% increase in preterm delivery, although there is no specific association with congenital abnormalities. These figures relate to Europe and North America, but in India and the Far East, fulminant hepatitis is more common with a reported maternal mortality of 72% for cases of third trimester infection. The reason for this geographical variation is thought to include ethnic differences in host immunity. There is also a geographical difference in the risk of vertical transmission by a mother who is a chronic carrier of hepatitis B surface antigen (HBsAg) throughout her pregnancy. This varies from a 7% risk of vertical transmission in Greece, compared to 73% in Japan. These differences seem to be directly related to the titre of HBsAg and also the presence of e antigen in maternal serum.

For infections acquired during pregnancy, the risk of vertical transmission to the fetus is determined by the gestational age at the time of maternal infection. A third trimester infection carries a 66% risk of transmission, compared to less than 10% if the virus is acquired earlier.

There is no evidence that any therapy given during pregnancy alters the risk of transmission or the maternal or perinatal morbidity. However, to prevent the risk of neonatal transmission, infants born of HBsAg-positive mothers should receive hepatitis B immunoglobulin and a dose of hepatitis B vaccine, at separate sites, within a few hours of birth.

HIV infection

Early reports that pregnancy in an HIV-infected woman resulted in an increased rate of progression to AIDS have not been substantiated. The immunological changes seen in uninfected women seem to be replicated (with postnatal recovery) in HIV-infected women, but at a lower absolute level.

Pregnancy outcome does not appear to be affected by HIV infection when compared to that of comparable HIV seronegative women from similar social groups (e.g. intravenous drug users in poor housing conditions).

Vertical transmission appears to occur in 15% of infants delivered to HIV-infected women in developed countries. Reports of transmission rates as high as 40% continue to be described from developing countries, particularly in sub Saharan Africa. Such differences highlight that there may be very different rates of transmission at different stages of an individual woman's disease. It appears that the risk of transmission is highest during periods of significant HIV viraemia, which is predominantly during and just after the seroconversion illness and then maximal in patients with significant immunosuppression leading to AIDS.

In reducing vertical transmission, antenatal AZT therapy, caesarean section and the avoidance of breast-feeding all have been shown to have a significant impact. Further studies are essential to examine the combined effects of these interventions in both developed and developing countries.

SUMMARY

The historical importance of syphilis as 'the great imitator' of other conditions is being superseded by the vast range of symptoms and signs associated with HIV infection. Currently 800 cases of HIV infection in the UK have occurred in women and this proportion is increasing. The majority of these women are intravenous drug users, but one-third of cases have been infected by heterosexual contact. With increasing numbers of women with HIV infection, the importance of a high level of clinical awareness and surveillance for this condition is essential.

40. Family planning

C. Watson

Expectations of the examiners

The candidate will be expected to have the following theoretical knowledge:

1. The factors influencing motivation for contraception and emotional/psychological factors related to fertility control.
2. The acceptability, effectiveness and safety of all available methods of contraception (including sterilization) with their advantages/disadvantages and risks/benefits.
3. How to provide counselling/advice to the couple choosing any contraceptive method and how to manage associated complications (including resuscitation if required at IUD insertion).
4. The organization of family planning services.

MOTIVATION FOR CONTRACEPTION

The following factors are known to be influential in determining whether an individual or a couple will seek contraception:

1. The personal/cultural ideal family size
2. The sex of the existing children in the family
3. Religious beliefs
4. Socioeconomic conditions
5. Expected dependency or assistance from children
6. Opportunities and education for women
7. The stage in family building
8. Age and marital status
9. The stability of the male/female relationship
10. The perceived risk of pregnancy
11. The availability of information about contraceptive services
12. Expectations about the confidentiality of services.

ACCEPTABILITY OF CONTRACEPTIVE METHODS

Even when a couple are motivated to use contraception, they may find their choice of method difficult and may finally opt for a method which is seen simply as the least of several evils. They will be influenced by the following factors:

1. Effectiveness of the method
2. Perceived safety of the method
3. Whether the method is used by the man or the woman
4. Convenience and simplicity in use
5. Whether action is required at the time of coitus
6. Freedom from forethought
7. Whether the method is well known or novel
8. Whether or not the method has religious approval
9. Availability of the method.

CONTRACEPTIVE CHOICE

In order to cater for as many needs and preferences as possible, it is important that couples are free to choose their source of advice and their method of contraception. Confidentiality may be of particular importance to some groups, e.g. young people. The role of the professional is to give information and after history/examination to advise the individual/couple of any factors which might influence the effectiveness or safety of the method(s) they may be contemplating. The final choice should be with the individual/couple, and is likely to be most successful when the couple are in agreement.

Commonly, a couple will opt to use more than one method during their reproductive life, changing their method to suit changing circumstances, e.g.:

1. First using the combined pill to delay onset of childbearing
2. Then using an IUD to space their children
3. Finally using sterilization when the family is complete.

EFFECTIVENESS

Definitions

Theoretical effectiveness is defined as what might be achieved under ideal circumstances but in practice is never achieved.

User-effectiveness is defined as that actually achieved in practice

Method-failure is defined as failure inherent to the method itself

User-failure is defined as failure due to using a method inadequately or not at all.

Some methods of contraception are particularly vulnerable to 'user-failure', e.g. oral contraceptives and condoms, while others are almost entirely vulnerable to 'method-failure', e.g. IUDs and sterilization.

Measurements of effectiveness

Pearl index

This method takes into account the length of time the woman has been exposed to the risk of pregnancy. It is expressed in terms of a rate per 100 woman-years (HWY) and is calculated as follows:

$$\text{Failure rate per HWY} = \frac{\text{Total no. of pregnancies} \times 1200}{\text{Total months of use for all those using method}}$$

Life-table analysis

This method takes into account the changing probability of pregnancy over a period of time and is therefore more accurate. Calculations are expressed in terms of a rate per 100 women after 'n' months or years of use.

The effectiveness of any method varies in practice with differences due to personal, social and cultural factors in the user, the provider, and the user–provider relationship. When user-failure is important, failure rates are highest in couples who are young or inexperienced. Fertility diminishes with age, particularly sharply in women after the age of 35 with a consequent lowering of failure rates.

For the purposes of counselling patients, methods may be usefully classified into three groups according to the 'best results that can be obtained in practice'. However, note that oral contraceptives, barrier methods and 'natural methods' have a much wider range of failure when used incorrectly or inconsistently.

1. Very highly effective (failures less than 1 per HWY)
    a. Sterilization (male or female)
    b. Combined oestrogen/progestogen pills (COC)
    c. Depot progestogen injections
    d. Subdermal contraceptive implants
    e. Intrauterine devices (high-dose copper)
    f. Intrauterine systems (high-dose progestogen)
2. Highly effective (failures 2–3 per HWY)
    a. Progestogen-only pills (POP)
    b. Diaphragm/cap with spermicide
    c. Male condom with spermicide
    d. Periodic abstinence (symptothermal method)
    e. Lactational amenorrhoea method
3. Moderately effective (failures may exceed 10 per HWY)
    a. Spermicide alone
    b. Periodic abstinence (calendar method)
    c. Coitus interruptus
    d. Home-made barriers and spermicides.

Further research is required on the effectiveness of the female condom, used with or without a spermicide, before it can be confidently assigned to the above classification.

SAFETY

Contraceptive safety should be assessed in comparison with the morbidity and mortality associated with pregnancy. Evaluations of absolute risk are dependent upon personal medical history (including age and smoking status), but also on the availability of high quality maternity services and safe, legal abortion. Where maternal mortality and morbidity are high, e.g. Latin America and Africa, the relative safety of contraceptive methods is very great. In developed countries where maternal mortality and morbidity rates are substantially lower, the risks of contraceptive use assume a relatively greater importance, but when the additional non-contraceptive health benefits of birth control methods are taken into account, most contraceptive practices will still yield a positive health benefit for most women. The careful selection of methods for women who may have particular risk factors can further improve the safety of fertility control and underlines the importance of having access to a full range of contraceptive methods. The simultaneous use of more than one contraceptive method may also benefit health, e.g. the use of male or female condoms as an additional protection may substantially reduce the risk of sexually transmitted infections including the human immunodeficiency virus.

STERILIZATION

Popularity

The General Household Survey (1993) revealed that in Great Britain 24% of women aged 16–49 relied on sterilization for contraception. Twelve per cent had been sterilized while 12% relied on sterilization of the male partner.

Methods

Bilateral vasectomy in the male and tubal procedures performed at laparoscopy or minilaparotomy in the female are the preferred methods. Clips or rings are now used in preference to diathermy for female sterilization. Interval sterilization has a better prognosis than sterilization carried out in association with pregnancy.

Advantages

1. Very highly effective
2. Needs no continuing motivation

3. One-time procedure with no ongoing costs
4. Safe: side-effects and health hazards are rare.

Disadvantages

1. Regret is possible. Reversal is expensive and cannot be guaranteed.
2. Needs surgeon/special equipment, i.e. relatively large capital outlay which tends to restrict availability.

Importance of counselling the couple

From the medicolegal point of view it is important to stress both the irreversibility of the procedure and the very small failure rate. Alternative contraception should be discussed as well as the implications of the male and female sterilization options (Table 40.1). Suggestions that tubal procedures in the woman predispose to later menorrhagia have not been substantiated. Recent suggestions that vasectomy has a causal relationship with an increased risk of prostatic and testicular cancers or renal calculi remain unproven and do not currently justify avoidance of the operation.

Table 40.1 Implications of the male and female sterilization options.

	Male	Female
Immediacy	Not immediately effective	Immediately effective
Failure	Less than 0.5% in first year	Less than 0.5% in first year
Mortality	1 in 100 000 (mostly under LA)	1 in 10 000 (mostly under GA)
Morbidity		
Early	Below 5% (bleeding, infection)	Below 5% (bleeding, infection, trauma)
Late	Sperm granuloma	Ectopic pregnancy
Reversibility	Chances dependent on extent of original procedure	
Availability	Marked regional/district variations	

HORMONAL CONTRACEPTION

Mechanism of action

The sex steroids (oestrogens and progestogens) used in available hormonal contraceptive preparations have the following actions:

1. Hypothalamus and pituitary inhibition of GnRH, FSH and LH via 'feedback' system.
2. Ovary — consequent inhibition of follicular activity, ovulation and luteal function.
3. Endometrium—inadequate secretory phase prejudices implantation.
4. Cervical mucus—progestogens render it resistant to sperm penetration.
5. Fallopian tubes—impaired function interferes with sperm/ovum transport.

Note: These actions are dose dependent and vary from one woman to another.

COMBINED OESTROGEN-PROGESTOGEN PILLS (COC)

Popularity

Currently used by over 60 million women worldwide, this method is also the most popular reversible method of contraception in Great Britain. Since first marketed in the early 1960s, the dose of oestrogen and then the dose of progestogen has been greatly reduced together with a trend since the early 1980s to introduce newer progestogens which have been claimed to produce more beneficial lipid profiles. This development received a setback in 1995 when several published studies reported evidence of an increased risk of venous thromboembolism associated with desogestrel and gestodene containing low-dose combined oral contraceptives when compared with levonorgestrel- and norethisterone-containing counterparts.

Advantages

1. Contraceptive benefits
   a. Very highly effective
   b. Convenient—no action required at time of coitus
   c. Reversible—do not cause subsequent infertility.
2. Non-contraceptive benefits
   a. Improvements in the menstrual cycle:
      i. Reduced blood loss and less iron deficiency anaemia
      ii. Reduced dysmenorrhoea
      iii. Reduced premenstrual problems
      iv. Prevention of 'mittelschmerz' (ovulation pain/bleeding)
      v. Increased regularity of bleeding (withdrawal bleeds)
      vi. Ability to manipulate the cycle, e.g. tri-cycle regime
   b. Reduction in gynaecological disease and need for surgery
      i. Reduction in benign breast tumours
      ii. Reduction in functional ovarian cysts, and probably fibroids and endometriosis
      iii. Reduction in pelvic inflammatory disease, therefore
      iv. Reduction in tubal infertility and ectopic pregnancy
      v. Reduction in ovarian and endometrial cancers (both duration of use and ex-use effects)
   c. Other possible or minor benefits
      i. Reduction in seborrhoeic conditions
      ii. Reduction in thyroid disease, peptic ulcer and rheumatoid arthritis.

Disadvantages

1. Requires continuous motivation to take the pill correctly.
2. Requires medical supervision.
3. Not immediately effective unless started on the first day of the cycle.
4. Minor side-effects may be experienced, especially in the early months of use, e.g. nausea, breast discomfort, weight gain, headache, (unusual with modern low-dose pills) or 'break-through bleeding'.
5. For a minority of women there may be serious health hazards and so screening for contraindications by a thorough history and appropriate examination and investigation should be understood before prescribing.

Cardiovascular disease

An observed increase in venous thromboembolic disease in current users has been attributed to oestrogen-induced changes in clotting factors, but it now seems likely that progestogens may also modify this effect.

An observed increase in arterial disease (ischaemic heart disease and cerebrovascular disease) in current users has been attributed to oestrogen-induced changes in clotting factors plus progestogen-induced changes in serum lipids (mainly HDL reduction). Recent epidemiological studies have confirmed that the absolute risk of myocardial infarction in women taking low-dose combined oral contraceptives is extremely small but significantly increased in smokers of cigarettes. The estimated excess risk of all types of stroke attributable to low-dose oral contraceptive use is also extremely low but greater for ischaemic than for haemorrhagic stroke. Smoking and hypertension increase these risks significantly and several studies point to a further association with migraine. Both arterial and venous clotting do not appear to be influenced by duration of use and there is no ex-use effect after the pill is discontinued.

Mean blood pressure rises slightly in COC users but remains within normal limits for most women. Asymptomatic, progressive, and reversible hypertension develops occasionally, necessitating cessation of pill-taking. Epidemiological studies have demonstrated some lowering of risks with lower dose pills and excess mortality and morbidity from arterial disease appears to be confined almost completely to women over the age of 35 who smoke.

Neoplasia

Carcinoma of the breast. Recent reanalysis of numerous studies suggests that women who are current users of combined oral contraceptives or who have used them in the past 10 years, are at a slightly increased risk of having breast carcinoma diagnosed, although the additional cancers diagnosed tend to be localized to the breast. There is no evidence of an increase in the risk of having breast cancer diagnosed 10 or more years after cessation of use, and the cancers diagnosed then are still less advanced clinically than the cancers diagnosed in never-users. There is no evidence at present that COC use increases mortality from breast cancers and the excess risk of diagnosis is very slight compared with the effect of other factors, e.g. positive family history.

Carcinoma of the cervix. There is some evidence of an association between COC use and an increased risk of CIN/invasive cancer with a duration-of-use effect. This has not been confirmed by all studies and confounding factors such as sexual behaviour need to be taken into account. A causal relationship is not yet reliably established.

Liver tumours. Benign and malignant tumours may be increased by long-term use of high-dose pills but are extremely rare in British women.

Contraindications to COC use

Absolute (but some not permanent)

1. Hormone-dependent tumours — breast, endometrial, trophoblastic.
2. Cardiovascular disease
   a. Venous — thromboembolism or thrombophlebitis
   b. Arterial ischaemic heart disease, cerebrovascular disease, peripheral vascular disease, Raynaud's disease, transient ischaemic attacks
   c. Valvular heart disease with risk of embolization or pulmonary hypertension
   d. Migraine which commences during COC therapy or is associated with aura
   e. Conditions predisposing to clotting, e.g. thrombophilias, immobility, elective major surgery and during treatment of varicose veins (sclerosant therapy or surgery).
3. Impaired liver or renal function including active hepatitis, cholestatic jaundice of pregnancy, certain rare inherited disorders, e.g. Dubin–Johnson and Rotor syndromes, hepatic tumours.
4. Serious conditions known to have been made worse by previous pregnancy or sex steroids, e.g. herpes gestationis, otosclerosis, chorea, porphyria, haemolytic-uraemic syndrome.

Relative (more than one in combination may be a very strong contraindication)

1. Age over 35 years
2. Current smoker
3. Hypertension
4. Hyperlipidaemia
5. Diabetes
6. Obesity
7. Family history of premature cardiovascular disease

8. Lactation
9. Puerperal psychosis/severe mood disorder
10. Homozygous sickle cell disease (not the trait)
11. Some diseases may be made worse by the COC, e.g. inflammatory bowel disease
12. Oligomenorrhoea/amenorrhoea should be investigated before prescribing the COC. Specialist advice may be required depending on the outcome.

Prescribing principles

Choose

1. Low oestrogen dose (20–35 µg ethinyloestradiol)
2. Low progestogen dose: e.g. 500 µg norethisterone or 150 µg levonorgestrel
3. Avoid pro-drugs (only pharmacologically active as metabolites)
4. Monophasic regimen which is simple for the patient
5. Low cost preparation.

Note: Newer progestogens (desogestrel, gestodene and norgestimate) have been developed to reduce the depressant effect on HDL cholesterol. Claims for the superiority of these more expensive preparations can only be substantiated by long-term epidemiological studies or randomized controlled trials, and at present must remain speculative. Women who wish to use desogestrel or gestodene containing combined pills (e.g. when the concomitant increase in sex hormone binding globulin may improve a tendency to acne) should be appraised of the possibly increased risk of thromboembolism, compared with other preparations.

Practical prescribing

1. The lowest dose monophasic preparation should be prescribed first and the patient warned to expect spotting or break-through bleeding for up to the fourth month of use. If cycle control is not attained by then, the dose of progestogen may be increased. (An increase in oestrogen is not usually practicable or desirable but some women may be helped by a triphasic preparation.)
2. The simplest regimen is to advise the patient to take her first ever pill on the first day of menstrual bleeding and to continue with 21 consecutive pills (one per day) followed by a 7-day break. The COC is then immediately effective, and a regular 28-day 'cycle' is the norm. The COC may be commenced immediately after therapeutic abortion or 3 weeks after childbirth.
3. Contraceptive efficacy may be lost if pills are forgotten (more than 12 hours late), malabsorbed, or subjected to drug interaction. An alternative contraceptive method should be advised during the lapse

and for 7 days after reinstitution of effective COC use, but when an enzyme inducing drug is used, contraceptive efficacy may not be regained until 8 weeks after cessation of therapy. If the 7 days extends into the 'pill-free' week, two packs of 21 pills should be taken consecutively without a break.

4. The most important drug interactions which may affect contraceptive efficacy are:
    a. Broad-spectrum antibiotics which may impair oestrogen reabsorption in the enterohepatic circulation (affects oestrogen only)
    b. Enzyme-inducing drugs (rifampicin, griseofulvin, some anticonvulsants) which interfere with oestrogen and progestogen metabolism in the liver (affects COC and progestogen-only methods). Patients wishing to use the COC and enzyme-inducers should be prescribed a COC with a high dose of oestrogen (50 µg) and progestogen.
5. COCs should be stopped 6 weeks in advance of elective major surgery if possible to allow clotting factors to normalize.
6. All patients need careful teaching about how to take the COC and careful counselling about what to expect. This information should also be given in writing. Free Contraceptive Education Service leaflets are available for this purpose.

PROGESTOGEN-ONLY PILLS (POP)

Mechanisms of action

Their effects on ovulation, the endometrium and tubal function are variable, hence there is difficulty in predicting menstrual patterns. They may be more effective if taken regularly about 4–6 hours before the likely time of intercourse to maximize the effect on cervical mucus when it is needed.

Advantages

1. No significant metabolic effects and they can therefore be used in lactating mothers, older women, diabetics, etc.
2. Can be used when oestrogens are contraindicated.
3. The continuous daily regimen may be simpler for patients to remember.

Disadvantages

1. As for disadvantages 1 to 3 of combined oestrogen/progestogen pills.
2. Less effective than COCs. The failure rate is age-related (0–4%).
3. Possible menstrual irregularity (spotting, short cycles or amenorrhoea) which may prove unacceptable to the patient.

4. Probably offer less protection against ectopic pregnancy than COCs.
5. Increased risk of developing functional ovarian cysts due to partial suppression of follicular development may cause diagnostic confusion with suspected ectopic pregnancy.

Contraindications to POP use

1. Hormone-dependent tumours (unless agreed with oncologist)
2. A past history of ectopic pregnancy is a relative contraindication, as methods which consistently prevent ovulation offer more protection against a recurrence.

Prescribing principles

There is no convincing evidence that any preparation is superior to another, therefore the cheapest should be prescribed.

Practical prescribing

1. Start the first pill on the first day of menstrual bleeding and continue with one pill daily at the same time of day. After pregnancy the POP may be started immediately (regardless of gestation) but bleeding patterns may be more acceptable if taking the first pill is postponed until 3 weeks postpartum.
2. Contraceptive efficacy may be lost if pills are forgotten (more than 3 hours late), malabsorbed or subjected to drug interaction from enzyme inducing drugs which may have an effect for up to 8 weeks from discontinuation. An alternative contraceptive method should be advised during the period at risk and for 7 days thereafter.
3. Instruction and counselling of the patient should be reinforced by written information (CES leaflets).

DEPOT PROGESTOGEN INJECTIONS

Mechanisms of action

The dose of progestogen is sufficiently large to inhibit ovulation fairly consistently. The endometrium tends to become atrophic with no secretory activity, and cervical mucus thickens.

Advantages

1. Very highly effective, and immediately if given in first 5 days of the cycle.

2. No user-failure between injections. Convenient, requiring no continuous motivation or action at time of coitus.
3. Safe—no mortality reported.
4. Reversible—does not cause permanent infertility.
5. Private—can be used unknown to uncooperative male partner.
6. Lactation not suppressed—may be enhanced.
7. Can be used when oestrogens contraindicated.
8. Erythropoiesis stimulated. Reduces crises in homozygous sickle cell disease.
9. Probable reduction in menstrual disorders as for COC (with exception of irregular bleeding but amenorrhoea usually supervenes with continuing use).
10. Protection from endometrial cancer.

Disadvantages

1. Cannot 'stop' in an emergency.
2. Some women dislike injections.
3. Requires medical supervision.
4. May be some delay in return of fertility after use (up to 2 years but usually about 6 months).
5. Bleeding irregularities may be unacceptable to the patient.
6. Weight gain affects some patients.
7. Measurable metabolic effects on glucose tolerance (reduced) and HDL-cholesterol (reduced) but significance unknown.
8. Theoretical risk of fetal masculinization if in pregnancy but unlikely in the dose used.

Contraindications

1. Pregnancy present or desired in near future.
2. Anxiety about possible menstrual disturbance.
3. Best avoided in early postpartum period (increases risk of heavy bleeding) and in breast-feeding mothers of premature infants (as excreted in small quantities in breast milk).
4. Acute or chronic liver disease (as for the COC).
5. Porphyria.
6. In view of the metabolic effects, caution should be exercised before use in women with impaired glucose tolerance or cardiovascular disease or risk.

Practical prescribing

Depo-Provera (DMPA-medroxyprogesterone acetate) and Noristerat (NET OEN norethisterone oenanthate) are both marketed in the UK and may be offered to patients after information and counselling. Manufacturer's information leaflets and audiotapes are available for Depo-Provera in English and a number of ethnic minority languages. Noristerat has a product licence for short-term use as a contraceptive, but doctors may assume responsibility for long-term prescribing. The usual doses are Depo-Provera 150 mg 12-weekly or Noristerat 200 mg 8-weekly. Both should be given by deep intramuscular injection into the gluteal muscle. In obese patients the deltoid may be a preferable site, to avoid subcutaneous injection.

Patients should be screened initially and at follow-up as for the COC and POP (BP, weight, breast and pelvic examination plus cervical smear). Excessive bleeding (defined as more than 7 days out of 21) should be actively managed after excluding other causes of bleeding. Unfortunately the efficacy of regimens of 'add back oestrogen' or shortening the intervals between injections have not been compared in randomized controlled trials and treatment remains empirical.

SUSTAINED RELEASE SYSTEMS

Long-acting sustained steroid releasing contraceptive methods are currently being developed. Those releasing progestogens alone are likely to be the first to reach the market in Great Britain. These methods all depend on the capacity of silastic rubber to release lipophilic drugs at a relatively constant rate and levonorgestrel releasing vaginal rings, intrauterine devices and subdermal implants have already been available in clinical trials.

With progestogen-only regimens, the mechanism of action is primarily on cervical mucus, although endometrial suppression must also contribute to the antifertility effect. Partial or complete ovarian suppression is also common and is responsible for menstrual disturbance and the occasional appearance of persistent functional ovarian cysts. Effectiveness is proportional to the daily dose of steroid released and is highest for subdermal implants when user-failure can be eliminated. The acceptability of all progestogen-only methods is mainly limited by the frequency of unpredictable menstrual bleeding patterns, but their safety and convenience are likely to assure them a place in overall contraceptive provision.

Currently only the subdermal implant (Norplant) and the levonorgestrel releasing intrauterine system (Mirena) are marketed in Britain.

Norplant subdermal implants

Norplant is a subdermal implant system providing long-acting, reversible, highly effective, low-dose contraception for 5 years. It was first marketed in Britain in 1993 and other implant systems may follow. Six silastic rubber capsules, each containing 36 mg of dry crystalline levonorgestrel, are placed subdermally on the medial aspect of the upper non-dominant arm. The system delivers approximately 80 µg of levonorgestrel per 24 hours during the first 6 months of use, declining to 30 or 35 µg daily after 12–18 months. The capsules are not biodegradable and should eventually be removed. Both insertion and removal (which can be more difficult) require local anaesthesia and aseptic technique and should only be undertaken by accredited practitioners.

Effectiveness is very high (approaching zero) in the first year and protects from both intrauterine and ectopic pregnancy, but failure may increase in later years when serum levels of levonorgestrel are significantly lower. No serious safety hazards have been identified. The acceptability in a UK population remains to be assessed but continuation rates in other countries have generally been favourable.

Discomforts are not rare but appear to be well tolerated, probably because women like the efficacy and convenience of the method. Irregular and unpredictable bleeding is the most frequent side-effect. Amenorrhoea is not common. Some women experience progestogen-related effects such as breast discomfort, abdominal bloating, headaches, and acne. As the method is very expensive, thorough counselling should be undertaken before a decision is reached to fit Norplant and great care should be exercised to avoid fitting it in a woman who is already pregnant.

Mirena — intrauterine system

This intrauterine system was first marketed in Britain in 1995. It is a modified Nova T/Novagard device with a silastic capsule fixed to the vertical stem containing 52 mg of levonorgestrel which is released into the uterine cavity at the rate of 20 µg/24 hours.

It is not suitable for emergency contraception but is highly effective in routine use and can be expected to reduce or eliminate menstrual blood loss after the first few months when irregular bleeding may occur. The progestogen released produces an endometrium unsuitable for implantation but ovulation is not usually inhibited and the effect on bleeding patterns is mainly due to the local effect of the levonorgestrel on the endometrium. This device can therefore benefit women with menorrhagia. The effect of levonorgestrel on cervical mucus is likely to increase the contraceptive effect and may also provide some protection from ascending infection in the genital tract.

The device is expensive and the diameter of the introducer is 4.8 mm (compared with 3.7 mm for the standard Nova T/Novagard). Local anaesthesia and dilatation of the cervix to Hegar 5 are sometimes required for successful insertion. Lack of attention to this factor may lead to failed insertions and considerable waste of resources. Progestogenic side-effects (breast discomfort, abdominal bloating, headaches, acne), functional ovarian cysts, irregular bleeding or amenorrhoea will lead some women to request removal. Careful preinsertion assessment and counselling should maximize continuation rates.

INTRAUTERINE DEVICES (IUD)

Popularity

Worldwide popularity exceeds that of oral contraceptives. An estimated 100 million women are current users of IUDs.

Mechanisms of action

The main method of action is believed to be alteration/inhibition of sperm migration, fertilization and ovum transport which lowers the fertilization rate, with the additional production of a sterile inflammatory response in the endometrium which inhibits implantation of the blastocyst. IUDs may therefore be used as an emergency method of contraception and should not be removed from the uterus within 7 days of coitus if pregnancy is not desired.

Advantages

1. Safe — mortality is very rare and there are no metabolic effects.
2. Highly effective and effective immediately or postcoitally.
3. Continuation rates are high as the method proves to be acceptable to the majority of women who choose it.
4. Reversible.
5. Requires no sustained motivation or action at time of coitus.
6. Can provide long-term contraception cheaply.

Disadvantages

1. Need for specially trained personnel to fit IUDs and give follow-up care.
2. Possible complications at time of insertion of the device include pain, bleeding, vagal inhibition, and perforation of the uterus.
3. Later complications may include pregnancy (including an increased relative risk of ectopic pregnancy), pain, bleeding, expulsion, displacement, infection or problems with the threads (lost threads or male dyspareunia).
4. The method provides no protection from sexually transmitted diseases.

Contraindications to IUD use

Absolute

1. Pregnancy
2. Acute or chronic pelvic infection
3. Certain congenital abnormalities of the uterus
4. Large fibroids which distort the uterine cavity
5. Wilson's disease or copper allergy (only for copper-bearing devices).

Relative

1. Menorrhagia
2. Malignant disease of the genital tract
3. Fixed retroversion of the uterus
4. Past history of ectopic pregnancy or pelvic inflammatory disease
5. Nulliparity
6. Congenital or rheumatic heart disease (may require antibiotic cover for insertion)
7. Compromised immune system
8. Lifestyle which exposes the woman to the risk of sexually transmitted infection.

Prevention and management of complications

Potential patients should be carefully screened for contraindications by history, examination and investigation if necessary. Insertion of the device should be carried out in a calm, relaxed manner with due attention to aseptic technique and analgesia for the patient if necessary, and precise adherence to the recommended fitting procedure, which differs for each device. Vagal inhibition resulting in bradycardia may be treated with i.v. atropine 0.6 mg. Facilities for basic cardiopulmonary resuscitation should be available whenever IUDs are fitted.

The device may have to be removed if menstrual pain and bleeding are unacceptable. Intermenstrual pain/bleeding may be due to infection or partial expulsion/displacement of the device. Suspected infection should be investigated and treated promptly in a department of genitourinary medicine, with follow-up of the partner.

Perforation may be suspected when threads are absent and may be investigated by ultrasound. If confirmed, laparoscopic removal of the device should be arranged without delay. If pregnancy occurs with the device in situ, the patient should be advised to have the device removed immediately while the threads are accessible. Previous expulsion is not a contraindication to the insertion of another device.

Practical prescribing

The devices currently recommended for use in Britain are:

1. Ortho Gyne-T 380 Slimline
2. Multiload Cu 250 (short and standard), Multiload Cu 375
3. Nova T/Novagard.

The choice of device may be made on the basis of its effectiveness and also on uterine size and tightness of the cervix as determined by sounding the uterus, but the choice of device is probably less important than the selection of the patient and the skill of the operator. IUDs may be fitted at any time in the menstrual cycle if contraception has been used effectively. After delivery it is customary to wait until 6 weeks postpartum for insertion but devices may be fitted at the time of delivery if appropriate and also at the time of termination of pregnancy.

Devices releasing the highest amounts of copper (the Ortho-Gyne T 380S and the Multiload 375) are the most effective but if the cervical canal is narrow it may be easier to fit a Nova T/Novagard device.

Despite the varying recommendations of the manufacturers it is likely that all devices can be left in utero for 5 years without loss of efficacy. Studies continue to define the optimal life of the more effective modern devices with data indicating the continued effectiveness of the Ortho-Gyne T 380S and Multiload 375 devices for at least 8 years. IUDs inserted in women over age 40 may be left in situ until after the menopause. It is probably advisable to remove them at about a year postmenopause before cervical/uterine atrophy makes the procedure problematical.

BARRIER METHODS OF CONTRACEPTION

Popularity

There has been renewed interest in barrier contraceptives in response to concern about HIV infection. Theory and clinical experience suggest that maximum contraceptive efficacy can only be obtained by using a barrier and spermicide together. The commonly used spermicide nonoxynol-9 has been shown to be active against HIV in vitro.

Advantages

1. Protection from sexually transmitted infection
2. Protection from carcinoma of the cervix
3. Instantly effective (after initial learning)
4. No systemic side-effects
5. Caps do not interfere with the sensation of either partner (although condoms are reputed to do so)
6. Available from non-medical sources.

Disadvantages

1. Need trained personnel to fit cap initially and check periodically

2. Require continuous motivation and supplies
3. Action required at time of coitus (for condom use)
4. User-failure can be high, e.g. the young/inexperienced
5. Couples may find barrier methods messy or distasteful
6. Small increase in cystitis/vaginal infections in cap users.

PRACTICAL PRESCRIBING

Caps

There are two types of cap:

1. Diaphragm (flat-spring, coil-spring and arcing types). These can be successful when the pelvic floor has good muscle tone. An arcing diaphragm is particularly useful when the cervix is difficult to cover.
2. Suction cap (cervical, vault and vimule types). These can be used when there is prolapse of the vaginal walls.

The patient should be fitted with a suitable cap and then taught how to remove and reinsert the device several times under supervision before she relies on the method. She should also be instructed in the correct use of spermicide and be given written instructions on the use of the method (see CES leaflet). Periodic checks of the fitting and correct placement of the cap should take place during use.

Sponges

Contraceptive sponges are no longer marketed in Great Britain.

Condoms

Male and female condoms are now available. These may be dispensed free of charge in hospitals, community health family planning clinics, and some general practices. Male condoms vary in shape, thickness, and lubrication. They may have features, e.g. texture or colour, designed to enhance their attractiveness to the user. Some brands now have a spermicide incorporated in the lubricant. There is a British standard for condoms and those without the 'kitemark' should not be used. There is also now a European standard for condoms which runs concurrently.

One type of female condom is now marketed in Great Britain. It is made of polyurethane rather than latex rubber and has an inner flexible ring to aid insertion and an outer ring to aid retention around the vulva. Further research is required to determine its user-effectiveness and initial experience suggests that its lack of acceptability will limit uptake. It is also more expensive than the male condom.

Clients should be given detailed instructions in the use of condoms and should also be made aware of the availability of emergency contraceptive methods (see CES leaflets.)

Spermicides

These are available as tubed creams, jellies or pastes, aerosol foam, soluble pessaries, foaming tablets, and water-soluble plastic film. High failure rates are to be expected if they are used without a barrier. The active ingredient is usually nonoxynol-9. Note: Oil-based spermicides or other products should not be used with caps/condoms as they can damage the tensile strength of the rubber.

PERIODIC ABSTINENCE

This method is also referred to as natural family planning, the rhythm method, or the safe period. It is based on the principle of avoidance of coitus during the 'fertile days' of a woman's menstrual cycle but in practice this is difficult to determine because:

1. Sperm may survive in the female genital tract for several days post coitus.
2. Ovulation cannot be predicted accurately in advance.

High effectiveness can therefore only be achieved by restricting coitus to the postovulatory phase of the cycle after the ovum is presumed to be incapable of being fertilized. The most accurate way of determining the 'infertile' days is to use various methods in combination — the 'symptothermal' method:

1. Observation from a menstrual calendar of the longest cycle length and calculation of the last fertile day by subtracting 10.
2. Observation of basal body temperature and reckoning on the infertile phase beginning on the third morning of elevated temperature readings following mid-cycle release of the ovum.
3. Observations of cervical elevation and softening at the time of ovulation; ovulatory pain, bleeding, or breast discomfort; and serial observations of cervical mucus. The infertile phase is reckoned to begin on the fourth evening after peak mucus production.

During 1996 a small device, incorporating a microcomputer and hormone assay system to measure LH and oestradiol from urinary dipsticks, was marked in Britain under the trade name 'Persona'. This expensive piece of technology provides an alternative method of determining the 'fertile' days of a woman's cycle by signalling 'safe' and 'unsafe' days with green and red lights. There are no randomized, controlled studies to compare its efficacy with other methods of identifying the fertile phase. Moreover, the successful use of periodic abstinence is also dependent on the couple's motivation to avoid intercourse on the 'fertile' days.

Advantages

1. Free of any known physical side-effects.
2. May be acceptable to couples whose religion or culture debars them from other methods.
3. Always available and cheap (after teaching).
4. The knowledge gained by couples practising the method may also assist them when planning conception.

Disadvantages

1. High user-failure rates which vary between six and 25 pregnancies per HWY.
2. The infertile period may be difficult to identify, e.g. during fever.
3. The couple have to accept considerable limitations on the days available for coitus. Sustained motivation and cooperation are essential to success.

Practical prescribing

Temperature charts and fertility thermometers are available on prescription in Great Britain. The couple should be counselled and taught effectively and offered on-going support. A CES leaflet is available.

LACTATIONAL AMENORRHOEA METHOD

Women who have delivered a baby in the preceding 6 months, who are breast-feeding fully (without giving any supplemental feeds), and who are amenorrhoeic have only a 1–2% chance of becoming pregnant. If these three conditions are fulfilled, it is reasonable to rely on them alone for contraceptive protection.

EMERGENCY CONTRACEPTION

A request for emergency contraception should lead to a review of the couple's on-going contraceptive strategy. In order that the method can be used at all, the population needs to be educated about its existence and availability. The method should be accessible on every day of the week. There are two methods:

1. *Hormonal.* The most popular regimen is the one recommended by Yuzpe: Ovran 50 (levonorgestrel 250 µg plus ethinyloestradiol 50 µg) two tablets stat followed by two tablets 12 hours later. This must be instituted within 72 hours of unprotected coitus. Prior exposure to conception in the current cycle outside the 72-hour period is a contraindication. The next menstrual period may occur on schedule,

early, or late. Nausea may affect up to 50% of takers. Caution should be exercised in prescribing for patients with a past history of thromboembolism and an alternative method would be advised for a patient with a history of migraine with aura who presented during a migraine attack. The overall failure rate is reported to be between one and five per 100 women per cycle. An alternative progestogen-only method, advocated by Ho and Kwan in 1993, involves taking levonorgestrel 0.75 mg (25 Microval tablets stat) within 48 hours of unprotected intercourse followed by a repeat dose 12 hours later.

2. *IUD insertion*. This is effective if fitted within 5 days of exposure to unprotected coitus. Nulliparity and rape are relative contraindications because of the greater susceptibility to sexually transmitted infection. A past history of ectopic pregnancy is a relatively strong contraindication. The method is virtually 100% effective and may be retained by the woman as her on-going method or removed with the next period if so desired.

ORGANIZATION OF FAMILY PLANNING SERVICES

Family planning services in Great Britain were mainly provided by the Family Planning Association (a charitable body) until they were transferred to the National Health Service during the 1974 reorganization. The intention was that all who needed advice and help with family planning (regardless of sex or marital status) should be able to choose a free service from the following sources (DHSS Circular HSC(l S) 32 May 1974):

1. Community health services
2. Hospital services
3. Family practitioner services.

These services should be seen as complementary to each other and liaison should be encouraged.

COMMUNITY HEALTH SERVICES

Family planning advice and supplies may be delivered by:

1. Community midwives and health visitors
2. Community family planning clinics
3. Special youth advisory centres
4. Domiciliary family planning services.

HOSPITAL SERVICES

Family planning advice and supplies may be delivered by:

1. Hospital midwives working in antenatal/postnatal clinics and parentcraft classes
2. Hospital outpatient family planning clinics
3. Hospital family planning 'visitors' who see patients in postnatal and postabortion wards
4. Hospital gynaecology clinics especially termination of pregnancy (TOP) request clinics
5. Hospital staff in any department may find it appropriate to advise or refer patients as part of their regular clinical care.

FAMILY PRACTITIONER SERVICES

General practitioners and practice nurses may choose to provide family planning services within normal surgery hours and/or in special 'sessions'.

41. Psychosexual counselling

C. Watson

Expectations of the examiners

The candidate will be expected to have an understanding of the principles involved in counselling patients with psychosexual problems.

Definition

Human sexuality involves gender identity, sexual object choice, sexual drive, and sexual function (behaviour). Individuals display wide variations in these parameters and therefore it is a general principle to assert that it is the client who decides whether any particular state is a 'problem'. Doctors should be sensitive to this issue and should not make assumptions about their patient's wishes.

Examples of these problems are:

1. Problem of gender identity—transsexualism
2. Problem of sexual object choice—fetishism
3. Problem of sexual drive—hypogonadism
4. Problem of sexual function—vaginismus.

Interesting facts

The true incidence of any aspect of human sexuality is not known but complaints about sexual problems are common and most relate to sexual dysfunction, i.e. problems of sexual function or interest. There is ample evidence, nonetheless, that many patients find it difficult to ask for professional help in this area and that of those who do, the sexual dysfunction may be associated with other more fundamental problems in the relationship or the personality. It is also likely that many patients experience sexual dysfunction but do not regard it as a problem.

Pathophysiology

Sexual dysfunctions which impede or prevent a couple from having or enjoying sexual intercourse include the conditions listed in Table 41.1.

375

Table 41.1 Sexual dysfunctions.

Disorders	In the woman	In the man
Initiation	Lack of interest	Lack of interest
Sexual arousal	Failure of lubrication and swelling response	Erectile failure
Penetration	Vaginismus	Erectile failure
	Dyspareunia	Dyspareunia
Orgasm	Failure of orgasm	Premature ejaculation
		Retarded ejaculation

Problems in one partner almost always affect the other and an individual or couple may have more than one coexisting difficulty. For example, it is common to find premature ejaculation in the male partner accompanied by orgasmic dysfunction in the female partner. Sexual dysfunctions may also be classified according to whether they are primary or secondary to a period of normal function.

Aetiology

Psychological factors always play a part in sexual dysfunction, even when physical factors are mainly responsible. Counselling the individual or couple is therefore an important element of management.

Physical causes of sexual dysfunction

Illness. Any physical or mental illness may be expected to interfere with sexual life. Chronic illness, stress, fatigue and depression may be associated with loss of sexual interest. Vascular disease and neuropathy, e.g. in diabetics, may prevent erection. Endocrine disorders which reduce free testosterone may be associated with lack of sexual drive. It is common for women to experience a loss of sexual interest after childbirth which may be attributed to a complex interaction of stressful life events, changing marital roles, fatigue, physical and hormonal changes (particularly in the lactating mother), and possible dyspareunia from an episiotomy scar.

Age. Although many individuals/couples enjoy sexual expression well into old age, most will have to adjust to changes in their sexual responsiveness as they become older. Erectile impotence is a common complaint in men over 50 which may simply reflect a general reduction in sexual responsiveness and the need for more tactile stimulation, but organic factors (as yet imperfectly understood) may also be important.

Drugs. Many drugs (both therapeutic and recreational) can affect sexual functioning. Alcohol probably inhibits sexual response through central nervous system effects. When assessing the possible role of therapeutic drugs in patients with sexual dysfunctions, it is often impossible to determine to what extent the drug therapy, e.g. antihypertensives or antidepressants, might be responsible for symptons which could also be attributed to the disease being treated, e.g. hypertension or depression.

Psychological causes of sexual dysfunction

Immediate causes

Learning difficulties. Sexual ignorance continues to play a small part in sexual problems. Unrealistic expectations may also contribute to sexual dissatisfaction (e.g. if 'vaginal orgasm' is believed to be the 'norm' for women). Couples sometimes do not relate their socioeconomic difficulties, e.g. living virtually without privacy, to the sexual problems they are experiencing.

Sexual anxiety. Sexual anxiety can prevent the physiological changes of sexual arousal and contribute to premature ejaculation in the man. Fear of failure contributes to erectile impotence in men who may feel that they are expected to 'perform'. Other men who experience premature ejaculation may have an excessive need to please their partner and may be so overconcerned about this that they are unable to focus on their own sexual pleasure.

Lack of communication between the sexual partners. Some couples find it difficult to talk about sexual matters and may therefore give less pleasure to each other than they could if they knew more about each other's preferences. Feelings of rejection and guilt may develop due to lack of understanding and can cause unnecessary distress.

Underlying causes

Relationship difficulties between sexual partners. Serious conflict, general communication difficulties, lack of commitment, lack of trust and disappointment in the partner may be associated with sexual problems which are unlikely to improve unless the basic relationship difficulties can be resolved.

Personal difficulties. Each partner may have difficulties which may relate to their upbringing, past experience and attitudes towards sexuality. They may experience conflict with the idea that sexual behaviour should be pleasurable and feel consequent guilt and shame. Negative sexual experiences such as childhood sexual abuse or rape are increasingly recognized as contributors to these difficulties.

Assessment

As most people still find it difficult to present their sexual problems, the attitude of the professional to whom they first unburden themselves is extremely important.

The attitude of the doctor is probably more important than any specific knowledge or skill in treating sexual problems. Many individuals/couples will be helped at a 'primary' level by the following features in the therapist:

1. Listening skills and the use of open-ended questions
2. Genuine concern about the patient

3. Lack of embarrassment—being at ease with sexual matters
4. A non-judgmental attitude and avoidance of 'standard-setting'
5. Avoidance of medical jargon and use of ordinary language.

As the problem unfolds it may become apparent that 'secondary' or specialist help is needed but it is important not to refer the patient on too quickly in case they may feel rejected and unable to contemplate the process of unburdening themselves a second time to another professional.

Because of the difficulties felt by patients, sexual problems may not be overtly expressed but may present covertly with another complaint which may well relate to the sexual organs, their function, or contraception. Doctors working in gynaecological situations need to be alert to complaints which may serve as a 'ticket of entry' to the 'real problem' which is a sexual one. Common presentations include complaints of dyspareunia, discharge, pelvic pain, or 'side-effects' from the contraceptive pill. These complaints will normally require a careful history, examination and possible investigation before it can be agreed that they have their origin in psychological distress. There is also the possibility that both a physical and psychological problem may coexist or that a physical problem may be the cause of sexual dysfunction, e.g. dyspareunia due to vaginal thrush.

Clinical examination can be an important part of the assessment of sexual problems. The main purpose may be to assess the part played by organic disease in any complaint but the examination may also serve to educate the patient or to increase his/her sexual confidence (e.g. in vaginismus).

Investigations

The urine should be tested for glucose in all men presenting with secondary impotence or late-onset ejaculatory problems. Superficial dyspareunia in women may indicate the need for a variety of tests such as a vaginal swab or full genitourinary screening. Pelvic ultrasound or laparoscopy may be needed in the assessment of deep dyspareunia. In men, measurements of erectile function such as nocturnal tumescence studies, measurement of penile blood pressure and blood flow, and more invasive procedures such as arteriography, intracavernosal injections of smooth muscle relaxants and peripheral nerve conduction tests are also specialist techniques.

It is customary to measure serum testosterone, FSH, LH and prolactin levels in men complaining of loss of sexual interest or erectile difficulties but the results are seldom outside normal limits.

Treatment

The general principles of treating sexual dysfunctions include:

1. Consider treating the couple irrespective of which partner presents.
2. Define the problem and what the couple would like to change.

3. Aim to reduce sexual anxiety by education and 'permission giving' which may modify unhelpful attitudes. Fear of unwanted pregnancy may be a source of anxiety and contraceptive counselling may prove to be therapeutic.
4. Facilitate communication between the partners.
5. Encourage new behaviour which will give mutual pleasure to the couple.
6. Specific problems may need specific treatment programmes, e.g. vaginismus.
7. Tackle more difficult interpersonal or intrapersonal problems if they appear to be 'blocking' progress.

Management of specific problems

Lack of sexual interest

The management of this problem will be the management of the underlying cause. Endocrine abnormalities will be rare and more often the lack of desire is secondary to stress, fatigue, depression, physical illness, drugs (e.g. alcohol), other sexual dysfunctions, or relationship difficulties.

Failure of sexual arousal

Failure of the lubrication/swelling response in women may result in dyspareunia, lack of enjoyment, resentment and withdrawal from sexual encounters. It may be treated as outlined in the general principles. It may be particularly beneficial to ban sexual intercourse for a limited time and to encourage graded pleasuring exercises as a substitute. Once sexual arousal and enjoyment have been re-established the couple may regain the confidence to enjoy intercourse again. Erectile difficulties may be treated successfully by the same means, provided there is no major organic deficit. When organic factors predominate, the couple may be motivated to try physical treatments such as mechanical aids to erection, intracavernosal injections of vasactive drugs (e.g. papaverine or alprostadil), vascular surgery (if appropriate), or a penile prosthesis as a last resort.

Vaginismus

This is an involuntary spasm of the pelvic floor muscles surrounding the lower part of the vagina which may prevent penetration or render it painful. It appears to be a learned response triggered by fear of penetration and although it is usually primary it may occur secondary to traumatic experiences such as childbirth. Treatment should aim to help the couple understand the nature of the problem (pictures and models are helpful).

The woman should be encouraged to tackle the avoidance which is usually exhibited in any phobic condition and helped to embark on a system of graded exercises (using fingers or dilators) while learning progressively to gain control and relax the pelvic floor muscles (Kegel exercises). The partner's involvement and encouragement in treatment are usually beneficial. Operative treatment should be avoided.

Dyspareunia

The management involves treating the underlying cause.

Male dyspareunia is rare but may be caused by lacerations from oversharp IUD threads or from candidal or other infections which may also affect the female partner.

Female dyspareunia. The causes of female dyspareunia which may require treatment (in addition to failure of sexual arousal or vaginismus) include:

1. Vulval conditions: candidal vulvitis, herpes genitalis, urethral caruncle, Bartholinitis.
2. Vaginal conditions: atrophic vaginitis, infective vaginitis (candidal or trichomonal), chemical vaginitis, vaginal scars.
3. Pelvic conditions: cystitis, pelvic inflammatory disease, pelvic pain syndrome, endometriosis, fibroids, ovarian tumours, constipation, inflammatory bowel disease.

Orgasmic dysfunction

Many women do not experience orgasm during sexual intercourse although some will subsequently 'learn' to do so. This knowledge may be therapeutic to women who regard themselves as 'inadequate' because they require additional clitoral stimulation to reach orgasm. The capacity to experience orgasm may be helped by encouraging a couple to increase their sexual arousal (by 'super-stimulation' and fantasy) and by learning to relax and 'lose control' when high levels of sexual arousal are reached.

Premature ejaculation

The complaint of premature orgasm appears to be limited to men. After orgasm an erection is lost rapidly and the man remains refractory to sexual arousal for a variable period. His orgasm therefore usually terminates sexual intercourse, whereas a woman is capable of multiple orgasms without a refractory period. Anxiety reduction and re-education to control the ejaculatory reflex are the basis for most therapeutic approaches for men who are distressed by premature ejaculation.

SUMMARY

Sexual problems are common and may be presented to doctors overtly or covertly. The patient will choose to present the problem because she/he believes the doctor has some expert interest, knowledge or skill and therefore problems are frequently aired in discussions about contraception, obstetrics, or gynaecology.

Concerned attention by the doctor at the first presentation may need to be followed by referral to a specialist but this should not be the initial response. The treatment of some conditions will be within the scope of the primary care doctor.

Appendix I

Obstetric terms and definitions

Amniotomy. Surgical rupture of the membranes to induce or enhance labour.

Android pelvis. A funnel-shaped male-type pelvis with diameters which decrease from above downwards.

Antepartum haemorrhage. Bleeding from the birth canal in the period from the 24th week of gestation to the birth of the baby.

Asynclitism. Tilting of the fetal head in labour so that the anterior or posterior parietal bone presents.

Attitude of the fetus. Relationship of fetal head and limbs to the fetal trunk, usually flexion.

Bregma. Anterior fontanelle.

Brow. The part of the fetal head between the root of the nose and the anterior fontanelle.

Caput succedaneum. Oedema from obstructed venous return in the fetal scalp caused by pressure of the head against the rim of the cervix or birth canal.

Cephalhaematoma. Collection of blood beneath the periosteum of a skull bone, limited to that bone by periosteal attachments.

Cervical dystocia. Difficult labour due to failure of the cervix to dilate, in spite of adequate uterine contractions.

Chloasma. The brown pigmented facial mask of pregnancy.

Couvelaire uterus. The uterus appears purple due to haemorrhage within its musculature, and occurs with severe placental abruption.

Crowning of the head. Phase in the second stage of labour when a large segment of the fetal scalp is visible at the vaginal orifice, the perineum being distended and the anus dilated.

Engagement. Engagement occurs when the widest diameters of the presenting part have passed through the pelvic inlet.

Erythroblastosis fetalis. Haemolytic disease of the newborn usually due to rhesus antibodies.

Fontanelle. Space at the junction of three or more skull bones, covered only by a membrane and skin.

Fourchette. The fold of skin formed by merging of the labia minora and labia majora posteriorly.

Funnel pelvis. (See Android pelvis.)

Hyaline membrane. A homogeneous membrane lining the alveoli, alveolar ducts, and respiratory bronchioles, and an important cause of death in premature infants.

Hydrops fetalis. Gross oedema of fetal subcutaneous tissues together with ascites, pericardial and pleural effusions, usually due to erythroblastosis.

Kernicterus. Yellow staining of the baby's brain due to high blood levels of inconjugated bilirubin causing severe neurological damage or death.

Lie of the fetus. Relationship of the long axis of fetus to the long axis of the uterus, usually longitudinal, but can be transverse or oblique.

Linea nigra. Brown or black pigmented line in the middle of the abdominal wall during pregnancy.

Lochia. The discharge from the uterus during the puerperium, initially red, then yellow, then white.

Lower uterine segment. The thin expanded lower portion of the uterus which forms in the last trimester of pregnancy.

Moulding. Alteration in shape and diameters of the fetal head during labour (the fontanelles and sutures permit the force of contractions to compress the head against the bony pelvis and adapt its shape to that of the birth canal).

Naegele's rule. To estimate the probable date of confinement add 9 months and 7 days to the first day of the menstrual cycle (correction is required if cycle not 28 days).

Neonatal death. A liveborn infant who dies within 28 days of birth.

Obstructed labour. There is no descent of the presenting part in the presence of good contractions.

Operculum. The plug of mucus that occludes the cervical canal during pregnancy.

Pawlik's grip. Suprapubic palpation with the outstretched hand to identify the presenting part of the fetus, its position, flexion, and its engagement.

Pelvic brim or inlet. The plane of division between the true and false pelvis. The plane passes from the upper border of the symphysis pubis, along the pubic crest to the iliopectineal eminence, then to the sacroiliac joint, along the wings of the sacrum to the centre of the sacral promontory.

Pelvic outlet. Runs from beneath the symphysis pubis along the ischiopubic ramus to the ischial tuberosity along the sacrotuberous ligament to the fifth sacral vertebra.

Pelvimetry. Measurement of the size of the pelvis.

Perinatal mortality. Stillbirths plus first week deaths expressed per 1000 total births.

Placenta accreta. Absence of decidua basalis, so that the chorionic villi are attached to uterine muscle.

Placenta circumvallata. Placenta with a double fold of amnion forming a ring on the fetal surface some distance in from the edge of the placenta.

Placenta increta. Chorionic villi are in the uterine muscle.

Placenta percreta. The villi are through the uterine muscle.

Placenta succenturiata. There is one or more accessory lobe of the placenta.

Position of the fetus. The relationship of a defined area on the presenting part (called the denominator) to the quadrants of the maternal pelvis.

Presenting part. That part of the fetus felt on vaginal examination.

Prolonged pregnancy. A pregnancy that lasts longer than term (37–42 completed weeks).

Puerperium. The period during which the reproductive organs return to their prepregnant condition (usually regarded as an interval of 6 weeks after delivery).

Show. A discharge of mucus and blood at the onset of labour when the cervix dilates and the operculum (cervical mucus plug) falls out.

Sinciput. That part of the fetal head in front of the anterior fontanelle.

Spalding's sign. Overlapping of the fetal skull bones, seen radiographically after fetal death.

Station. The level of the presenting part within the mother's pelvis (the ischial spines are the reference points on vaginal examination).

Symphysiotomy. Division of the pubic symphysis to enlarge the diameters of the bony pelvis.

Third degree tear. A perineal laceration passing through the anal sphincter.

Vasa praevia. Fetal vessels lying in the membranes in front of the presenting part (there must be an associated velamentous insertion of the cord, succenturiate lobe, or bipartite placenta).

Velamentous insertion. The umbilical cord inserts onto the membranes over which the vessels course to reach the fetal surface of the placenta.

Vernix caseosa. Produced by sebaceous glands and prevents waterlogging and maceration of the fetal skin by the amniotic fluid.

Vertex. The area between the anterior and posterior fontanelles and the parietal eminences.

Wharton's jelly. The mucoid connective tissue supporting the umbilical cord vessels.

Appendix II

Risk factors in obstetrics

General factors
Age less than 18 years
Age more than 36 years
Nullipara of 35 or more
Parity greater than 4

Menstrual history uncertain
Last period more than 2 weeks
Pill stopped within 3 months of last period
Cycle length before last period more than 30 days
Intrauterine device in situ
Vaginal bleeding since last period

Previous obstetric history
Stillbirth or neonatal death
Small baby, less than 2.5 kg
Large baby, more than 4.0 kg
Fetal congenital abnormality
Significant antibodies (defined by haematologist)
Hypertension or proteinuria
Eclampsia
Two or more legal abortions (less than 13 weeks)
Two or more miscarriages (less than 13 weeks)
Late miscarriage or legal abortion (13 weeks or more)
Preterm delivery (less than 37 weeks)
Cervical suture
Caesarean section, hysterotomy, or myomectomy
Postpartum haemorrhage or manual removal of placenta
Labour less than 2 hours
Labour more than 12 hours
Operative vaginal delivery
Postnatal depression

Maternal health
Relevant medical condition
Pelvic abnormality (including fibroids)
Smoking more than 10 per day at booking
Social factors
Problems with housing
Family history of diabetes
Family history of congenital abnormality
Haemoglobinopathy
Risk of transmissible viral factors
Drinking more than 10 units of alcohol per week at booking
Current drug abuse by woman or partner
Not fluent in English

Booking examination   Blood pressure more than 140/90
Proteinuria
Weight more than 90 kg
Weight less than 45 kg
Height less than 1.52 m
Cardiac murmur
Uterus large or small for dates
Other pelvic or abdominal mass
Blood group rhesus negative

City and Hackney District Health Authority system (from Carroll et al 1988 Journal of Obstetrics and Gynaecology 8: 222–227).

Appendix III

The fetal skull

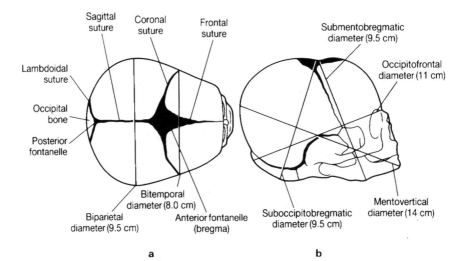

Fig. III
Frontal suture—between the two frontal bones
Coronal suture—between the frontal and parietal bones
Sagittal suture—between the two parietal bones
Lambdoidal suture—between the occipital bone and the parietal and temporal bones.

Anterior fontanelle (bregma)—large diamond-shaped depression where the frontal coronal and sagittal sutures meet. Closes at 18 months of age.
Posterior fontanelle—smaller triangular-shaped depression where the sagittal suture meets the lambdoidal sutures.

Diameters of the fetal skull
Biparietal diameter: 9.5 cm (vertex presentation)
Submentobregmatic: 9.5cm (face presentation)
Occipitofrontal: 11 cm (deflexed head, usually occipitoposterior)
Mentovertical: 14cm (brow presentation)
Suboccipitobregmatic: 9.5cm (vertex presentation).

Appendix IV

Diameters of the normal female pelvis

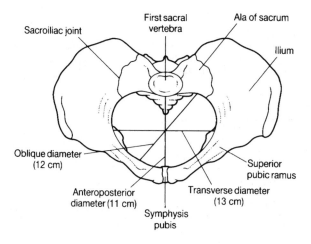

Fig. IVA: The pelvic brim
The outline of the brim follows the upper border of the first sacral vertebra, the alae, the sacroiliac joint, the ilium, the superior pubic ramus and the symphysis pubis.

Anterioposterior diameter: 11 cm
Oblique diameter: 12 cm
Trasverse diameter: 13cm.

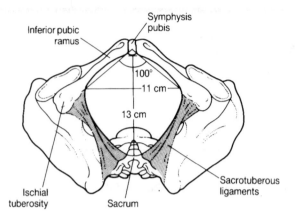

Fig. IVB: The pelvic outlet
The boundary of the outlet passes from the symphysis pubis, down the inferior rami of the pubic bones to the ischial tuberosities, and then obliquely upwards and posterior along the sacrotuberous ligaments to the tip of the fifth sacral vertebra.

Anteroposterior: 13cm
Transverse: 11 cm
Oblique diameter: 12cm.

Appendix V

Normal values in pregnancy

Haemoglobin concentration:	12 weeks	12.0 g/dl
	36 weeks	11.1 g/dl
White cell count:	12 weeks	8.1×10^6
	36 weeks	10.2×10^6
Packed cell volume		< 0.35
Platelets		$< 175 \times 10^6$
ESR	32 weeks	44–114
Serum urate:	32 weeks	< 0.35 mmol/l
	36 weeks	< 0.40 mmol/l
Serum glucose (fasting)		< 5.5 mmol/l
Serum glucose (random)		< 8.7 mmol/l
Glomerular filtration rate		170 ml/min
24 hour urinary protein		< 0.3 g/24 h

Appendix VI

Partograms—the graphic description of labour

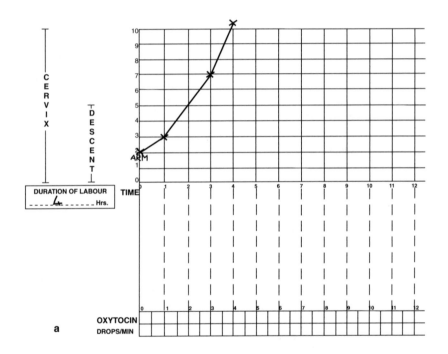

Partograms showing **a.** normal labour and **b.** inefficient uterine action corrected with oxytocin, overleaf.

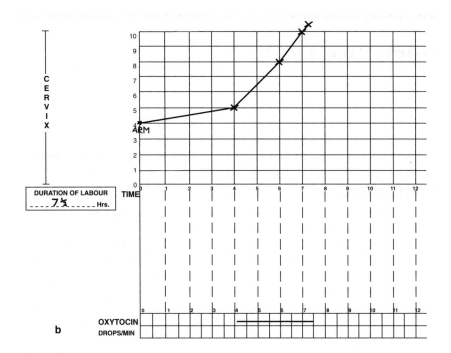

b

Suggested reading

J. Rymer

OBSTETRICS

Beischer N, Mackay E 1997 Obstetrics and the newborn, 2nd edn. W. B. Saunders
Magowan B 1996 Churchill's pocketbook of obstetrics and gynaecology. Churchill
 Livingstone, Edinburgh
McDonald M 1996 Loss in pregnancy — guidelines for midwives. Baillière-Tindall
Report on confidential enquiry into maternal deaths in the United Kingdom 1991–1993.
 HMSO, London
Studd J (ed) 1981–98 Progress in obstetrics and gynaecology, vols 1–13. Churchill
 Livingstone, Edinburgh

GYNAECOLOGY

Loudon N (ed) 1995 Handbook of family planning, 3rd edn. Churchill Livingstone,
 Edinburgh
Magowan B 1996 Churchill's pocketbook of obstetrics and gynaecology. Churchill
 Livingstone, Edinburgh
Shaw R W, Soulter W P, Stanton S L 1997, Gynaecology, 2nd edn. Churchill Livingstone,
 New York
Studd J (ed) 1981–98 Progress in obstetrics and gynaecology, vols 1–13. Churchill
 Livingstone, Edinburgh
Whitfield C R (ed) 1995 Dewhurst's textbook of obstetrics and gynaecology for
 postgraduates, 5th edn. Blackwell Scientific Publications, Oxford (for reference).

SEXUALLY TRANSMITTED DISEASES

Holmes K, King K 1990 Sexually transmitted diseases, 2nd edn. McGraw-Hill, London
 (for reference)
Willcox R, Willcox J 1982 Venereological medicine. Blackwell, Oxford

PSYCHOSEXUAL MEDICINE

Spence S H 1991 Psychosexual therapy. Chapman and Hall, London

NEONATAL MEDICINE

Rennie J M, Roberton N R C 1997 Textbook of neonatology, 3rd edn. Churchill
 Livingstone, Edinburgh

Index

Abdominal circumference 198, 199
Abdominal examination
  antenatal booking visit 163–164
  antenatal routine visits 168
  ectopic pregnancy 89
  endometriosis 56
  first stage of labour 219, 220
  objective structured clinical examination
    (OSCE) 30–31
  pelvic pain 62
  spontaneous abortion 79
  stress incontinence 128
Abdominal mass, neonate 327
Abdominal wall endometriosis 56
Abnormal lie 236, 247–248
ABO incompatibility 322
Abortion Act (1967) 85, 297
Abortion, spontaneous 77–80
  biochemical pregnancies 77
  chromosomal abnormalities 153
  congenital infections 178
  maternal mortality 304
  rhesus incompatibility 194
  statistics 296
  tubal 90
  see also Recurrent miscarriage
Abstinence contraception methods 371–372
Achondroplasia 198
Active management of labour 222
Acute abdomen 100
Acyclovir 345
Adenomyosis 45, 54
Adhesions 49, 65, 340
Adrenal dysfunction 51
Age of viability 287
AIDS see HIV infection
Alcohol as tocolytic 186
Alpha-fetoprotein 12, 298
  antenatal screening 155, 164
  multiple pregnancy 250
α-1–antitrypsin deficiency 323
Ambiguous genitalia 74, 328
Amenorrhoea 51–52
  ectopic pregnancy 89
  with hirsutism/virilism 74
  hydatidiform mole 92

Amenorrhoea (contd)
  menopause 38, 51, 52
  primary 51
  secondary 51
  uterine congenital abnormalities 70
Amniocentesis 156, 161, 164, 178, 298, 299
  rhesus isoimmunization 194, 195
Amniotic fluid embolism 229, 278–279
  maternal mortality 303
Anaemia 168, 207–209
  multiple pregnancy 251, 252
Anaesthesia 254
  hepatic drug metabolism 255
  maternal mortality 304, 306
  placental drug transfer 255
Analgesia 254
Androblastoma 74
Androgen-secreting tumours 74, 75
Androgens 118
  corpus luteum 38
  hirsutism/virilism 73, 75
  menopause 118
  polycystic ovarian syndrome 49, 50
Anencephaly 198
Ankle-crown length 313
Anovulatory bleeding 42–43
Antenatal
  care 160–173, 300
  booking visit 161–167
  diabetes mellitus 212–213
  diagnostic methods 156–158
  education 172–173
  epilepsy 213–214
  multiple pregnancy 250
  objectives 160
  pain relief in labour 255
  screening 154–155, 161, 299
  visits
    advice for parents 171–173
    fetal growth/well-being assessment
      169–171
    hospital fares 292–293
    investigations 168–169
    see also Booking visit
Antepartum haemorrhage 185, 202–206,
  276–277

Antepartum haemorrhage (*contd*)
  perinatal mortality 299
  rhesus incompatibility 194
Anterior colporrhaphy 129
Antibiotic therapy
  pelvic inflammatory disease 342
  puerperal infection 266, 268
Anticardiolipin antibodies 81
Anticoagulation 45, 84, 215
  in puerperium 269
Anticonvulsants 121, 193, 214
  congenital abnormalities 213
  pre-eclampsia 191, 192
Anti-D immunoglobulin 80, 169, 193, 196, 273
Antiphospholipid antibodies 81, 288
Antisperm antibodies 60, 68
Antithyroid drugs 216
  neonatal effects 332
Aortocaval compression 221
Apgar score 309, 310
Arcuate uterus 70, 71
Artificial insemination with donor semen 67
Artificial rupture of membranes 237, 248
Ascending genital tract infection 178
Asherman's syndrome 52, 80, 88
Aspiration of gastric contents (Mendelson's syndrome) 261, 263
Asymmetrical growth retardation 197, 198, 200, 201
Atrophic vaginitis 118
Auscultation
  fetal heart 31, 230
  neonatal examination 327
Autoimmune disease, recurrent miscarriage 81, 84
Azoospermia 66, 67

Backache 176, 254
Bacterial vaginosis 337, 338
  treatment 339
Bacteroides 341
Barlow's test 329
Barrier contraception 369–371
Bartholin's gland adenocarcinoma 105
Bartholin's gland swellings 97
Basal cell carcinoma of vulva 105
BCG vaccination, neonate 330
Bearing down reflex 223
Beckwith-Wiedemann syndrome 326
Benign genital tract conditions 95–102
Bereavement counselling 80
  intrauterine death 290
Bicornuate uterus 45, 70
Biochemical reference values 389
Biparietal diameter (BPD) 198, 386
Birth canal trauma 240
Birth plans 172–173

Birth rate 296
Birth trauma 299, 300
  forceps delivery 240
  limbs 328
  macrosomia 211, 331
Bishop's score 237
Bladder drill 131, 132
Blighted ovum 78
Blood group antibodies screening 195, 299
Blood pressure monitoring
  antenatal care 167
  pre-eclampsia 191
Body temperature chart 66–67
Bonding 313
Bone density measurement 120
Bonney's test 129
Booking visit 161–167
Brachial plexus injury 328
Brandt-Andrews method 227
Breast abscess 272, 319
Breast atrophy, menopausal 118
Breast cancer 120
  hormone replacement therapy association 123
  oral contraceptive pill association 359–360
Breast engorgement 271, 319, 320
Breast milk
  composition 270–271, 316–317
  drugs secretion 317, 318
Breast-feeding 172, 270–273, 313, 316–317
  antenatal preparation 271
  contraceptive effect 272, 372
  contraindications 317
  initiation post-partum 271
  problems 271–272, 319
  technique 319
Breast-milk jaundice 323
Breech presentation 13, 168, 244–246, 329
  epidural analgesia 258

CA 125 115, 116
Caesarean section 224, 241–243
  epidural analgesia 260–261
  maternal mortality 306, 307
  method 242–243
  prophylactic antibiotics 304
Candida albicans
  pruritus vulvae 95
  treatment 339
  vaginal discharge 337, 338, 339
Caps 369, 370, 371
Caput succedaneum 324
Cardinal ligaments 136
Cardiotocography 13, 230, 231
  first stage of labour 219
  intra-uterine growth retardation 200
  preterm labour 185

Cardiovascular disease 209–210
  epidural analgesia 258
  maternal mortality 305
  menopause 119, 123
  oral contraceptive pill association 359
Carpal tunnel syndrome 176
Cavernous haemangiomata (strawberry
  naevi) 322
Cephalhaematoma 241, 322, 324
Cephalopelvic disproportion 168, 221,
  224–225, 236, 242
Cerebral haemorrhage, maternal 189
Cerebrovascular disease 258, 305
Cervical carcinoma 19, 53, 109–111, 202
  oral contraceptive pill association 360
  staging 110
Cervical cerclage 72, 84–85
Cervical dilatation 217, 219, 223
Cervical ectropion 98–99, 202
Cervical effacement 217, 218
Cervical incompetence 70, 80, 88, 185
  recurrent miscarriage 82, 84
Cervical intraepithelial neoplasia (CIN)
  104, 106–109
  grades 107–108
  progression to invasive carcinoma
  106–107
Cervical malignancy 106–111
Cervical polyp 99, 202
Cervical ripening 217–218
  induction of labour 236
Cervical shock 80, 280–281
Cervical smear 21, 108, 163
Cervical stenosis 52, 277
Cervical trauma 228
Cervicitis 99
Cervix
  benign conditions 98–99
  menstrual cycle changes 40
  in puerperium 264
  transformation zone 107
Chancroid 345
Chemical vaginitis 336
Chest shape abnormalities 327
Child benefit 294
Chlamydia trachomatis
  lymphogranuloma venereum 345
  pelvic inflammatory disease 340, 341,
  342, 343
  vaginal discharge 337
Choanal atresia 320, 325
Choledochal cyst 324
Cholestasis in pregnancy 177
Chordee 327
Chorioamnionitis 185
Choriocarcinoma 94
  hydatidiform mole association 91, 92, 93,
  94
Chorionic villus sampling 13, 156–157,
  161, 298

Chorionic villus sampling (*contd*)
  rhesus incompatibility 194
Chromosomal abnormalities 153, 197, 288,
  298
  maternal age 163
  recurrent miscarriage 82, 84
  spontaneous abortion 78
Chromosome analysis 157
Chronic hypertension 189
Chronic pelvic pain syndrome 59, 61, 62,
  340
Chronic renal disease 189
Clam cystoplasty 132
Classical abdominal Semm hysterectomy
  (CASH) 147
Clavicle fracture 326, 328
Cleft lip 326
Cleft palate 320, 326
Climacteric 18, 117
  menorrhagia 46
Clitoromegaly 95
Clue cells 338
Coagulation defects
  postpartum haemorrhage 228
  pre-eclampsia 190, 191
Coelomic epithelium metaplasia 55
Coloboma 326
Colostrum 270
Colporrhaphy 139
Colposcopy 18, 108
Colposuspension 129, 130, 136
Combined oestrogen-progestogen oral
  contraceptive pill 358–362
  cardiovascular disease association 359
  contraindications 360–361
  neoplasms association 359–360
  prescribing 361–362
Communication skills 32
Community health family planning services
  373
Complete abortion 77
Complete hydatidiform mole 91, 92
Condoms 369, 370, 371
Condylomata lata 346, 347, 348
Cone biopsy 108, 111
Confidential Enquiry into Maternal Deaths
  (England and Wales) 15–16, 88, 226,
  301
Confidential Enquiry into Stillbirths and
  Deaths in Infancy (CESDI) 287, 301
Congenital abnormalities 153, 185, 245,
  247, 288, 332
  antenatal screening 161
  anticipatory neonatal care 309
  anticonvulsant medication 213
  at risk groups 156
  epilepsy association 213
  female genital tract 69–72
  maternal diabetes mellitus 211, 331
  multiple pregnancy 250, 251

Congenital abnormalities (*contd*)
  perinatal mortality 298
  prevention 300
  spontaneous abortion 78
  ultrasound detection 165
Congenital adrenal hyperplasia 74, 75, 328
Congenital cataracts 326
Congenital dislocation of hips 329–330
Congenital glaucoma 325
Congenital heart disease 154
  maternal 209, 210
Congenital infections 153, 178
Conjunctival haemorrhages 325
Connective tissue disease 78
Constipation
  overflow incontinence 132, 133
  in pregnancy 175
  uterovaginal prolapse 136
Continuous fetal heart monitoring 230
  see also Cardiotocography
Contraception 353–374
  acceptability of methods 353–354
  choice of method 354
  effectiveness 354–356
    measurement 355
  emergency 372–373
  method-failure 354
  motivation 353
  multiple choice questions 22–23
  organization of services 373–374
  puerperium 272, 273
  safety 356
  user-failure 354
Contraceptive history 162
Contraceptive sponges 370
Cord care 315–316
Cord compression, fetal heart rate patterns
  233, 234
Cord examination, neonate 327
Cord prolapse 242, 274–275
  multiple pregnancy 252
  transverse lie 248
Cordocentesis 157, 169, 171, 200, 299
Cornual implantation 245
Corpus luteum 38
  lifespan 38
  visualization for ovulation detection 67
Corpus luteum cyst 102
Counselling
  hormone replacement therapy 121
  premenstrual syndrome 125
  sterilization 357
  therapeutic abortion 86
Cracked nipples 272, 319
Craniosynostosis 325
Crigler-Najjar syndrome 323
Cushing's syndrome 74
Cyanosis, neonate 321
Cystic fibrosis 154, 323
  neonatal screening 330

Cystic hygroma 326
Cystocele 136, 137
  surgical repair 139
Cytomegalovirus 180–181
  congenital infection 17, 153, 180, 323
  spontaneous abortion 78
  see also TORCH syndrome

Deep dyspareunia 60
Deep vein thrombosis 214, 215, 306
  in puerperium 268, 269
Delayed gastric emptying 221, 261
Delivery
  breech presentation 246
  fetal distress 234
  multiple pregnancy 251–252, 258
  placenta praevia 205
  placental abruption 203–204
  pre-eclampsia 191
  preterm birth 187
  rhesus isoimmunization 194, 196
  transverse lie 248
Dental treatment 292
Depot progestogen injections 363–365
  contraindications 364
  prescribing 364–365
Depression, puerperal 269
Dermal sinus, spine 328
Dermoid cyst 61
Descent of head 218, 219
Detrusor hypotonia 132
Detrusor instability 127, 130, 132
  see also Urge incontinence
Dexamethasone 76
Dextrocardia 327
Diabetes mellitus 12, 210–213, 325
  antenatal care 212–213
  congenital abnormalities 331
  insulin-dependent 211
  intra-uterine growth retardation 197
  neonatal problems 331
  non-insulin-dependent 211
  perinatal mortality 16, 299
  prepregnancy care 212
  recurrent miscarriage 82
  see also Gestational diabetes
Diaphragm 370
Diaphragmatic hernia 327
Diet, antenatal advice 171
Dihydroepiandrosterone (DHEA) 73
Dihydrotestosterone (DHT) 73–74, 75
Dilatation and evacuation 87
Diplomas Examination Regulations 3
Disseminated intravascular coagulation
  antepartum haemorrhage 276
  placental abruption 203
  pre-eclampsia 190
Dizygotic twins 249
DNA analysis 157–158

'Domino' care 167
Down syndrome (trisomy 21) 153, 325
    antenatal screening/diagnosis 155, 161,
        164
    eyes 325, 326
    fontanelles 324
    head shape 324
Drug-induced abortion 78
Drug-induced hirsutism 74
Drug-induced sexual dysfunction 376
Drugs secreted into breast milk 317, 318
Dural puncture 260
Dysfunctional uterine bleeding 21, 45, 100,
        101
    treatment 46–47
        acute arrest 47
Dysmenorrhoea 48–49, 61, 99
    endometriosis 56, 58
Dyspareunia 58–60, 376, 378, 379
    endometriosis 56, 59
    management 380
    pelvic inflammatory disease 340

Early pregnancy bleeding 77–94
Eclampsia 192–193, 242
Ectopic pregnancy 18, 59, 61, 88–91
    diagnosis 89, 341
    following endometrial ablation/resection
        143
    laparoscopic treatment 145–146
    maternal mortality 304, 306
    pelvic inflammatory disease 340
    recurrence risk 88–89, 91
    rhesus isoimmunization 194
    rupture 280
    surgery 89–90
    symptoms 88
Edward syndrome (trisomy 18) 153
    feet 329
    head shape 324
Eisenmenger's syndrome 210
Emergency contraception 372–373
Employment, antenatal advice 172
Endocervical swabs 342, 343
Endometrial ablation/resection 47, 142–144
    with laparoscopic sterilization 143
Endometrial biopsy 46
Endometrial cancer 18, 53, 111–113, 120
    hormone replacement therapy association
        123
    staging 112
Endometrial menstrual cycle changes 38–40
    luteal phase 38
    menstrual phase 40
    proliferative phase 38–39
    secretory phase 39–40
Endometrial polyps 45, 99
Endometrial suppression 142

Endometriosis 19, 54–58
    dysmenorrhoea 48, 49
    dyspareunia 56, 59
    treatment 57–58
        laparoscopic 145
Engagement of head 218
    antenatal monitoring 168
    failure 168
Enterocele 136, 138
Entonox 256
Enzyme defect detection 157
Epidural analgesia 257–261
    complications 259–260
Epidural catheter insertion 258, 259
Epidural space 257
Epilepsy 213–214
    maternal mortality 305, 307
Episiotomy 224, 240
Epistaxis 175
Epithelial dystrophies of vulva 96–97
Epithelial (Epstein) pearls 326
Erb's palsy 276, 328, 329
Erectile impotence 376, 377, 378, 379
Erythema toxicum (urticaria neonatorum)
        321
Erythromycin 268, 342, 346
Escherichia coli 183
Essential hypertension 193
Ethnic variation
    maternal mortality 302
    perinatal mortality 298
Etoposide 115
EXAMINATION FOR DRCOG 3–34
    addresses 7
    appointment certificate 3–4
    dates 4–5
    Diplomas Examination Regulations 3
    diplomates 7
    eligibility 3
    examples
        appointment certificate 4
        computer answer sheet 11
        OSCE clinical skills station 31
        OSCE communication station 33
        OSCE knowledge/factual station 28
    format 5
    multiple choice questions 5, 10–26
        answer sheet 11
        answers 23–26
        family planning 22–23
        gynaecology 17–21
        neonatal medicine 16–17
        obstetrics 10, 12–15
        sexually-transmitted diseases 21–22
        statistics 15–16
    objective structured clinical examination
        (OSCE) 5, 27–34
    preparation 8–9
    Report of the DRCOG Working Party 9
    results 6–7

EXAMINATION FOR DRCOG (*contd*)
syllabus 5–6
gynaecology 6
neonatal medicine 6
obstetrics 5–6
written paper 5, 10–26
Extended (frank) breech 244, 245
External cephalic version 194
External rotation (restitution) 218, 224
Extrahepatic biliary atresia 315, 323

Facial palsy 326
Fallopian tube development 69
Familial hypertrichosis 74
Family credit 292, 293, 295
Family planning services organization
373–374
Family practitioner family planning services
374
Fatigue in pregnancy 176
Feeding difficulties 319–321
preterm baby 334
Feet, dysmorphic features 329
Femur length 198, 199
Ferning 40
Fetal biophysical profile 169, 170
Fetal blood sampling 195, 234, 235
Fetal blood tests 157
Fetal breathing movements 185
Fetal circulation 17
Fetal distress 233–235, 242
anticipatory neonatal care 309
multiple pregnancy 252
Fetal drug metabolism 255
Fetal growth assessment
antenatal monitoring 168, 169
ultrasound parameters 198
Fetal growth chart 200
Fetal heart auscultation 31, 230
Fetal heart rate
decelerations 232–233, 234
monitoring
fetal growth/well-being assessment 169,
170
induction of labour 237
partogram 219
patterns 231–233
Fetal hypoxia 230
Fetal monitoring 230–235
pre-eclampsia 191
Fetal movement charts 169, 191
Fetal movements
fetal growth/well-being assessment 169
first stage of labour 219
intra-uterine growth retardation 200
Fetal skull 386
Fetal well-being assessment
antenatal monitoring 169
first stage of labour 219
intra-uterine growth retardation 200

Fetishism 375
Fetomaternal haemorrhage 194
Fetoplacental blood flow assessment 169,
170
Fetoscopy 157, 178
Fibroid polyps 99
Fibroids 45, 78
Flexed (complete) breech 244, 245
Fluid/electrolyte imbalance, preterm baby
334
Folic acid deficiency 208
Folic acid supplements 151, 168, 208
Follicle stimulating hormone (FSH)
menopause 38, 118, 120
menstrual cycle 37, 38
ovulation induction 41
pulsed release 37
Follicular cyst 102
Follicular phase 37–38
Fontanelles 29, 34, 324–325, 386
Footling breech 244, 245
Forceps delivery 15, 224, 238–240
epidural analgesia 260
pudendal block 261
Formula feeds 318
Formula-feeding 316
feeding practice 318
Fothergill (Manchester) repair 139
Frequency of micturition 100, 115, 177
Fructosaemia 323
Functional incontinence 134
Fundal height measurement
antenatal visits 168
fetal growth/well-being assessment 169
intra-uterine growth retardation 198
Fundal placenta 247

Galactosaemia 317, 323, 326
Gamete Intra Fallopian Transfer (GIFT) 68
Gardnerella vaginalis 339
Gastroschisis 327
Gender identity problems 375
Genetic counselling 158–159
Genital herpes *see* Herpes simplex
Genital tract
atrophy at menopause 118
congenital abnormalities 69–72
sepsis, maternal mortality 304, 307
support structures 136
Genital ulceration 343–346
Genital warts 104, 346–348
treatment 347–348
General anaesthesia 261–263
complications 263
induction 262
Gestational age assessment 161, 165
Gestational diabetes 211
antenatal screening 212
multiple pregnancy 251
risk factors 212

Gestational hypertension 189
Glucose tolerance, antenatal screening 169, 212
Glucose-6–phosphate deficiency 323
Gluococorticoids, fetal lung maturation 187
Glycosuria 211, 212
    antenatal monitoring 168
GnRH analogues 42, 57, 76
Goitre, neonatal 326, 332
Gonadotrophin releasing hormone (GnRH) 37, 42
    see also GnRH analogues
Gonadotrophin releasing hormone (GnRH) agonists 84
Gonadotrophins
    at climacteric 117, 119
    ovulation induction 41–42, 68
    pulsed release 37
Gonorrhoea 104
Graves' disease 216
    neonatal problems 332
Guthrie test 330
Gynaecological emergencies 274–282
Gynaecological malignancy 103–116
    cervix 106–111
    ovary 113–116
    pelvic pain 61
    screening 103
    uterus 111–113
    vulva 103–106
Gynaecology
    examination syllabus 6
    multiple choice questions 17–21
    objective structured clinical examination (OSCE) 28
    'physiological' treatments 41–43
    suggested reading 392

H₂-receptor blockers 221, 262
Haematological values in pregnancy 389
Haematuria 56
Haemoglobin S (HbS) 208
Haemolytic disease of newborn
    blood tests at delivery 196
    neonatal jaundice 322
    rhesus isoimmunization 194
Haemophilus ducreyi 345
Haemorrhage
    abortion 80, 87
    early pregnancy bleeding 77–94
    ectopic pregnancy 89
    hydatidiform mole 92
    prolonged bleeding 43
Haemorrhoids 175, 269
Haemostatic mechanisms
    changes in pregnancy 214
    delivery of placenta 226
Hands, dysmorphic features 329

Harlequin change 321
Hashimoto's thyroiditis 216
Head circumference 198
Head compression, fetal heart rate patterns 232
Head shape 324
Headache in pregnancy 176
Heart rate, neonate 314
Heartburn 175
HELLP syndrome 193
Heparin 215, 269
Hepatitis A 323
Hepatitis B 14, 22, 164, 348–350, 351
    congenital infection/vertical transmission 323, 351
    immunization 349
    neonate 330–331
Hepatitis C 349
    congenital infection 323
Hereditary spherocytosis 323
Herpes neonatorum 16
Herpes simplex 104, 110, 181–182, 188, 345
    antiviral therapy 345
    congenital infection 181, 182, 323
    prevention 182, 345
    genital ulceration 343–346
    pelvic inflammatory disease 341
    vaginal discharge 337–338
    see also TORCH syndrome
Hips, congenital dislocation 329–330
Hirschsprung's disease 315
Hirsutism 20, 73–76
    androgens metabolism 74
    polycystic ovarian syndrome 49, 50
HIV infection 21, 164, 343, 348, 350, 369
    pregnancy 351–352
    vertical transmission 350, 351–352
Home deliveries 165, 167, 283–286
    assessment of suitability 283–285
Hormonal contraception 42, 357–358
    combined oestrogen-progestogen pill 358–362
    depot progestogen injections 363–365
    emergency contraception 372–373
    progestogen-only pill 362–363
    sustained release systems 365–367
Hormone replacement therapy 20, 117–123
Hormone-releasing IUD 47, 89, 122
Hospital family planning services 373–374
Hot flushes 118
Human chorionic gonadotrophin (hCG) 38
    choriocarcinoma 94
    hydatidiform mole 92, 93
    ovulation induction 41, 42
    polycystic ovarian syndrome 84
Human menopausal gonadotrophin (hMG) 41
Human papilloma virus (HPV) 105
    cervical carcinoma 109

Human papilloma virus (HPV) (*contd*)
  cervical intraepithelial neoplasia (CIN) 346
  genital warts 346
Human placental lactogen 270
Human T-lymphotrophic virus-1 (HTLV-1) 349
Hyaline membrane disease (respiratory distress syndrome) 333
Hydatidiform mole 20, 91–93, 94
  complete 91
  invasive 92
  partial 91, 92
Hydrocele 328
Hydrocephalus 168
Hydrops fetalis 194
Hypercoagulable state 269
Hyperemesis 92, 250
Hyperinsulinaemia 49, 50
Hypertension 120, 188–193
  definition 189
  epidural analgesia 257
  maternal mortality 303, 306
  multiple pregnancy 251
  see also Pre-eclampsia
Hyperthyroidism 216
Hypogonadism 375
Hypopituitarism, neonate 323, 327
Hypospadias 327
Hypotension with epidural analgesia 259–260
Hypothalamic dysfunction 51
Hypothalamus-pituitary-gonad axis 37
Hypothermia 310–311
  preterm baby 334
  small for gestational age baby 333
Hypothyroidism
  maternal 216
  neonatal 323, 326
Hysterectomy
  cervical carcinoma 111
  cervical intraepithelial neoplasia (CIN) 108
  choriocarcinoma 94
  dysfunctional uterine bleeding 47
  endometrial adenocarcinoma 113
  hydatidiform mole 93
  laparoscopic 146–148
  ovarian cancer 115
  uterine fibroids 101
  uterovaginal prolapse 139
Hysterosalpingogram 67
Hysteroscopy 141, 142
Hysterotomy 87

Immunologically-mediated abortion 78, 82, 84
Imperforate anus 327
In vitro fertilization (IVF) 41, 42, 67, 68

Inborn errors of metabolism 153, 317
Income support 292, 293, 295
Incomplete abortion 77, 79–80
Incoordinate uterine action 70, 72, 252
Induction of anaesthesia 262
Induction of labour 236–238
Inefficient uterine action (primary dysfunctional labour) 221
Inevitable abortion 77, 79–80
Infection
  intrauterine 288
    abortion 80, 87
    preterm premature rupture of membranes 188
  maternal 178–183
    breast-feeding contraindication 317
  neonatal jaundice 322, 323
  preterm baby 333
Infertility 19, 20, 64–68
  ectopic pregnancy risk 89, 91
  endometriosis 54, 56, 58
  male 64, 65, 66
  polycystic ovarian syndrome 50
  post-abortion 80, 87, 88
  treatment 41–42, 67–68
Inguinal hernia 327
Inhalation agents 256
Insomnia 177
Instrumental delivery 224
  anticipatory neonatal care 309
Insulin therapy 212
Intermenstrual bleeding *see* Irregular vaginal bleeding
Intersex state 95
Intestinal obstruction 315, 324
Intracranial haemorrhage
  forceps delivery 240
  maternal mortality 305
  preterm baby 333–334
  ventouse delivery 241
Intracranial pressure elevation 325
Intra-cytoplasmic Sperm Injection (ICSI) 67
Intrahepatic biliary hypoplasia 324
Intrapartum death 290
Intrauterine contraceptive device (IUCD) 22, 45, 367–369
  complications 368
  contraindications 368
  ectopic pregnancy risk 89
  emergency contraception 373
  hormone-releasing 47, 89, 122
  infertility 65
  misplaced 48
  prescribing 368–369
Intra-uterine death 185, 289–290
Intra-uterine growth retardation 14, 185, 196–201
  definition 196
  maternal diabetes mellitus 211

Intra-uterine growth retardation (*contd*)
  multiple pregnancy 251
  pre-eclampsia 189, 190
  uterine congenital abnormalities 70, 72
Intrauterine insemination (IUI) 41
Intrauterine system (IUS) 122
Intrauterine transfusion 196
Intraventricular haemorrhage 333–334
Invasive hydatidiform mole 92
Inverted nipples 172, 317
Iron deficiency anaemia 207–208
Iron status 44, 46, 101, 164
Irregular vaginal bleeding 42–43, 52–53,
      99, 110, 112, 118
Irritable bowel syndrome (IBS) 61, 62

Jarisch-Herxheimer reaction 346
Jaundice *see* Neonatal jaundice
Jitteriness 331, 332, 333

Kegel exercise 380
Kernicterus 194, 322
Kjelland's forceps 224, 238, 239, 240
Kleihauer test 196, 288
Klumpke's palsy 328

Labour 14–15
  active management 222
  definition 217
  diabetes mellitus 213
  diagnostic criteria 218–219
  fetal monitoring 230–235
  first stage 217–222
  normal mechanism 218
  oxytocic drugs 227
  second stage 223–225, 255
  third stage 226–229
Lactation 264
  antenatal advice 172
  contraceptive effect 272, 372
  physiology 270
  suppression 272–273, 291
  see also Breast-feeding
Laparoscopic hysterectomy 146–148
Laparoscopic minimally invasive surgery
      144–148
Laparoscopic oophorectomy/ovarian
      cystectomy 146
Laparoscopic pelvic lymphadenectomy 146
Laparoscopic sterilization with clips 28, 34
Laparoscopically assisted vaginal
      hysterectomy 147
Laparoscopy and dye instillation 67
Laser endometrial ablation 142, 144
Leiomyomata *see* Uterine fibroids
Leiomyosarcoma 100
Let down reflex 270, 271

Leukoplakia 96
Levator ani muscles 136
LHRH analogues 50, 68, 125
Lichen sclerosis 105
Lichen sclerosus et atrophicus 96
Life-table analysis 355
Liquor volume assessment 168
Listeria monocytogenes 183
Listeriosis 78, 153, 183, 288
Liver enzymes in pre-eclampsia 190
Liver tumours 360
Local anaesthetics 258
  toxicity 260
Locked twins 252
Low birth weight 184
Lower genital tract
  endometriosis 56
  menstrual cycle changes 40
Lupus anticoagulant 81
  perinatal mortality 299
Luteal phase 38
Luteinizing hormone (LH)
  menopause 118, 120
  menstrual cycle 38
  mid-cycle surge 38
  monitoring for ovulation detection 67
  ovulation induction 41
  pulsed release 37
Lymphogranuloma venereum 345

McDonald suture 85
Macroglossia 326
Macrosomia 211, 331
Major pregnancy complications 184–216
  antepartum haemorrhage 202–206
  hypertensive disorders 188–193
  intra-uterine growth retardation 196–201
  maternal systemic disorders 207–216
  preterm labour 184–187
  preterm premature rupture of
      membranes 187–188
  rhesus isoimmunization 193–196
Male dyspareunia 380
Male infertility 64, 65, 66
Malnutrition 288
Malposition 168, 242
Malpresentation 168, 242
  anticipatory neonatal care 309
  multiple pregnancy 250, 251
  uterine congenital abnormalities 70, 72
  uterine fibroids 102
Manchester (Fothergill) repair 139
Manual removal of placenta 194
Marfan's syndrome 326
Mastitis 271, 319
  neonate 327
Maternal mortality
  abortion 304
  amniotic fluid embolism 303

Maternal mortality (*contd*)
  anaesthesia 304, 306
  aspiration of stomach contents 261
  caesarean section 242, 306, 307
  cardiac disease 209, 210
  direct deaths 302–304
  ectopic pregnancy 280, 304, 306
  epilepsy 305, 307
  fortuitous deaths 305
  genital tract sepsis 304, 307
  hypertensive disease 303, 306
  indirect deaths 304–305
  infections 305
  late deaths 305
  placenta praevia 303, 307
  placental abruption 303
  postpartum haemorrhage 226, 303, 307
  pre-eclampsia 189
  prevention 306–307
  pulmonary embolism 302–303, 306
  statistics 301–307
  substandard care 301
  thromboembolic disease 214
  uterine rupture 304
Maternal mortality rate 301
Maternity benefits 292–295
Mean cell haemoglobin concentration
    (MCHC) 207
Mean cell volume (MCV) 207
Meconium 314, 315
  aspiration 310
Meconium-stained liquor 219, 230, 234
  anticipatory neonatal care 309
  neonatal resuscitation 310
Medical disorders 162–163, 287
  sexual dysfunction 376
Megaloblastic anaemia 208
Mendelson's syndrome (aspiration of gastric
    contents) 261, 263
Menopause 117–123
  gonadotrophins 38
  oestrogen deficiency 118–119
  presenting symptoms 119
  uterovaginal prolapse 136
Menorrhagia 44–47, 99, 100
Menstrual blood loss 44, 45
Menstrual cycle 17–18, 37–43
  endometrial cycle 38–40
  follicular phase 37–38
  lower genital tract changes 40
  luteal phase 38
  menstrual phase 40
  ovarian changes 37–38
  ovulation 38
  proliferative phase 38–39
  secretory phase 39–40
Menstrual disorders 44–53
  amenorrhoea 51–52
  dysmenorrhoea 48–49
  hirsutism/virilism 74

Menstrual disorders (*contd*)
  intermenstrual bleeding 52–53
  menorrhagia 44–47
  postcoital bleeding 53
Menstrual history 162
Menstrual phase 40
Mentovertical diameter 386
Mesonephric (Wolffian) duct 98
Micrognathia 320, 326
Micropenis 327
Microphthalmia 325
Migraine 176
Milia 321
Milk stools 314, 315
Minimally invasive surgery 141–149
Minor pregnancy disorders 174–177
Mirena intrauterine system 366–367
Miscarriage Association 80
Missed abortion 77, 79–80
Mittelschmerz 65
Mobiluncus 339
Molluscum contagiosum 346, 347
  treatment 348
Mongolian blue spots 321
Monozygotic twins 249
Moro reflex 330
Moulding of head 313, 324
Moulding in utero 328
Mouth, neonate 326
Müllerian (paramesonephric) duct 69
Multiload Cu 250 369
Multiload Cu 375 369
Multiple pregnancy 12, 165, 168, 185, 198,
    242, 245, 247, 249–253, 288
  anticipatory neonatal care 309
  delivery 251–252, 258
  perinatal mortality 298
Mumps 114
Muscle tone, neonate 330
Mycoplasma hominis 341
Myelomeningocele 329

Nabothian follicles 98
Narcotic analgesia 256–257
  anticipatory neonatal care 309
Narcotics abuse 288
  neonatal problems 332
Natural family planning (periodic
    abstinence) 371–372
Nausea/vomiting 174
  narcotic agent side effects 257
Neisseria gonorrhoeae
  gonorrhoea 104
  pelvic inflammatory disease 340, 341,
    342, 343
  vaginal discharge 337
Neonatal care facilities 300
Neonatal death rate 297
Neonatal feeding problems 319–321

Neonatal hepatitis 324
Neonatal hypoglycaemia 333
  maternal diabetes mellitus 211, 331
Neonatal immunizations 330–331
Neonatal jaundice 194, 315, 322–323
  maternal diabetes mellitus 211
  phototherapy 322, 323
  preterm baby 334
  prolonged 323–324
Neonatal medicine 309–334
  anticipatory care 309
  care of normal baby
    delivery room 310–313
    postnatal ward 313–331
  congenital abnormalities see Congenital
    abnormalities
  examination of newborn 321–330
  examination syllabus 6
  multiple choice questions 16–17
  objective structured clinical examination
    (OSCE) 29
  pre-existing maternal disease 331–332
  suggested reading 392
Neonatal physical examination 321–330
Neonatal resuscitation 16–17, 309–310
  advanced 312
  basic 311
Neonatal routine observations 313–315
Neonatal screening tests 330
Neonatal temperature control 310–311, 313
Neonatal thyrotoxicosis 332
Neoplasia, maternal mortality 305
Neural tube defects 151, 154
  antenatal screening 155, 164, 166
Neutral thermal environment 311
Neville Barnes forceps 238, 239
Niemann-Pick disease type 3 324
Night sweats 118
Nipple problems 272, 319
Nipple shields 172
Non-rotational forceps 238
Norplant subdermal implants 365–366
Nova T/Novagard 369

Obesity 112, 212, 214, 284
Oblique lie 247–248
Obstetric analgesia/anaesthesia 254–263
Obstetric emergencies 274–282
Obstetric history 162, 195, 285, 287
Obstetric intervention 236–241
  caesarean section 241–243
  forceps delivery 238–240
  induction of labour 236–238
  ventouse deliveries 240–241
Obstetric risk factors 165, 384–385
Obstetrics
  examination syllabus 5–6
  multiple choice questions 10, 12–15
  suggested reading 392
  terminology 382–383

Occipitoanterior position 224
Occipitoposterior position 221, 224, 254
Oestrogens
  bone loss prevention 122
  climacteric/menopause 117, 118–119
  corpus luteum 38
  hormonal contraception 357
  hormone replacement therapy 120–121,
    122
  plasma lipid effects 119
Oligohydramnios 198, 245, 328, 329
Oligospermia 66, 67
Omphalocele 327
One parent benefit 294
Oophorectomy, laparoscopic 146
Operculum release ('show') 218, 219
Oral contraceptive pill 22, 42, 46, 109,
    113–114
  combined oestrogen-progestogen
    358–362
  contraindications 81, 93
  dysfunctional uterine bleeding
    management 46, 47
  dysmenorrhoea management 48
  endometriosis management 57
  hirsutism management 76
  intermenstrual bleeding management 53
  polycystic ovarian syndrome management
    50
  post-partum use with breast-feeding 272
  premenstrual syndrome management
    125
  see also Progestogen-only pill
Orgasmic dysfunction 376, 380
Oropharyngeal suction 224
Ortho-Gyne T 380S 369
Ortolani's test 329
Osteoporosis 118–119, 122–123
Ovarian cancer 21, 113–116
  screening 115–116
  staging 114
Ovarian cyst 102
  laparoscopic cystectomy 146
Ovarian follicles 37–38
Ovarian hyperstimulation 281–282
Ovarian mass torsion 281
Ovarian neoplasms 48, 59
Ovary
  benign conditions 102
  fetal development 37
  menstrual cycle changes 37–38
Overflow incontinence 127, 132–133
Ovulation 37, 38
  cervical changes 40
  infertility investigations 66–67
  post-partum 265, 272, 273
  signs/symptoms 65
  temperature chart 66–67
Ovulation induction 41–42, 68, 114, 250
Ovulatory bleeding 45, 53

Pain in labour 254–255
Pain relief 254, 255–263
    epidural analgesia 257–261
    general anaesthesia 261–263
    inhalation agents 256
    narcotic agents 256–257
    physical methods 255–256
    pudendal block 261
    spinal analgesia 261
Palatal clefts 320, 326
Palpation
    abdominal examination 30
    first stage of labour 219, 220
Paramesonephric (Müllerian) duct 69
Paraurethral injectables 130
Parent-child bonding 313
Parentcraft 316
Partial hydatidiform mole 91, 92
Partogram 219, 390, 391
Parvovirus 288
Pearl index 355
Pediculosis pubis 348
Pelvic abnormalities 168
Pelvic diameters 387–388
Pelvic examination
    antenatal booking visit 164
    dyspareunia 60
    ectopic pregnancy 89
    endometriosis 56
    first stage of labour 219
    menopause 119
    objective structured clinical examination
        (OSCE) 31
    pelvic pain 62
    spontaneous abortion 79
    stress incontinence 128–129
    uterine fibroids 100
    uterovaginal prolapse 138
Pelvic floor 136
Pelvic floor exercises 129, 139
Pelvic haematocele 90
Pelvic inflammatory disease 45, 49,
        340–343
    definition 340
    dyspareunia 59, 340
    ectopic pregnancy 88, 340
    infertility 65, 340
    pelvic pain 61, 340
    treatment 342
Pelvic lymphadenectomy, laparoscopic 146
Pelvic pain 60–63
    ectopic pregnancy 89
    endometriosis 54, 56
    pelvic inflammatory disease 61, 340
    uterine fibroids 101, 102
Pelvic venous congestion 61, 62
Peptococcus 341
Percussion 30
Perinatal mortality 16, 287
    aetiology 298–300

Perinatal mortality (*contd*)
    antepartum haemorrhage 299
    congenital abnormalities 153, 298
    epidemiology 297–298
    maternal diabetes mellitus 210, 211, 299
    placenta praevia 299
    placental abruption 299
    pre-eclampsia 190, 299
    preterm labour 184
    prevention 300–301
    rhesus incompatibility 299
    statistics 297–301
Perinatal mortality rate 297
Perineal innervation 255
Periodic abstinence 371–372
Peripheral cyanosis 321
Peripheral paraesthesiae 176
Persistent patent ductus arteriosus 334
Persistent patent urachus 327
Pfannenstiel incision 242
Pharmacokinetics 255
Phenylketonuria 317
    neonatal screening 330
Phototherapy 322, 323
Physiological jaundice 322
Pinard stethoscope 230
Pituitary microadenoma 51
Place of delivery 165, 167
Placenta praevia 168, 202, 204–205, 236,
        242, 245, 247, 276
    caesarean section 307
    maternal mortality 303, 307
    multiple pregnancy 251
    perinatal mortality 299
Placental abruption 202–204, 242, 276
    intra-uterine growth retardation 197
    maternal mortality 303
    perinatal mortality 299
Placental delivery 194, 226, 227
Placental drug transfer 255
Placental margin bleeding 202
Placental site determination 165
Plasma volume 207
Plasmapheresis
    rhesus isoimmunization 195
Pneumothorax 327
Polycystic ovarian syndrome 19
    amenorrhoea 52
    anovulatory bleeding 42
    hirsutism 74, 75
    infertility 41, 50
    laparoscopic treatment 146
    menstrual disorders 49–50
    recurrent miscarriage 81, 84
Polycythaemia 322
    small for gestational age baby 333
Polyhydramnios 168, 185, 245
    diabetes mellitus association 211, 212
Port-wine stains 322
Postcoital bleeding 53, 99, 110

Postcoital test 66
Posterior urethral valves 314
Postmenopausal bleeding 110, 111, 112
Postnatal examination 273
Postpartum blues 269
Postpartum collapse 229
Postpartum depression 269
Postpartum haemorrhage 15, 226, 228–229,
    240, 264
    maternal mortality 303, 307
    multiple pregnancy 252
    risk factors 227
    secondary 265–266
    uterine fibroids 102
Postural hypotension 176
Posture during labour 221
Potter's syndrome 198
Pre-eclampsia 14, 185, 189–192, 242, 300
    assessment 190
    diabetes mellitus association 211
    hydatidiform mole 92
    intra-uterine growth retardation 197
    management 191–192
    perinatal mortality 299
    see also Hypertensive disorders
Premature ejaculation 376, 380
Premature menopause 118
    infertility treatment 41
Premature placental separation 252
Prematurity 12–13, 245, 247, 333–334
    anticipatory neonatal care 309
    complications 17
    definition 184, 333
    feeding problems 319
    maternal diabetes mellitus 211
    multiple pregnancy 251
    survival 184
    see also Preterm labour
Premenstrual syndrome 124–126
Prenatal diagnosis 152–159
    at risk groups 163
Preoperative medication 262
Prepregnancy care 151–152
    asymptomatic infection diagnosis 350
    diabetes mellitus 212
    epilepsy 213
Presacral neurectomy 58
Prescription charges 292
Presentation 168
Preterm labour 184–187
    ascending infection 178
    diabetes mellitus 211
    intraventricular haemorrhage prevention
        334
    management 186–187
    prevention 187, 304
    risk factors 185
    uterine congenital abnormalities 70
Preterm premature rupture of membranes
    187–188

Primary dysfunctional labour (inefficient
    uterine action) 221
Primitive reflexes assessment 330
Procidentia 137, 138
Progesterone
    corpus luteum 38
    endometrial response 39
    hormonal contraception 357
    measurement for ovulation detection 67
    menstrual cycle 38, 40
Progestogen therapy
    dysfunctional uterine bleeding 46, 47
    hormone replacement therapy 121, 122
    infertility treatment 41
    premature menopause 41
Progestogen-only pill 362–363
    contraindications 363
    ectopic pregnancy risk 89
    prescribing 363
Progress in labour 221
    partogram 219
Prolactin 270, 272
Prolactin-secreting tumour 51
Proliferative phase 38–39
Prostaglandins
    cervical ripening 218
    dysmenorrhoea 48
    hydatidiform mole treatment 93
    induction of labour 237
    menstrual blood loss 44–45
    menstrual cycle 38
    pelvic pain 61
    therapeutic abortion 87
    uterine contractions 218
Proteinuria
    antenatal monitoring 167–168
    pre-eclampsia 189, 190
Pruritus gravidarum 177
Pruritus vulvae 95–96, 104, 106
Psychosexual counselling 375–381
    suggested reading 392
Psychosexual dysfunction 48, 49, 58, 59,
    60, 375
Puberty
    cervical transformation zone changes 98,
        107
    hypothalamus-pituitary-gonad axis 37
Pudendal block 261
Puerperal fever 266
Puerperal infection 266–268
Puerperal psychosis 15, 269
Puerperal pyrexia 264
Puerperium 264–269
    contraception 272, 273
    haemorrhoids 269
    psychiatric complications 269
    thrombosis 269
Pulmonary embolism 214, 215, 279–280
    maternal mortality 302–303, 306
    in puerperium 269

Pulmonary hypertension, primary 210
Pulmonary metastases, hydatidiform mole 92, 93
Pyruvate kinase deficiency 323

Radiofrequency endometrial ablation 142, 144
Rectal bleeding 56
Rectocele 136, 137–138
  surgical repair 139
Recurrent miscarriage 81–85
  first trimester 81–82
  second trimester 82–83
  uterine congenital abnormalities 70
  uterine fibroids 102
Red cell enzyme abnormalities 323
Red cell structural abnormalities 323
Reference values in pregnancy 389
Renal disease 78, 197, 299
Renal tract anomalies 69
Renal transplantation 299
Respiratory distress 320, 325, 327
  causes 314, 315
  signs in neonate 314
Respiratory distress syndrome (hyaline membrane disease) 187, 211, 333
Respiratory rate, neonate 314
Resuscitation
  fetal distress management 235
  see also Neonatal resuscitation
Retained placenta/products 228, 229
  postpartum haemorrhage 265
  uterine congenital abnormalities 70, 72
Retinopathy of prematurity 334
Retracted nipples 319
Retrograde menstruation 55
Rhesus incompatibility 12, 80, 193–196, 288, 300, 322
  antenatal care 169
  anticipatory neonatal care 309
  anti-D antibodies 194
  anti-D prophylaxis 80, 169, 193, 194, 196, 273
  blood tests at delivery 196
  isoimmunization prevention 196
  perinatal mortality 299
  screening at booking visit 195
Rheumatic heart disease 209, 210
Rheumatoid arthritis 81
Rhythm method (periodic abstinence) 371–372
Ring pessary 130, 139
Risk factors, obstetric 384–385
  antenatal assessment 165
Rotational forceps 238, 240
RU486 87
Rubella 179–180
  congenital infection 153, 179, 323, 326
  immunization 180
    post-partum 273

Rubella (contd)
  maternal immune status 67, 155
    antenatal screening 164, 179–180
  spontaneous abortion 78
  see also TORCH syndrome
Rudimentary uterine horn 70
Rupture of membranes 219
  ascending infection 178
Russell viper's venom test 81

Sacrococcygeal pits 328
Safe period (periodic abstinence) 371–372
Salpingo-oophorectomy 115
Sarcoma
  uterus 111
  vulva 105
Scabies 348
Scalp abrasion/laceration 325
Screening
  antenatal 154–155, 161, 299
  cervical intraepithelial neoplasia (CIN) 108
  ovarian cancer 115–116
  test criteria 103
Secondary arrest of labour 221
Secretory phase 39–40
Semen analysis 66
Semen preparation 67
Septic abortion 77, 79, 80
Sex hormone binding globulin (SHBG)
  androgens binding 74, 75
  polycystic ovarian syndrome 49
Sexual abuse history 48, 62
Sexual activity, antenatal advice 171
Sexual arousal problems 379
Sexual dysfunction 375–378
  attitude of therapist 377–378
  investigations 378
  physical causes 376
  psychological causes 377
  treatment 378–379
Sexual interest problems 379
Sexually transmitted infection 335–352
  asymptomatic/systemic infections 348–350
  definition 335–336
  genital lesions 343–348
  genital warts 346–348
  infestations 348
  multiple choice questions 21–22
  pelvic inflammatory disease 340–343
  suggested reading 392
  vaginal discharge 336–340
Shared care 165
Sheldon Report (1971) 300
Shirodkar suture 84
Shock 89, 90
Shoulder dystocia 275–276, 331

'Show' (operculum release) 218, 219
Sickle cell disease 163, 164, 197, 208–209
  antenatal screening 155
Single gene defects 153
Single umbilical artery 327
Skin atrophy, menopausal 118
Skin care, neonate 316
Sleep, antenatal advice 172
Sling procedures 129
Small for gestational age baby 332–333
Smoking 109, 151, 162, 175, 197, 202,
  203, 287, 300
Social fund maternity payment 293
Sonar pulse detector (sonicaid) 230
Sore nipples 272, 319
Spermicides 371
Spina bifida 328
Spinal analgesia 261
Spinal hairy patch 328
Spinnbarkeit 40
Spiral arterioles 39, 40
Stamey procedures 129
Statistics 296–307
  multiple choice questions 15–16
Status epilepticus 305
Statutory maternity allowance 294
Statutory maternity pay 293
Sterilization 22, 356–357
Sternomastoid tumour 326
Sticky eyes 325–326
Stillbirth 287–291
  benefit entitlements 294
  definition 287
  discharge 291
  management following delivery 290–291
  risk factors 287–288
  support for parents 291
Stillbirth certificate 290
Stillbirth and Neonatal Death Society
  (SANDS) 291
Stillbirth rate 297
Stork marks 322
Strawberry naevi (cavernous
  haemangiomata) 322
Streptococcal infection 188, 266, 288
  maternal septicaemia 305
  neonatal sepsis 314
Stress incontinence 100, 127–130
  cystocele 137, 138
Sturge-Weber syndrome 322
Subgaleal haematoma 241
Subseptate uterus 70
Substandard care 301
Suck reflex 319
Sucking blisters 326
Sucking problems 319–320
Suckling 270, 271, 272
Suction cap 370
Suction evacuation 86–87
  hydatidiform mole 93

Superficial dyspareunia 58, 59, 104
Superovulation 41
Support during labour 222
Sustained release systems 365–367
  Mirena intrauterine system 366–367
  Norplant subdermal implants 365–366
Sutures 29, 34, 324–325, 386
Symmetrical growth retardation 197, 198
Symptothermal contraception method 40,
  371
Syphilis 22, 164, 288, 348, 349
  condylomata lata 346, 347, 348
  congenital infection 153
  genital ulceration 344
  serology 344
  spontaneous abortion 78
  treatment 346
  vertical transmission prevention 350–351
Systemic disease, maternal 207–216, 285
  breast-feeding contraindication 317
  spontaneous abortion 78
Systemic lupus erythematosus 13–14, 81
  perinatal mortality 299

Talipes calcaneovalgus 328
Talipes equinovarus 328
Tay-Sachs disease 163
Temperature, neonate 314
Teratoma 74
Testosterone
  hirsutism/virilism 74, 75
  polycystic ovarian syndrome 49
Testosterone implants 74, 121
Thalassaemia 163
  antenatal screening 155
Theca lutein cysts 93, 102
Therapeutic abortion 19, 85–88, 194
  counselling 86
  maternal mortality 304
  methods 86–87
  statistics 296–297
Threatened abortion 77, 79
Thromboembolism 120, 214–215
  multiple pregnancy 252
  in puerperium 269
  risk factors 214, 359
Thyroid dysfunction 45, 46, 215–216
  amenorrhoea 51, 52
  neonatal problems 332
  recurrent miscarriage 82
Thyrotoxicosis, neonatal 332
Thyroxine therapy 216
Tocolytics 186–187
TORCH screen 288
  intra-uterine growth retardation 198
TORCH syndrome 178, 179
Total spinal block 260
Toxoplasma gondii 181

Toxoplasmosis 178
  congenital infection 153, 181, 323, 326
  spontaneous abortion 78
  see also TORCH syndrome
Transcervical resection of endometrium
    (TCRE) 142, 144
Transexualism 375
Transient tachypnoea of newborn 314
Transplacental infection 178
Transvaginal ultrasound
  menorrhagia 46
  polycystic ovarian syndrome 75
Transverse lie 247–248
Traumatic cyanosis 321
Treponema pallidum 344
Trichomonas vaginalis 21, 104, 340
  treatment 339
  vaginal discharge 337, 338, 339
Trisomy 18 see Edward syndrome
Trisomy 21 see Down syndrome
True incontinence 133–134
Tubal abortion 90
Tubal infertility 64, 65, 68
  laparoscopic treatment 145
  pelvic inflammatory disease 340
Tubal patency assessment 67
Tuberculosis 330, 341
Turner's syndrome (45XO) 153, 326, 329
Twin pregnancy see Multiple pregnancy
Twin-to-twin transfusion 251, 299
Tyrosinaemia 323

Ultrasound
  abnormal lie 247
  antenatal screening 154–155, 156, 161,
      165, 166
  breech presentation 245
  congenital dislocation of hips 330
  ectopic pregnancy 90
  fetal growth/well-being assessment
      169–170, 198, 200
  hydatidiform mole 93
  intra-uterine growth retardation 198
  multiple pregnancy 250
  ovarian cancer screening 116
  ovulation detection 67
  ovulation induction monitoring 41
  placenta praevia 204, 205
  placental abruption 203
  placental site detection 205
  pre-eclampsia 190, 191
  preterm labour 185
  spontaneous abortion 79
  stillbirth 288
  uterine fibroids 101
Umbilical flare 327
Umbilical hernia 327
Ureaplasma urealyticum 341
Ureteric ectopy 133

Urethral caruncle 97–98
Urethrocele 136
  surgical repair 139
Urge incontinence 130–132
Uridine diphosphate glucuronyl transferase
    deficiency 323
Urinary fistula 127, 133–134
Urinary frequency 100, 115, 177
Urinary incontinence 127–134
Urinary tract infection 177, 183, 185, 268
Urinary urgency 18–19
Urodynamic investigations 129, 130, 131,
    133
Urogenital sinus 69
Urticaria neonatorum (erythema toxicum)
    321
Uterine abnormalities 69, 70, 185, 244, 247
  recurrent miscarriage 83
  spontaneous abortion 78
Uterine atony 228–229
Uterine contractions 217, 218
  fetal heart rate patterns 232–233
  labour pain 254
  partogram 219
  second stage 223
  third stage 226
Uterine fibroids 100–102
  degenerative change 100
  malignant change 100
  in pregnancy 102
Uterine inversion 228, 229, 278
Uterine malignancy 111–113
Uterine perforation 80, 87
Uterine polyps 99
Uterine prolapse 59, 136–137
Uterine retroversion 59
Uterine rupture 228, 229, 240, 277, 299
  management 277
  maternal mortality 304
  uterine scar 277
Uterine sarcoma 111
Uterine scar 242, 258, 285
  uterine rupture 277
Uteroplacental insufficiency
  fetal heart rate patterns 233
  intra-uterine growth retardation 200
Uterosacral ligaments 136
Uterovaginal prolapse 135–140
  surgical repair 139
Uterus
  benign conditions 99–102
  development 69
  in puerperium 264
  support structures 136
Uterus didelphys 70, 71

Vaccination in pregnancy 13
Vacuum extraction 224
  pudendal block 261
  see also Ventouse deliveries

Vagina 20–21
  benign conditions 98
  development 69
  menopausal changes 118
  menstrual cycle changes 40
  ovulation-associated changes 65
  support structures 136
Vaginal anomalies 70
Vaginal cysts 98
Vaginal discharge 99, 110, 111, 112,
      336–340
  neonate 328
Vaginal examination *see* Pelvic examination
Vaginal septum 70, 71, 72
Vaginal smear 40, 338
Vaginal trauma 228
Vaginal vault prolapse 137
Vaginal wall prolapse 136
Vaginismus 60, 379–380
Varicella (primary herpes zoster;
      chickenpox) 182
Varicose veins 175–176
Vasa praevia 202, 205
Vascular naevi 321–322
Vasomotor instability, menopausal 118
Ventouse deliveries 240–241
Very low birth weight 184
Virilism 73–76
Virilized female genitalia 74, 328
Vitamin B6 therapy 125

Vitamin K supplements 214
Vitamin K_1 prophylaxis 313
Vomiting
  neonate 320–321
  see also Nausea/vomiting
Vulval benign conditions 95–98
Vulval carcinoma 105–106
Vulval carcinoma in situ 104
Vulval epithelial dystrophies 96–97
Vulval intraepithelial neoplasia (VIN)
      103–104
Vulval irritation 105, 106
Vulval lumps/swellings 97–98
Vulval malignancy 103–106
Vulval melanoma 105
Vulval sarcoma 105
Vulvectomy 104, 106

Widow's mother's allowance 295
'Wind' 320
Wolffian (mesonephric) duct 98
Wolman's disease 324
Wrigley's forceps 238, 239
Wrist drop 328

X-ray pelvimetry 246

Zellweger's disease 324